menopause

EVERYTHING
you need to know

T0150271

Praise for Nicole Jaff's work

'Ms Jaff takes complicated topics and explains them in clear language with attention to evidence … She reviews the medical literature and is able to take the key messages and discuss them in ways that are meaningful to the lay reader. At the end of each chapter, she offers what she calls "empowerment points", or take-home messages that are often referred to in medicine as "clinical pearls". Ms Jaff does an excellent job of debunking anecdotal medicine, unlike many other books available on the market. This is a worthwhile read and I definitely recommend it to women looking to be informed about menopausal health. This book will allow them to have more informed discussions with their own healthcare practitioners.'

Dr Marla Shapiro, Associate Professor, Department of Family and Community Medicine, University of Toronto, *Menopause Flashes*, North American Menopause Society

'My computer tells me that this is the 100th book that I have reviewed over the past years. It is the best written with the most clear English of any that I have received.'

John McGarry, *Journal of the British Menopause Society* (now Menopause International)

'This is a worthwhile read and I definitely recommend it to women looking to be informed about menopausal health. This book will allow them to have more informed discussions with their own healthcare practitioners.'

Dr Tobie de Villiers, President, International Menopause Society

'Nicole Jaff has braved the highways of conflicting information about hormone replacement therapies to bring us *Menopause Today*. Her book goes a long way to cutting through the mumbo jumbo of myth and fear that has accumulated around the "change" … Jaff lays the responsibility of women's bodies squarely at the feet of women themselves. She inspires readers to approach their health with diligence and intelligence. Women who are at this stage of their lives owe it to themselves to read this book.'

Maureen Isaacson, *Sunday Independent*

'*Menopause Today* is essential reading not only for those women approaching the menopause but also for those who have experienced the menopause and who want clarity of the changes that occurred during this inevitable period in their lives. A must read.'

Professor Derick Raal, Head of the Division of Endocrinology and Metabolism, University of the Witwatersrand

'*Menopause: The Complete Guide* is a must read for every woman … It is an extremely useful and encouraging book.'

Puja Rajkumari, *Poise*, Indian Menopause Society

'I could not put your book down. How readable is that! The simplest most understandable, absolutely up-to-date and informative book on the menopause and women's health that I have ever read … I think the empowerment focus is intelligent, welcome, and uncommon.'

Elizabeth Barret-Connor, MD, Distinguished Professor and Chief, Division of Epidemiology/Family and Preventive Medicine, University of California

NICOLE JAFF

menopause

EVERYTHING
you need to know

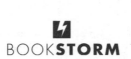

For my family, Nicholas, Sophie and Elizabeth, for their unwavering love and support. And to my mother, Joan Bernitz, who showed me a wider world.

ISBN 978-1-920434-20-5

First edition 2011

Published jointly by

Bookstorm (Pty) Limited	and	Pan Macmillan South Africa
Suite 10		Private Bag X19
Private Bag X12		Northlands 2116
Cresta 2118		Johannesburg
Johannesburg		South Africa
South Africa		**www.panmacmillan.co.za**
www.bookstorm.co.za		

Distributed by Pan Macmillan
Via Booksite Afrika
Edited by Catherine Murray
Cover design by René de Wet
Cover photo by Patrick Toselli
Typeset by Lebone Publishing Services
Printed and bound by Ultra Litho (Pty) Limited

Acknowledgements

Both editions of this book could not have come into being without the help and dedication of a host of medical experts. With humour and endless patience, Dr Merwyn Jacobson, medical director of Vitalab, Centre for Assisted Conception, Vice Chairperson of the South African Society of Reproductive Medicine and Gynaecological Endoscopy (SASREG) gave huge amounts of his time to helping and encouraging me; teaching me about the intricacies of the female reproductive system and guiding me around the many pitfalls of trying to explain the complex process of menopause. He forced me to pay minute attention to detail and curbed my tendency to make sweeping statements. To him I owe the title of Chapter 5: 'If I shake you, will you rattle?'

Professor Derick Raal, Head of the Division of Endocrinology and Metabolism, University of the Witwatersrand, took time out of his very busy life to explain to me, using wonderful metaphors, the medical mechanics of the endocrine system, cardiovascular disease and diabetes. Consistently helpful and considerate, he never failed to return my calls and answer my queries, even late at night.

Other professionals who gave me the benefit of their expertise and offered invaluable help and advice were: Dr Michael A Abrahams, gynaecologist and menopause practitioner in New York City, Dr Carol-Ann Benn, senior consultant at Chris Hani Baragwanath Hospital, lecturer in the Department of Surgery at the Faculty of Health Sciences, University of the Witwatersrand, and national director of Netcare Breast Care, Centre of Excellence; Ria Buys, registered dietician; Dr Susan Brown, Faculty of Health Sciences, University of the Witwatersrand; Professor Linda Cardozo, professor of urogynaecology and consultant gynaecologist at King's College Hospital in London; Professor Demitri Constantinou, director of the Centre of Exercise Science and Sports Medicine, Faculty of Health Sciences, University of the Witwatersrand; Jannie Claassen, Kinesiologist; Nigel J Crowther, associate professor and head of research, Department of Chemical Pathology, National Health Laboratory Service, Faculty of Health Sciences, University of the Witwatersrand; Dr Paul Dalmeyer, reproductive specialist; Dr Michael Davey, gynaecologist, founder member and president of the South African Menopause Society; Dr Jenny Edge, surgeon at the Christiaan Barnard Memorial Hospital in Cape Town; Dr Gereth Edwards, plastic and reconstructive surgeon; Dr Gillian Keast, friend and general practitioner; Dr Gary Levy, dermatologist; Dr Stanley

Lipschitz, specialist physician and specialist geriatrician; Professor Marilyn Lucas, PhD, clinical psychologist, Chair of Neuropsychology Cognitive Neuropsychology, University of the Witwatersrand; Professor Shane Norris (PhD), director and associate professor, MRC/WITS Developmental Pathways for Health Research Unit, Department of Paediatrics, School of Clinical Medicine, Faculty of Health Sciences, University of the Witwatersrand; Dr Joanne Miller, ophthalmologist; Ms Shira Moch, part-time lecturer in the Department of Pharmacology, Faculty of Health Sciences, University of the Witwatersrand; Dr Jody Pearl, specialist neurologist; Dr Naomi Rapeport, specialist physician; Dr Kogie Reddi, pathologist, Lancet Laboratories; Dr Russell Seider, director of screening and diagnostic mammography Donald Gordon Wits University Medical Centre; Dr Trudy Smith, principal specialist and senior lecturer, Department of Obstetrics and Gynaecology, Johannesburg Hospital and University of the Witwatersrand; Tracy Snyman, medical scientist, Development Laboratory, Department of Chemical Pathology, Faculty of Health Sciences, University of the Witwatersrand; Dr Michael Suzman, clinical assistant in surgery at the Weill Medical College of Cornell University and director of plastic surgery at Westchester Medical Group, White Plains, New York; Dr Susan Tager, CEO at the Wits University Donald Gordon Medical Centre; Anne Till, registered dietician and director of Anne Till and Associates; Professor Lizette van Rensburg, professor of human genetics and cancer genetics, University of Pretoria; Dr Daniel A Vorobiof, medical oncologist, director Sandton Oncology Centre, Johannesburg.

Medical experts may have different opinions based on different interpretations of medical research. In this book, after careful study, I have chosen those conclusions which in my opinion best reflect the available evidence, but these opinions may not always be the same as those of the experts who have advised me. Any errors are mine alone.

Contents

How to make the most of the book

I've tried to use as few technical terms as possible. Different countries use different units of measurements; those used in the USA are in brackets after each measurement. The medical terms are usually in italics next to the more down-to-earth word or phrase. There's a lot of additional information as well as a full glossary at the end of the book. So next time the doctor talks about 'hyperplasia' you'll know he means that the lining of your womb is thickened. Some sections of the book are drier and more technical than others, but I've included them so you'll understand how your body works and you can make responsible health choices.

You can use the book as a reference, dipping into it when you need a particular piece of information, or you can read it right through. You can use the index to find a specific topic. It's written in such a way that by the time you reach the end, all the pieces of the puzzle should have fallen into place and most of the mysteries of menopause will have been unveiled. Each chapter ends with a series of empowerment points, which you can glance at before you visit your healthcare practitioner. If you find an issue that you would like to discuss with your doctor at your next visit, keep a notebook handy and jot down the point. Always make notes before you visit your healthcare practitioner, to help you remember all the questions you need to ask during your appointments, when you may feel rushed and anxious.

There are hundreds of references for each chapter in the bibliography at the back so you can also refer your doctor to these, if he or she asks you the source of your information. It is very important that you understand that because of the vast body of research, different doctors will have read different publications and will have different opinions about what they learn. Just look at the heated and varied reactions from various experts to the Women's Health Initiative in Chapter 3. Your specialist may not agree with another medical expert, often with good reason, and the issues I discuss in this book may be subject to change as soon as new research is published – remember in menopause, as in all branches of medicine, the body of knowledge is constantly evolving. The information you will find in this book is my interpretation of the current available research in language that makes it easier to understand what's going on during this time of your life.

Introduction

Whether you are one of the lucky ones who believe that menopause is a 'passage to power, enabling you to become a wise woman or shaman', or someone who dreads it, believing it is the path to a miserable, estrogen-deficient old age, women who don't struggle during the menopause transition are rare. We know our bodies are ageing and we feel less attractive than we used to. Our weight is often skyrocketing and many of us struggle with exhausting physical symptoms like hot flushes, night sweats, mood swings and memory loss. There are tremendous changes taking place in our lives and in our psyches during this time. Our children leave home and we start to question our life choices; we're uncertain about our future and afraid of ageing and death.

In 1996 I was plunged into an early menopause after unnecessary surgery and my own transition was traumatically abrupt. I understood so little about my body or my health that I felt I had 'betrayed' myself through my lack of knowledge and my inability to take responsibility for my health. I was sure that my life was over and I was in despair. At the age of 46, I bought into the menopause stereotype that many of us Western women have been taught to believe. I felt old, dried up, wrinkled, unsexy and useless. But my training as a trauma counsellor came to my rescue and I stopped blaming myself. As I read and learnt about menopause I saw that I could reframe; that my experience might be a way of helping others.

For two years I immersed myself in medical literature and research, trying to understand the complexities of menopause, so that other women would not battle as I had. Writing a book about menopause was cathartic for me. It helped me reframe my experience and forgive myself. I watched the 'birth' of the first edition with extreme anxiety – I was daring to challenge the experts, to write as an ordinary woman about one of the most controversial and confusing areas of medicine; to speak out for women so that they would feel there was someone they could identify with in their corner.

When my first book on menopause was published in 2005, the response was both humbling and heartening. My readers discussed it with their doctors, shared it with their friends, kept it next to their beds and gave it to their mothers. They consulted it to answer the numerous questions that arose in their daily lives in relation to peri- and postmenopause. Many wrote to me saying how happy and relieved they felt that they were not alone.

The responses of academics and clinicians were equally positive. Far from objecting to a non-medical person writing about this subject, they were incredibly receptive. Many of them congratulated me, reviewed the book with insight and generosity, recommended it to their registrars and kept it in their consulting rooms, suggesting their patients read it. Nowadays I often find myself sharing a platform or conducting workshops with these doctors. When I'm invited to address their congresses or debates, I am eager to do so, believing that if I can learn new information, discuss certain confusing issues about menopause and reach a better understanding of medical perspectives which I can clarify, I may be helping other women.

When the first edition of *Menopause* was published I felt that I had come to the end of a long and painful journey. Six years later, as I sit at my computer screen, rewriting, revising, adding sections and updating this new comprehensive guide, I realise my journey has just begun. Menopause is a vast subject, the scientific evidence is constantly changing, and opinions surrounding it are dynamic and diverse. In the years since I began writing about menopause, a huge volume of new research has emerged. There are exciting developments in diagnosing and treating breast cancer, and fascinating information on genetic testing. Treatments, which are more sophisticated and easier to use, have become available for osteoporosis but problematic areas that also need to be addressed have emerged.

The information from the Women's Health Initiative (WHI) acted as a huge catalyst in the medical world and the pharmaceutical industry (Chapter 3), because it turned so much conventional wisdom about Hormone Therapy (HT) upside down. However, it hasn't convinced many doctors that they should practise evidence-based medicine. These clinicians are still sceptical about the results of the WHI and some continue to advocate HT to all women instead of assessing each individual case. They suggest that menopausal women, with few exceptions, should be on HT at all costs since, according to them, we need HT to live happy, productive lives even if we don't have symptoms. In spite of the recommendations of many prominent menopause societies, who advise that women should only take HT to treat moderate to severe menopause symptoms that compromise our quality of life or to help prevent bone loss in certain postmenopausal women, these clinicians still prescribe the use of HT as a protection against a wide range of diseases.

In addition, many of them do not fully explain the risks and benefits of HT to their patients, despite the research, nor do they regard their patients as individuals who should be carefully informed before they use HT. I'm troubled by the increase in the number of doctors using bioidentical hormones that haven't been approved by the various medical regulatory bodies in different countries. There's a tendency for these healthcare practitioners to prescribe HT as 'anti-ageing' medicine, so that many women find themselves spending exorbitant amounts of money on a cocktail of hormones they've been told will keep them young, sexy and disease-free; claims that aren't based on rigorous research.

Initially when I wrote about menopause, I said 'knowledge is power', because I believe that once we're armed with the correct information, a visit to the doctor's office won't be so traumatic. We won't feel bullied into making a decision that might prove to be wrong for us. Because there's so much complex, conflicting information about menopause and it's expressed in incomprehensible medical terminology, we may be afraid to ask relevant questions and if, and when, we get answers, we aren't able to decipher them so we can make important decisions about our health. Although we're paying for the consultation, we often feel that we're not really entitled to information or have the right to understand what's going on in our bodies and to make good decisions. Even those of us who are most confident are strangely diffident when questioning our doctors' opinions or asking them for explanations and recommendations.

It's vital for us to work together with our healthcare practitioners, and not to leave the doctor's office feeling confused and anxious. If we want to know more about menopause, we should be able to read about it in user-friendly language that's informative and simple to understand. We should feel comfortable discussing the latest research with our medical practitioners and be able to comprehend the different options available to us, to understand our choices. We should feel empowered to make the right decisions for ourselves.

In my late fifties, I feel more alive than I did in my thirties. I give workshops where midlife women can hear the latest information and feel comfortable sharing their experiences and fears with other women. I've passed a board exam and become a licensed healthcare practitioner; I've written a three-hour exam earning me the prestigious certification from the North American Menopause Society as a NAMS Certified Menopause Practitioner, allowing me to use the initials NCMP after my name. I'm doing my PhD – investigating the effects of the menopause transition on the health of a group of 1 000 black South African women. I managed, with a lot of sweat and tears, but without HT, to study for the exams, to remember what I had learnt and retrieve it when I needed it in the stressful setting of the exam room, where I was by far the oldest candidate. I welcome the challenges of academic research and love working with other research fellows, many of whom are 20 years younger than I am. Far from being over, my menopausal life is full of excitement and promise.

This new, comprehensive book is for those women who battle through perimenopause, and for those who have finally reached menopause but are overwhelmed by the huge amounts of information with which they're bombarded by the media and the Internet. It's for all the women who write to me hoping for a 'miracle cure', and for some unravelling of the confusing and conflicting information they're getting from their different healthcare practitioners and advertisers so they can live happy, healthy lives. It's for women who call me in tears asking for help; wondering what will happen if they choose a different path from their doctor's recommendations – whether they will get dementia if they don't take HT or breast cancer if they do. It's for women who want to take responsibility for their health and who are wary of being sold treatments that may benefit the seller more than the buyer. It's for women who believe they have the right to up-to-the-minute information, which will inform their choices and the decisions they make about their health in menopause. It's for women who want to be in partnership with their doctors. It's for all women who believe that menopause is not an ending but the beginning of some of the best years of their lives.

1
What is menopause?

Prue is tall and slim. She is an ardent sportswoman in her early forties, matter of fact and organised in her daily life, self-contained and extremely down to earth. So it was out of character for her to be laughing hysterically and describing her anxiety and distress during the past few weeks. 'I am so relieved this morning,' she said, 'I've just got my period. I'd missed two months, had unbelievably sore boobs and felt emotional, even slightly sick. I was absolutely sure that I was pregnant – it felt just like it. But it's back again and really heavy.

'The reason I was so freaked out,' she explained, 'apart from my age [she has two children in high school] is that my husband's had a vasectomy and there's no possible way I could be pregnant!'

We all laughed, but what Prue had just experienced could happen to any woman of her age. She is perimenopausal. The symptoms of perimenopause vary widely and may come out of the blue. For some women there are clear, unambiguous signs; for others, the transition from being a fertile woman in the menstrual cycle to being menopausal is so gradual that they hardly even notice.

Because there is so much research into the subject of menopause at this time and because the findings of the Women's Health Initiative (WHI) in 2002 turned the accepted ideas about menopause on their heads, it is vital that women understand what is happening to their bodies in the years before the actual moment of menopause so that they are better able to micromanage this often tumultuous time and will be able to look back on those years as fulfilled, healthy and productive.

WHAT DOES PERIMENOPAUSE MEAN?

The term menopause actually means the last day of your last period ever. From that point, in medical terms, you are considered menopausal. Until then, your body – as it moves from being fertile, able to produce eggs and bear children, to the moment of menopause when you no longer ovulate – is in a transition period known as the *climacteric*, a word meaning a critical stage in human life; a period that is especially likely to be connected with a change in health. During this time when you are moving towards menopause, the changes taking place in your body cause certain symptoms, physiological (physical) and psychological changes that are happening to you as the levels of estrogen in your body fluctuate and the levels of progesterone start to decline. We use the word **peri**, which comes from the Greek word meaning 'around, round about and about', in conjunction with the word 'menopause', because it is a useful way to describe all the things that are going on in your body before, during and after the actual moment of menopause.

Before I describe what happens in perimenopause, there is a very important point that you need to understand. Each woman is an individual so her menopause is unique and specific to her and her own body or biochemistry. It is pointless to compare yourself, your perimenopausal symptoms and the way you choose to manage your menopause with anyone else. As a friend of mine who is a preschool teacher points out, 'You always have to remind parents that each child develops differently. I tell parents that just because Jenny is catching a ball at four years old doesn't mean that Susie's ready to do so; she will in time, but she is developing at her own pace.' Don't forget this when you're sitting around discussing your perimenopause with your friends.

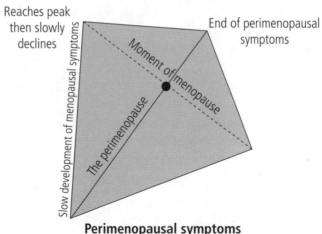

Perimenopausal symptoms

Much of the confusion arising from menopause is caused by the fact that for decades women were lumped together as a species and treated as if they were all the same, with no understanding that what was great for one woman might be disastrous for another. The old adage (slightly altered from a feminist perspective) holds good here: 'One woman's meat is another woman's poison.' It is vital to remember that the time leading up to menopause is different for every woman, just as the symptoms listed below are different for every woman.

The changes of perimenopause usually begin in the most subtle way, two to 14 years before the actual onset of menopause, depending on your own body chemistry, unless you have undergone a surgical or chemical menopause. The diagram of the perimenopause shows how these symptoms build up over a period of time and then slowly decline after the actual moment of menopause. For some women the good news is that they will hardly experience any symptoms, or only some of them for a very short time, while other unfortunate women will experience the full range of symptoms. These symptoms may continue for several years after the moment of menopause. So, as you read through the list and recognise some or all of these symptoms, remember that there are millions and millions of women out there going through a similar experience; you are not alone and what is happening to you is part of your life process as a woman. This stage will resolve itself, as did all the other stages in your life.

Some of the main symptoms of perimenopause

- Hot flushes (you may see books written in America describing them as hot 'flashes')
- Night sweats
- Forgetfulness
- Undefined anxiety
- Inability to concentrate
- Mood swings
- Weight gain
- Sleep pattern changes
- Loss of libido (sexual desire)
- Change in the type of PMS
- Headaches or migraines
- Irregular periods – either too often or with months in between
- Changes in the type of menstrual periods
- Symptoms that mimic pregnancy: sore breasts, ravenous hunger, tearfulness, fatigue

Symptoms that may persist after the other symptoms have abated

- Vaginal dryness
- Persistent loss of libido
- Urinary problems

The list of perimenopausal symptoms is long, varied and often specific to you alone, so although I have only listed the most common symptoms in this chapter, on pages 304–305 at the end of the book you will find a list of almost every possible symptom that women complain about during perimenopause, which may reassure you that you are not going mad or suffering from some obscure and life-threatening disease.

The symptoms of perimenopause may mostly be blamed on your changing hormone levels. Your levels of estrogen are fluctuating and you don't have adequate progesterone to balance the estrogen. In fact, when the levels of estrogen stop fluctuating, many of the symptoms that have plagued you throughout the perimenopause will stop. Estrogen is an extremely potent hormone and in Chapter 2, I will explain the physiology of estrogen and why it has such a powerful effect on you.

YOUR MENSTRUAL CYCLE

Once you understand the process of your menstrual cycle and the roles that estrogen and progesterone play in it, it is much easier to understand what is happening to your body during perimenopause. Look at the diagram of the womb below so you have a picture of what your reproductive system looks like.

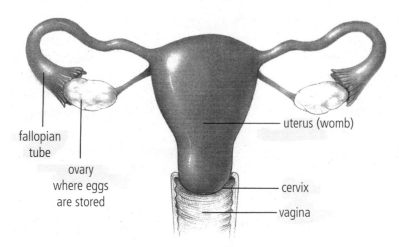

Simple diagram of the womb

You are born with two ovaries containing eggs. Each egg is surrounded by a sac-like structure called a *primordial follicle* (this means that the follicle is in a primitive state). The egg and follicle are often called the *egg unit* and are in a resting state. When you start puberty your ovaries contain about 500 000 eggs, but by the time you reach menopause only about 3 000 eggs remain. The diagram of the reproductive cycle will help you understand how the ideal 28-day menstrual cycle works. This is also a good place to remind you that only about 12 per cent of women have a 28-day cycle, so your cycle may normally be between 24 days and 35 days, or you may be one of those women who has always had irregular periods.

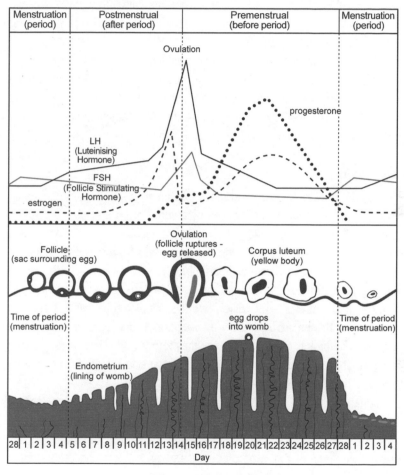

The menstrual cycle

The build-up to ovulation

Your menstrual cycle begins on the first day of your period (the first day of a full bleed). The *pituitary gland* in your brain produces a hormone called *follicle stimulating hormone* (FSH). This is one of the important hormones to note when understanding what is happening to your body, because when women become perimenopausal or go to their doctors complaining about some of the symptoms I have listed above, they often have blood tests which show that their FSH levels are raised.

The FSH causes the egg units to produce estrogen and this increased production level of estrogen causes the lining of the womb (*endometrium*) to thicken. During this time up to 1 000 egg units begin to mature. By day nine, one of these egg units starts to grow much more quickly than the others and becomes the dominant (leader of the pack) follicle. The other egg units, having done their work in supporting the *dominant follicle*, start to degenerate.

As this follicle matures its estrogen production increases and on about day 13 it reaches a level which tells the *hypothalamus*, the part of the brain involved with your endocrine system and thus your menstrual cycle, to send a message to the pituitary gland to reduce the FSH production and to secrete *luteinising hormone* (LH).

Ovulation

On day 14, which is called mid-cycle in our ideal 28-day cycle, the ripening follicle develops a weak spot caused by a surge of LH and the contents of the follicle are slowly pushed out through this weakened area. This process creates a chemical change around the ovary, which attracts the finger-like extensions at the end of the fallopian tube. These behave very much like the waving fronds of a sea anemone and create a current that draws the egg and the fluid that was in the follicle into the fallopian tube, which leads into your womb. This process is known as *ovulation*. It may pass unnoticed or it may be painful and many women say they know when they have ovulated because of the physical sensation or pain on one side, which may come from the rupturing follicle.

Sometimes the small amount of fluid or blood spilled when the follicle releases its contents may irritate the pelvic lining, which may cause tenderness. Often women can tell when they have ovulated because they experience some of the symptoms that are caused by rising progesterone which is released during this time. These may be a sudden very bad headache or migraine, a craving for chocolate, tender or very sensitive breasts, or an outbreak of acne or one huge pimple that always seems to appear in the same place.

The ruptured follicle is now known as the *corpus luteum* (Latin for yellow body) and begins to produce small amounts of estrogen and increasing amounts of progesterone, which stabilises the thickened lining of your womb or uterus, so that if the egg is fertilised the lining will be lush and ready to receive the fertilised egg. If you do not become pregnant the corpus luteum begins to degenerate and the levels of progesterone and estrogen it produces begin to drop. Since the lining of the womb needs progesterone to sustain it, when the levels of progesterone and estrogen have dropped far enough the lining begins to crumble and within a couple of days it separates from the wall of your womb and you start to menstruate approximately 14 days after ovulation. This menstrual cycle generally continues in more or less the same way during your fertile years unless you are pregnant, or until you begin to get older, which is when things start to change.

WHAT HAPPENS TO YOUR MENSTRUAL CYCLE AS YOU BECOME PERIMENOPAUSAL?

As I have discussed above, the ovary is a hormone-producing organ that becomes less effective as you age, but it doesn't just shut down and stop producing hormones. This is where so many doctors were so mistaken in their determination to explain to women how they had 'run out' of estrogen and why they needed hormone replacement therapy (HRT). During your fertile years, the main hormones produced by your ovaries are two types of estrogen (estradiol (E2), which is very potent, and estrone), progesterone and small amounts of androgen (see Chapter 2). As you approach menopause your changing ovaries produce estrogen in lower amounts and increased amounts of androgen. (Testosterone, the main male hormone, is an androgen.) At the same time the balance of the types of estrogen being produced changes and you begin to produce larger amounts of estrone and smaller amounts of estradiol. Your ovaries are still functioning, but less efficiently.

From your late thirties onwards an ageing process takes place. This varies widely among women. Each of us has a biological clock and the rate at which it ticks depends on the different biochemistry of each woman. This means that it may tick faster for some women, so their egg units become less efficient earlier, or more slowly for others, in whom the symptoms and signs of perimenopause appear later. The process may happen in your mid-thirties or in your late forties and may take from two to 14 years.

As you age your remaining egg units become progressively less efficient, regardless of the rate of your biological clock. Because the egg unit is becoming inefficient, which means that it is less responsive and less functional, the hypothalamus and pituitary gland respond accordingly. The pituitary has been doing its job month in and month out for many years, producing FSH, which means that there is a consistent level of hormones rising and falling during your most fertile years. When the pituitary 'recognises' that the remaining follicles are not responding to FSH as they used to, it increases the FSH production to try to force the follicles to respond, a process that may be slow and subtle in some women, and precipitous in others. This is the reason why so many doctors tell women they believe to be perimenopausal to have a blood test to see if their levels of FSH are rising.

WHY DO HORMONES FLUCTUATE DURING PERIMENOPAUSE?

So, why do levels of estrogen rise and fall so erratically during the peri-menopausal years? It's quite simple really. The follicles in your ovaries are starting to show their age and are less effective, so their response at the beginning of your 28-day cycle is poorer. The pituitary, responding to the fact that the follicles aren't doing their job, pumps out higher levels of FSH in a desperate effort to stimulate them and some follicles respond by pushing out large amounts of estrogen, sometimes much higher than average. If this happens you may ovulate and experience exaggerated symptoms of ovulation like sore breasts, heightened emotional responses and sugar cravings. If you have ovulated, your levels of progesterone rise and fall and you get a period, which because the high amounts of estrogen have made your womb lining thicker than usual, the period is very heavy and may be accompanied by large clots.

On the other hand, your follicles may respond to the raised amounts of FSH by producing unusually large amounts of estrogen but you don't ovulate because the maturing egg cannot complete the process. This means that the lining of your womb gets thicker and thicker but you don't have a period because there is no ovulation so the follicle hasn't become the corpus luteum and doesn't produce the progesterone which helps to control menstruation. This is why you don't have your period at the usual time.

But now, just to add to your confusion, your estrogen level may drop suddenly and this thickened lining may become unstable and shed, causing a heavy bleed, which is not a period, at a time that is entirely unrelated to your 'normal' cycle, perhaps out of the blue after several months of having no period. Or the lining of your womb may thicken just a bit and then become unstable because of the fluctuating levels of estrogen and you have a funny, light bleed when you least expect it. Or you may have continued estrogen production without ovulation, which means that the endometrium becomes so thick that it cannot be maintained and partially breaks down, causing bleeds that are heavier and last longer than usual.

Another point to remember is that even if you have irregular periods, if your ovaries are still ovulating, even only occasionally, you may still get pregnant, so until you have been confirmed as fully menopausal and haven't had a period for at least 12 months you should still use contraception (unless your husband or partner has had a *vasectomy*).

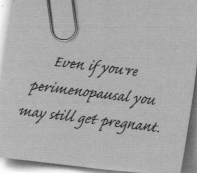

Even if you're perimenopausal you may still get pregnant.

These irregular bleeds or 'periods' are signs of perimenopause and are caused by fluctuating levels of high and low estrogen that are no longer balanced by progesterone. In a normal menstrual cycle these two hormones balance each other out but now they are out of sync because the levels of progesterone are steadily declining while estrogen production may remain normal or become higher.

Remember, it is these changing levels of estrogen and not simply low levels that cause many of the symptoms of perimenopause: hot flushes, memory lapses, exhaustion one day because the estrogen level has dropped, or wild irritability and tearfulness, bloating and sore breasts on another, because it has risen or you have ovulated. So blood tests showing high FSH and low estrogen may not be useful at the start of perimenopause.

Let's assume that you are showing signs of perimenopause so you go to your doctor, who recommends that you have a blood test. The test results show that you have raised levels of FSH and lowered levels of estradiol (E2). The doctor then recommends additional estrogen in the form of estrogen therapy (ET) but despite this, the next week, because your raised levels of FSH affect your remaining egg units and your estrogen levels rise suddenly, you may ovulate and because of the ET you are taking, your body will have too much estrogen and you will suffer the associated symptoms of excess estrogen.

The problem with relying on blood tests at the start of perimenopause is that a woman may continue to menstruate for a long time in spite of raised levels of FSH. Some doctors may recommend a low-dose contraceptive pill, which inhibits ovulation and controls your fluctuating estrogen. But as with all hormone therapy, it is important to find out whether this treatment suits your individual body chemistry and whether it is absolutely necessary.

The prospect of these rising and falling levels of hormones and their consequences may be very depressing, but there is some good news. As you approach menopause the drastic changes in hormones level out and you will probably have the same high levels of FSH and LH and the same levels of estrogen for the rest of your life, if you lead a balanced life. However, estrogen levels may be affected by an increase in or loss of weight, by chemicals or stress, and they may fluctuate. If they are stable though, most of the symptoms of perimenopause will eventually stop and the only symptoms that may remain are those of postmenopause: vaginal dryness, low libido and, sometimes, urinary problems.

Most experts do not believe that a blood test by itself is useful in diagnosing the menopause.

HOW CAN YOU TEST FOR MENOPAUSE?

By now you must be thinking, 'How on earth can I confirm that I am actually menopausal?' Today most experts do not believe that a blood test by itself is useful in diagnosing the menopause. This is because a single blood test which looks at your levels of FSH, LH and estradiol, especially in the first few years of perimenopause while you are still menstruating, may not be accurate due to the fluctuating levels of these hormones. In peri-menopause, your FSH levels may react to the fluctuations of your estrogen levels. So when your estrogen levels drop, your FSH may be high, but a few days later the FSH may be lower again as your estrogen levels rise. If you have a blood test only to determine your levels of estradiol (E2) and they are less than 50 pmol/L (13.6 pg/ml), there may still be some doubt as to whether or not you are menopausal.

There are two reasons for this. The first, as we know, is because estrogen levels may fluctuate madly during the early years of perimenopause. The second is that estrogen, progesterone and testosterone are bound to something called *sex hormone-binding globulin* (SHBG), a protein produced by the liver which binds the main hormones and decreases their biological effectiveness. The only hormones that are really relevant are those that are not bound to the SHBGs because these are the hormones that can easily enter the body tissues. They are called *bioavailable*.

Some manufacturers of 'natural' or *bioidentical* hormones, and healthcare practitioners who recommend these products, will tell you that a salivary assay is the only accurate way to test the baseline of hormones, including estradiol, progesterone and testosterone. They may tell you that they can determine what the 'normal' levels of your hormones should be for your age. There is no efficacy evidence that this type of testing is accurate or reliable and so far 'normal' levels of hormones in menopausal women have not been established. Another problem with this kind of testing is that in order to establish serum hormone levels from your saliva you need *at least* five daily saliva samples because hormone levels vary greatly in each individual woman throughout the day and from one day to the next. Your doctor will tell you that even the hormone levels in your blood as opposed to those in saliva vary from day to day.

If you are in your late thirties or your early forties, have irregular periods and are experiencing some of the symptoms discussed above, your best bet may be to have a blood test which shows your FSH and your E2 levels. There is some discussion about when this test should be done and whether it is an accurate predictor of menopause because FSH levels may remain high despite the fact that estradiol levels appear adequate in blood tests. Two other hormones, *inhibin B* and *Anti-Müllerian Hormone* (AMH), are involved in FSH levels. Inhibin B is produced by the ovaries to help with the recruitment of eggs. As women age, their ovaries produce lower levels of inhibin B, causing the pituitary to produce higher levels of FSH.

AMH is also produced by the developing follicles in the ovaries and there is now a lot of interest in new research suggesting that this hormone may also be useful in determining whether a woman still has an adequate number of functioning eggs in her ovaries. So, if you combine levels of inhibin B, AMH and FSH you will probably have a fairly accurate idea of whether or not you are menopausal. However, currently these tests for levels of inhibin B and AMH are not usually done on peri- and postmenopausal women, so your doctor should test your FSH levels. Ideally you should have the test between day two and day five of your menstrual cycle while you are menstruating regularly so that you have a baseline level with which to compare any future results.

If you are already perimenopausal and your periods are irregular, it will be more difficult to pinpoint when you should have your test, and you could have the FSH levels tested in conjunction with your E2 levels. If the test shows that your FSH is high and your E2 is low, it probably means that you are perimenopausal. However, although there are norms for the hormone levels, results may vary greatly depending on the individual. Also remember that the actual hormone measurements may vary slightly depending on the methodologies used by different labs.

As a rule of thumb, if you haven't had a period for 12 months and you have FSH levels that are greater than 20 IU/L(20mIU/ml) and E2 levels lower than 50 pmol/L (13.6 pg/ml), you can be pretty confident that you are now menopausal. These results should be interpreted by a healthcare practitioner who understands the subtle changes that are taking place in your body during the time of perimenopause.

THE DIFFERENT STAGES OF PERI- AND POSTMENOPAUSE

Because it can be difficult to obtain accurate hormone levels during the perimenopause, and because this time in the reproductive cycle is often marked by changes in bleeding patterns or in menstrual flow, a group of researchers, clinicians and organisations involved in women's health sponsored the Staging of Reproductive Aging Workshop (STRAW) in 2001 to help describe the different stages in a woman's reproductive cycle as she ages, and to standardise the terms doctors and researchers use in relation to this. STRAW suggested a standardised set of criteria and terminology, which have become internationally accepted when describing the stages of the menopause transition. STRAW described seven stages of menopause. But remember, since all women are different, the stages and irregularities in bleeding that you may experience will be specific to you and the STRAW definitions should only be used as a road map to help you understand what's happening to you during your peri- and postmenopausal years.

Premenopausal means you have had a period in the past three months and there have been no changes in regularity over the past 12 months. **Perimenopausal** is divided into two stages: *early perimenopausal* – when you've had a period in the past three months but have had some changes in your regularity over the past year, and *late perimenopausal*, meaning you haven't had a period for the past three months but have had some bleeding during the year. **Postmenopausal** is described as any time after your last period ever, and is divided into two stages: *early postmenopause*, which is also divided into two parts, the first being the year after your last period and the second being the next four years; and *late postmenopausal*, meaning from five years after your last period until your death.

STRAW has been extremely useful in ongoing menopause research and is incorporated into many different studies examining menopause. Recent studies are investigating endocrine (hormone) changes before and during the menopause transition in conjunction with the criteria used by STRAW.

Before your doctor says you are menopausal, you should have had a thorough physical examination. Also remember that a transvaginal ultrasound, which allows your doctor to evaluate more clearly what is happening in your womb and your ovaries, is now considered an integral part of your gynaecological physical. Using this technique your doctor can rule out any major abnormalities in your womb and ovaries. Depending on the results of that examination, your doctor will probably recommend tests to establish your levels of FSH, E2, prolactin and your thyroid function.

The reason I suggest that you have a physical examination and check prolactin levels and your thyroid function is that there may be factors other than the decline of normal ovarian functioning that are influencing your menstrual cycle. So if you don't think that you are perimenopausal, ask your doctor to check your thyroid function; note whether you are on any new medication for other conditions and exclude the possibility of illnesses that may affect menstruation. Excessive weight loss and lifestyle habits like too much alcohol and heavy cigarette smoking may cause menstrual changes, as will chronic or acute stress and sometimes just travelling through different time zones.

By now you should have a better understanding of how your body works and how you've reached this perimenopausal stage. You also know why you start getting strange symptoms and what the changes signal. Unlike Prue, you won't be freaked out when your periods suddenly stop and think that you are pregnant!

EMPOWER YOURSELF

- **Ask your doctor to explain:** It is entirely reasonable and sensible for you to ask your doctor to explain your symptoms and the results of your tests in a way that is clear and easy for you to understand. You should never feel rushed or stupid or that you are wasting their time. You have paid for the consultation and this is your time. If your doctor does not do so in a manner that is acceptable to you, then you must seriously question whether he or she is the correct practitioner for you.
- **Insist on testing your hormone levels:** Don't accept it when your doctor tells you that they think you are too young to be perimenopausal or that you will get your menopause when you're 40. Doctors aren't psychic. Insist that you have your FSH tested if you think you may be perimenopausal. There is no harm in being sure. Even if you aren't experiencing the symptoms of menopause you may want to have a record of your levels as a baseline comparison for the future.
- **Ask for clarification:** Never feel awkward about asking questions or asking for information to be clarified.
- **Discuss test results in detail:** If you have had tests, the practice should phone you with the results as soon as possible and you should be able to discuss these results in detail with your doctor at a follow-up appointment.

2
All about hormones

I had just started writing this chapter when my phone rang and a woman asked to speak to me. She told me she was in her sixties. She was obviously well educated, articulate and informed, and had made it her mission to research osteoporosis, with which she had been diagnosed.

She refused to take osteoporosis medicine (bisphosphonates) because she is a firm believer in alternative and complementary medicines. She told me that she had consulted experts in America and the UK, where she had spent time with one of the so-called gurus of natural progesterone, a disciple of Dr John Lee, who practises in London. This doctor had recommended natural progesterone, which she was to apply to her skin in a 'small dollop … about the amount you would put on a toothbrush'.

She asked me what I thought of natural progesterone. I took a deep breath. It is very confusing when women talk about natural progesterone. What does the word 'natural' mean? Natural progesterone is a product that has been formulated to be biologically identical to the progesterone that is found in your body. Like all the other hormone replacement products, it has been synthesised in a laboratory. Yet this woman, who is very opposed to conventional HT, was quite happy to put an arbitrary amount of progesterone on her body, without any real understanding of the strength and potential side effects of this hormone, which is, in its own way, as powerful and potentially harmful as too much estrogen.

In Chapter 1, I discussed several hormones that play a large part in a woman's peri- and postmenopausal life. But when you do not understand how these hormones work, it is hard to appreciate just how much they can affect you during the transition to menopause. If you grasp how they function, you can, together with your doctor, make an informed decision about whether or not you want to use hormone therapy.

Hormones are chemical substances that act like messengers. They travel through your body in your bloodstream to different tissues, where they send out signals for organs to react in a certain way. The hormones come from a series of glands that form something called the *endocrine* system. There are many different kinds of hormones and they behave in a most complex and subtle way to affect our bodily functions. However, I will only write about a few of the main hormones that will affect you most during your menopausal process and the last few decades of your life.

SEX STEROID HORMONES – ESTROGENS, PROGESTERONE AND TESTOSTERONE

Estrogens, progesterone and testosterone, which I mentioned in Chapter 1, are called sex steroid hormones. All the sex steroid hormones originate from cholesterol and are controlled by the functions of the hypothalamus and the pituitary. In females, many of the sex steroid hormones are produced in the ovaries in a very specific order but some are produced in the adrenal glands, which are the small structures situated on top of your kidneys, and in the fatty tissues of your body. Doctors may refer to these fatty tissues as *adipose tissue*. Most of the hormones that are important to women are produced via a series of steps or pathways known as the *adrenal cascade*. Hormones and their actions are intricately woven into the functioning of your body. They are like the players in an orchestra. The hypothalamus is the musical director, the pituitary is the conductor and the various hormones are the members of the orchestra. As in an orchestra, if one player is out of tune, the whole piece of music is out of tune; so, if a hormone is not functioning at its appropriate level, the body is out of tune.

A hormone called *pregnenolone*, made from cholesterol, is the basic building block of the sex steroid hormones. The pregnenolone hormone produces *progesterone*, which as you will remember is secreted by the corpus luteum after ovulation. Other hormones that are derived from pregnenolone and progesterone are the *androgens* and the *estrogens*. I only discuss two of the androgens, namely testosterone and DHEA (*dehydroepiandrosterone*).

One of the above-mentioned estrogens, estradiol, is produced mainly in your ovaries and, to a lesser extent, in your fatty tissues. This estradiol is called *17β-estradiol* and is the most potent estrogen circulating throughout your body during your fertile years. *Estrone*, which is the principal circulating estrogen in your menopausal years, comes from the metabolism of estradiol but is produced chiefly by the conversion of an androgenic hormone called *androstenedione* in your fatty tissues and muscle cells and is stored there. A third estrogen called *estriol* is produced by the placenta in pregnant women and is the major estrogen in pregnancy. It is also an end product of estrone and estradiol produced in small amounts in normally menstruating women but it is not particularly

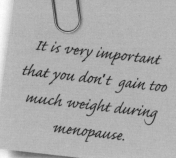

It is very important that you don't gain too much weight during menopause.

important in menopause. Some research suggests that estriol, which is known as free because it is not bound to a storage or carrier hormone and because it does not convert back into estradiol and estrone, may be a good hormone therapy (HT) option (see Chapter 4), though its safety has not been established.

Since the main source of estrone is your fatty tissues, the fatter you are the more estrone you will produce even if you have become menopausal. Raised levels of estrone are associated with stroke, breast cancer and cancer of the lining of the womb. It is therefore very important that you do not gain too much weight during this time.

In discussing estrogens I should mention an enzyme called *aromatase*, which is probably one of the most important enzymes responsible for the formation of estrogen in your tissues. You will read more about this hormone in Chapter 8 when I discuss breast cancer. The aromatase enzyme is found in your fatty (*adipose*) tissues, adrenal glands, muscles and skin. After menopause, when the ovaries stop secreting estrogen, the activity of this enzyme usually increases and becomes one of the main ways you continue to produce estrogen when you are postmenopausal. Aromatase can cause your estrogen levels to increase to a degree where your body shows all the effects of excess estrogen, such as thickening of the lining of the womb, bleeding and even estrogen-positive cancers. Aromatase is also present in our brains and bones, which may be the reason why our cognitive function and bone mass can be maintained after menopause even without HT.

The levels of hormone production are controlled by a feedback loop which resembles a thermostat: when the temperature drops, the thermostat will stimulate the heating so that the temperature rises. This is very similar to what happens with your hormone levels. In Chapter 1 I discussed how the hypothalamus sends a message to the pituitary, which initiates the secretion of two hormones, follicle stimulating hormone (FSH) and luteinising hormone (LH). The action of these two hormones leads ultimately to the production of estrogen and progesterone.

Because these major hormones are produced in the ovaries, many women believe that when they reach menopause they no longer produce them, but as I explained in Chapter 1, the ovaries don't stop functioning at perimenopause and menopause, they just operate differently. There are other areas in your body besides the ovaries that can produce estrogens, albeit in smaller amounts.

There is a very good reason why this happens. The hormones in your body give messages to different organs and tissues to behave in a certain way. They are able to do this because all these areas have special groups of cells which are called *receptors*. Receptors are all different, so the estrogen receptors will respond only to estrogen, while the progesterone receptors respond only to progesterone. A similar process takes place with all the hormones; there are specific receptors for specific hormones, much like locks and keys. The wrong key cannot open the lock.

Each hormone that I have mentioned has carefully defined functions and this is why when the levels of these hormones drop or rise and the receptors are deprived of their specific hormone or inundated with it, there will often be a profound effect on your body.

But here is the good news – because the precursors of the sex steroid hormones are also made in the adrenal glands, and because there are specific hormone receptor sites throughout your body, these hormones continue to be produced, just in smaller amounts. For example, as I mentioned, even though levels of estradiol drop during the menopause transition, you continue to produce estrone, some of which is converted to estradiol. So although there are often very noticeable changes in your body during perimenopause and menopause, the small amounts of sex steroid hormones that are still being produced allow your body to adjust to the different hormonal levels and this is when the most aggressive symptoms of the perimenopause will generally tail off.

Each hormone has its own unique function and once you see how it works you will begin to understand that if the amount of a particular hormone drops below or rises above its normal levels, certain symptoms will occur.

Estrogens

Estradiol is the most potent of all the estrogens and is a vital hormone in maintaining a healthy fertile cycle. There are two types of estrogen receptors: ER alpha and ER beta. ER alpha is found mainly in the breast, womb and bone, while ER beta is found mostly in the ovaries (in the testes and prostates of men), lungs and certain areas of the brain.

There are estrogen receptors throughout your body – your brain, skin and hair follicles, your breasts, your skeleton, the fatty tissues of your thighs and buttocks, and other body areas. Thus estradiol adds fatty tissue to your breasts, thighs and hips, mainly during puberty, but this can continue throughout the rest of your life. There are also estrogen receptors in your vagina and your uterus, so estradiol is involved in the growth of your uterus and thickens the lining of your womb in preparation for pregnancy. It also keeps your vagina moist and plump. One of the reasons for this is that the walls of the vagina and the outer areas of the urethra are very rich in estrogen receptors. It makes sense, therefore, that during perimenopause, when the levels of estrogen are fluctuating, or when they stabilise and become lower than the levels experienced during your reproductive years, the lining of the walls may change, become thinner and less elastic. There will also probably be less lubrication, because estrogen stimulates the secretion of vaginal and cervical mucus. Several changes to your vagina during perimenopause can affect your sexuality, but not all of these are the result of reduced levels of estrogen, as I will explain when I discuss sexuality and menopause.

Since there are estrogen receptors in the skin, you can see how lowered levels of estradiol may impact on your skin's youthful appearance. There are also estrogen receptors in the smooth-muscle cells of your arteries and it is believed that estrogen might play a protective role in preventing heart disease. The issue of estradiol and heart health will be discussed in Chapters 4 and 7. The estrogen receptors in your brain appear to interact with different brain chemicals (*neurotransmitters*), so the fluctuating levels of estradiol in perimenopause may cause some of the mood swings and erratic emotions that I discussed in Chapter 1. These interactions are very complicated and further research needs to be done to improve our understanding of estrogen's role in both your brain and your heart.

Estrogen is also very helpful in reducing the risk of fracture in peri- and postmenopausal women because it stimulates the activity of the osteoblasts or bone builders in the bones.

Like the other hormones, estrogen can have some adverse effects on your body. Breast cancer and cancer of the lining of the womb can be caused by excess estrogen, which overstimulates the estrogen receptor cells in these areas, but I will discuss these in detail in Chapter 8.

Progesterone

Progesterone is the sex steroid hormone responsible for sustaining a pregnancy by maintaining the thickened lining of the womb. Progesterone comes from the ovaries but is also produced in small amounts in the fatty tissue of the brain and nervous system. One of the main roles of progesterone is to balance the effects of estrogen on the female body. Progesterone helps to limit your blood loss during menstruation. This is one of the reasons why during perimenopause bleeding may be heavy and you may have longer periods than usual.

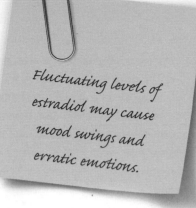

Fluctuating levels of estradiol may cause mood swings and erratic emotions.

Progesterone may cause fluid retention during the second half of your menstrual cycle and often causes weight gain and adult acne. Raised progesterone levels also stimulate the breasts so that they feel heavy and sensitive. The progesterone receptors in the brain and nervous system may react to falling levels of this hormone by causing heightened levels of anxiety and depression. It is also interesting to note that excess amounts of progesterone can unmask and enhance depression. Too little progesterone may affect your body's production of cortisol because, as I mentioned above, progesterone is a building block for cortisol.

Progesterone has sedative properties, which may help to calm you and to promote deeper sleep. So when levels of progesterone drop during perimenopause your sleep patterns may change and you may experience 'panic attacks' or palpitations. Progesterone helps to build and maintain bone, and it can affect your thyroid function. A lack of progesterone may cause endometrial cancer because there is uncontrolled stimulation of the lining of the womb by estrogen.

Testosterone

Testosterone is an important male hormone that is also produced in small amounts in women. Like the other sex steroid hormones, it is derived from cholesterol and is produced in the ovaries and the adrenal glands. It can also be produced from estradiol in the liver and fatty tissues. It is one of the male androgenic hormones. In puberty, the effect of testosterone on girls is similar to the effect it has on boys, though to a lesser extent, causing increased body odour, pubic hair, an oilier skin (which can lead to acne), and bone growth. Testosterone may be intricately intertwined with a woman's libido (sexual desire), but as I will discuss further on, there are many other issues that affect your sex drive in perimenopause. And since there are testosterone receptors in areas other than your ovaries, even if you have had a hysterectomy you will still produce small amounts of this hormone.

Testosterone also affects the quality of your muscle tone and energy levels. If your estrogen levels drop below your levels of testosterone, this imbalance can affect your hair growth, and the hair on your head may become thinner, sometimes mimicking the way men go bald on the top and front of their heads. You may also develop facial hair and an oilier skin, which can lead to adult acne.

OTHER IMPORTANT HORMONES

Cortisol

Another group of hormones called *glucocorticoids* is produced in our adrenal glands. These also have pregnenolone and progesterone as their building blocks, but cortisol is the only one that is really relevant to menopausal women.

Cortisol comes from the adrenal cortex in the adrenal glands and is one of the hormones most important to maintaining a healthy body. A hormone called *adrenocorticotropin* or adrenocorticotropic hormone *(ACTH)* is secreted by the pituitary gland and stimulates the adrenal glands to produce cortisol. If you are stressed, either physically or emotionally, the pituitary gland increases its production of ACTH, resulting in raised levels of cortisol, which cause all sorts of problems. This is why, later in the book, I will discuss the importance of dealing sensibly with your stress levels.

Cortisol is a very powerful hormone; it is the watchdog of your immune system because it helps it to respond to stress, extreme temperature changes and allergic reactions, and has a strongly protective effect in slowing down the inflammatory reactions of your body. It plays a vital role in helping to maintain blood pressure and cardiovascular activity. Because it is instrumental in balancing the action of insulin in breaking down sugar, it helps raise your energy levels and ensures the appropriate metabolism of protein, fats and carbohydrates, which is why raised or lowered levels of cortisol can alter this delicate balance. Higher than normal levels of cortisol slow down your metabolism, which means that you gain weight. Too little causes you to lose appetite and weight and feel sluggish, exhausted and weak.

Normal levels of cortisol help to stabilise your emotions because certain sections of your brain that are involved in your emotional functioning are rich in cortisol receptors. However, extreme emotional stress appears to raise levels of cortisol and the effect of these higher levels is often to cause emotional upheaval and impaired memory function. Your cortisol levels rise and fall daily over 24 hours. Levels are usually highest between 6 – 8 am, and lowest around midnight.

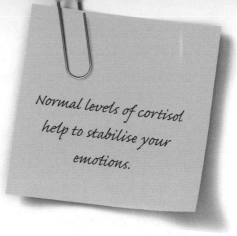

Normal levels of cortisol help to stabilise your emotions.

Cortisol can fluctuate because of raised levels of stress, illness and fever, and although it plays such an important role in maintaining the intricate hormonal working of your body, cortisol levels that are raised over a length of time because of factors such as long-term stress can have some very undesirable effects. These include the weight gain that I mentioned earlier, extreme fatigue, very low levels of energy, and a lowered immune system (all the cells, tissues and organs that work together to protect you from disease). Raised levels of cortisol can also lead to the suppression of the hormone known as DHEA.

DHEA

Dehydroepiandrosterone (DHEA) is an essential precursor (a substance from which another substance is formed) for the formation of all natural androgens and estrogens in humans. It is secreted by the adrenal glands and converted in the tissues and muscle cells to active androgens and/or estrogens, where it, and a similar hormone called d*ehydroepiandrosterone sulfate* (DHEA-s) can be building blocks for both testosterone and estrogen.

Levels of DHEA are highest in women at around the age of 30 and then drop quite dramatically, so they are about 60 per cent lower at the time of menopause. This reduction happens at the same time that levels of androgens and estrogens fall. In menopausal women, once the ovaries have stopped secreting estrogen, about 80 per cent of all androgens and estrogens come from DHEA from the adrenals. Recent research has shown that levels of DHEA in women vary widely, in both women who have kept their ovaries and those who have had them removed, though women without ovaries have 18 per cent less DHEA. This wide range of DHEA levels may partly explain why some women don't battle with menopausal symptoms. Studies show that 25 per cent of women who don't seem to suffer from menopausal symptoms, including dry vaginas, may have higher levels of DHEA, even though their estrogen levels are as low as those women who are battling with symptoms.

There is great interest in the role DHEA plays in the health of menopausal women, since it is thought that DHEA helps to strengthen the immune system, maintains bone density, helps you sleep normally and is involved in protecting heart health by controlling the levels of LDL cholesterol (the more dangerous or 'bad' cholesterol). It may also protect against type 2 diabetes, weight gain and muscle loss. Research shows that DHEA improves levels of vitality and energy, the ability to cope with stress, and the general sense of well-being and of being on the ball. Levels of DHEA-s drop as you age and new research is investigating whether low levels of DHEA-s can put you at greater risk for heart disease.

Thyroid hormones

Thyroid hormone is one of the most significant hormones in the menopausal process because so many middle-aged women suffer from some kind of thyroid dysfunction, which can cause symptoms that may mimic those that you may experience during your perimenopause.

There are two main thyroid hormones, thyroxine (T4) and triiodothyronine (T3), which are produced in the thyroid gland when the pituitary secretes a hormone called thyroid stimulating hormone (TSH). The best way to describe the action of thyroid hormones is to compare the functioning of your body to the idling of a car engine. If the engine idles too quickly (an overactive thyroid – hyperthyroidism) or too slowly (an underactive thyroid – hypothyroidism) we can expect engine problems. Thyroid hormones are essential to the promotion of healthy cell functioning in the human body; they help your body to function well and healthily.

The reason thyroid dysfunction is an important factor to be aware of in perimenopausal women is that many of the symptoms of too much or too little thyroid hormone may mimic the symptoms of perimenopause. If you have too little thyroid hormone circulating through your body you may experience, among others, the following symptoms, which are very similar to those experienced in perimenopause: fatigue, sensitivity to cold, memory problems, depression, menstrual disturbances (irregular or erratic periods) and weight gain. These menstrual problems may be caused by raised levels of prolactin, which can result from an underactive thyroid. If you are producing too much thyroid hormone you may find that you are very hyped-up, anxious, have palpitations, lose weight and experience irregular periods. This is why, in Chapter 1, I wrote that if you are having symptoms of perimenopause you should ensure that they are not, in fact, signs of thyroid problems.

Prolactin

Prolactin is secreted in the pituitary gland in response to high levels of estradiol and nipple stimulation during breastfeeding. It is responsible during pregnancy for helping to prepare your breasts to produce milk. Another of its functions is to repress ovulation after your baby is born. However, some women find that if they are not pregnant or breastfeeding and their prolactin levels are higher than normal, they may not menstruate. High levels of prolactin are called *hyperprolactinemia*. There are several reasons why prolactin levels may be inappropriately high, including a small tumour on your pituitary gland (*microadenoma*), medications like certain tranquillisers, antidepressants and blood pressure medication, greater amounts of estradiol, extreme stress and an underactive thyroid.

Insulin

Insulin is a hormone secreted by the area of the pancreas known as the islets of Langerhans. By maintaining steady levels of glucose in your body, insulin ensures that the sugars and the fats you eat are properly broken down (metabolised) and used to supply energy to your body's cells. Insulin ensures that these foods are used efficiently and that food energy that is not needed is properly stored and then released when it is needed. It also controls the way fat is stored in your body. However, if your insulin levels are raised, all sorts of problems can be expected and, as many women gain weight in midlife, they may start to experience them.

When you are overweight, eat the wrong foods and/or don't exercise, your insulin doesn't work as well as it should. Your doctor may call this *insulin resistance*. There is a lot of talk among menopausal women about insulin resistance and type 2 diabetes. Many healthcare practitioners suggest that insulin resistance causes obesity, but it's actually the other way around. So take care! It has become fashionable when a woman has insulin resistance to diagnose her as having something called the 'metabolic syndrome'. Many midlife women think that taking a medicine called Glucophage, which acts to make insulin work better, will keep their weight down, but as with all magic bullets, there are problems related to this. The best way to prevent insulin resistance is not to gain weight, or if you are already overweight, to lose weight. This is a very complicated and important subject, and I will discuss it at length in Chapter 10.

The way in which hormones send instructions to the various tissues and organs and keep our bodies working at optimum levels of health is miraculous. It is important to remember that this process is incredibly intricate and complicated. You can see from the extremely simplified description I have given of the major hormones involved in perimenopause that an imbalance in these hormones can cause all sorts of physical and psychological changes, illnesses and problems. This is why you need to be both educated and exceptionally careful before you make decisions about hormone therapy, so that you don't upset this delicate balance.

- **Thyroid dysfunction:** Because so many women in their fifth decade suffer from some kind of thyroid dysfunction, it is vital to eliminate this possibility when you experience what you and your doctor may assume are the symptoms of perimenopause. If your doctor does not recommend that your thyroid function be tested, ask for a test.
- **Check your cortisol levels:** In midlife many women find that their lives have become exponentially more stressful for a wide variety of reasons: the 'empty nest' syndrome, changing relationship patterns, bereavement, self-doubt and angst over lifestyle choices, and a partner who may also be suffering from a midlife crisis. As a result of these stressors, you may be suffering from raised levels of cortisol. If you know that you are unduly stressed and have been for any length of time, ask your doctor to prescribe a test to check your cortisol levels. Raised levels of cortisol can cause huge physiological and emotional problems. If you think that you have these symptoms you are probably not imagining them.

3
A brief history of hormone ~~replacement~~ therapy

'I need to see you!' Jenny sounded furious. I asked her what was wrong and she replied, 'I'm so angry I can hardly talk.' She explained that she had gone for her annual gynaecological check-up and had been informed by her doctor that she was now menopausal and that he would like to have a consultation with her and her husband.

Slightly mystified and more than a little anxious at this turn of events, Jenny and her husband came to the appointment. The doctor proceeded to list the woes of menopause, ending with these dire words: 'I'm not prepared to sleep with a dried-out old woman and that is why my wife is on HRT and you should be too!'

Jenny was appalled at this thunderbolt. Apart from the fact that she had no menopausal symptoms, she was not particularly keen to go on HRT and she and her husband enjoyed a happy and fulfilled sex life. She felt that this little interview had thrown a spanner into the works of their relationship and made her feel anxious and guilty. Was she in some sense shirking her wifely duty by not agreeing to take HRT?

She was also furious that the doctor had felt it necessary to tell her husband what she should be doing, as though she was an errant, rather ignorant child who could not make up her mind about her own treatment. She felt that if she had needed her menopause explained to her husband she would have been quite able to either explain the options to him herself or to make an appointment for him to meet her doctor on her own initiative.

In the past 40 years, many women have been 'bullied' by their doctors in similar ways. This particular doctor probably thought it was his duty to help this poor estrogen-deprived woman; to prevent her from becoming a miserable, dried-out old crone who would cease to be attractive to her husband. For the doctor, the benefits of estrogen replacement therapy were so apparent that he literally couldn't understand why a woman wouldn't feel the need to be on it.

HRT OR HT?

I think it is very important to be careful about the terminology we use when discussing this subject. The phrase *hormone replacement therapy* (HRT) was once used to describe hormone therapy but is now dated and has been replaced by the words *hormone therapy* (HT). Many menopause societies throughout the world and academic publications use the term HT, though others, especially in Europe and the UK, still use HRT. Others use the words *menopausal hormone therapy* (MHT). I prefer to use the term HT because as we saw in Chapter 1, you don't actually need to replace your estrogen, although you might need to balance it. Therefore the phrase HRT may emphasise the commonly held misconception that women in peri- and postmenopause are estrogen deficient and need to have their estrogen replaced. So when you see a doctor who uses the phrase HRT ask yourself why they are doing this and be careful that they are not expressing outdated views. In this chapter I use the term HRT when I am discussing the historical perspective, but when referring to the present I use HT.

This is probably the most complicated chapter in the book. But if you want to understand why this subject is so bewildering and why it seems so difficult to get simple answers to your questions, it is necessary to plough through some of the history and see why we have reached the confusing point we are at today. Understanding the dynamics surrounding the controversy about HT is really empowering, so persevere. In writing this chapter I have chosen the bits that seem most significant to me and have focused on the main issues.

Of all the topics surrounding the perimenopause, hormone therapy is the most controversial and difficult for women to grasp. There are so many factors that need to be taken into consideration, so much conflicting research and, it must be said, huge commercial interests at stake. So in the interests of understanding this subject better, here is a brief history of hormone replacement therapy; how we got to this place and why the whole topic has been turned on its head in the past few years.

FEMININE FOREVER – A FLAWED GOSPEL

In 1966 a book called *Feminine Forever* by Dr Robert Wilson radically changed the medical profession's perspective of menopause. The book, which was a paean of praise to the virtues of estrogen, became the gospel for those who touted the theory that menopause was a disease; that menopausal women were hapless victims, deprived of miraculous youth-providing estrogen, doomed to live as miserable, embittered, old women. The book was written in a powerfully smug, didactic and hectoring style. Women were described as 'de-sexed, unstable, frigid, cow-like, castrates'. Dr Wilson saw the state of menopause as a kind of purgatory: 'no woman can be sure of escaping the horror of this living decay'. And secure in his belief in his role as saviour of these desperate middle-aged women, he set out to save them from their fate. So deep was his conviction that estrogen would be the salvation of women that he managed to convince not only the average woman of the validity of his theory – over 100 000 copies of his book were sold in the first year of publication – but many of the most respected members of the medical fraternity agreed with him, particularly after he had published several articles on the subject in medical journals.

Dr Wilson's sexist and paternalistic views might have died a natural death if the doctors of the time had not agreed with them so wholeheartedly. His opinions gathered such momentum that the unappealing image he drew of menopausal women was perpetuated and the ensuing 35 years spawned a plethora of research, all showing the extraordinary benefits of estrogen replacement.

While in the past, advertising for HT exploited women's fear of estrogen deficiency, I notice that major pharmaceutical companies have radically changed their message since the first edition of this book was published in 2005. Their websites stress the importance of a healthy lifestyle, describing a much wider range of choices to help women in menopause feel better. They offer low and ultra-low-dose treatments and discuss the option of local vaginal estrogen. They still show a bevy of extremely pretty, glowing 'older' women, slim and vital with abundant hair, blowing in the breeze, but their HT recommendations are much more measured.

PREMARIN

The most popular of these magical antidotes to the 'disease' of menopause was a hormone treatment called Premarin. This wonder drug had been synthesised

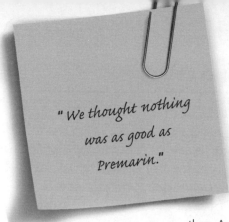

" We thought nothing was as good as Premarin."

from the urine of pregnant mares, hence the name *pre*gnant *mares'* uri*ne*, and the main estrogens in Premarin are estrone, equilin and equilenin. The estrogens in Premarin are known as *conjugated equine estrogens* (CEE). It was the gold standard of HRT, as it was called then. And although, as I explain in Chapter 2, estrone is the predominant estrogen found in postmenopausal women, equilin is not present in women.

A gynaecologist friend of mine, recalling lecturing medical students in the 1970s, says ruefully: 'We thought that nothing was as good as Premarin.' Because Premarin appeared to solve all the problems of menopause, it was accepted throughout much of the Western world. However, in December 1975 a dark cloud appeared on this rosy horizon. The prestigious *New England Journal of Medicine* published an article stating that there was a greatly increased risk of cancer of the lining of the womb in women who were taking Premarin.

In Chapters 1 and 2, I explained how estrogen is responsible for the build-up of the lining of the womb (*endometrial hyperplasia*) and that if there is no progesterone present to control menstruation, the presence of unopposed estrogen (estrogen used by itself without other agents to balance it) causes the womb lining (*endometrium*) to become thicker and thicker, increasing the presence of abnormal cells, which means that cancer may develop. So it is logical that peri- and postmenopausal women who are taking high levels of unopposed estrogen without shedding that thickened lining are going to be prone to endometrial cancer.

As you can imagine, there was a tremendous outcry about the article and, in spite of the fact that the main pharmaceutical companies tried to show that the statistics were overstated, the research that followed thick and fast on the heels of the original results not only confirmed the findings, but also showed that the risks of endometrial cancer if you were taking a hormone like Premarin were even greater than had originally been suggested. So, it was decided to add synthetic progesterone to the treatment and Provera, which is medroxyprogesterone acetate (MPA), saved the day. Doctors felt that if they prevented the build-up of the uterine lining they could continue to give women all the miraculous benefits of estrogen.

Over the past 40 years there have been literally thousands of publications devoted to explaining why HT is so beneficial to women – it protects our bones, our hearts, our brains and our colons; it keeps our skins young and glowing; and gives us plump, moist vaginas and superb memories. In short, it seems that there is no reason, apart from some concern about the risks of breast and endometrial cancer, why women should not be taking HT. The statistics showed that of the hundreds of thousands who took HT, only very few were at greater risk for breast cancer than their counterparts who were not on HT, and appropriate doses of progestogen for women with wombs solved the problem of endometrial cancer. However, this attitude changed radically with the results of the Women's Health Initiative (WHI), as we shall see below, and to their credit, the pharmaceutical company Pfizer, which bought Wyeth in 2009, issued a statement in October 2010 saying: 'We stand behind the current, science-based guidance in Prempro's label, which advises doctors to prescribe the medicine at the "lowest effective dose and for the shortest duration consistent with treatment goals and risks for the individual woman", and patients to "talk regularly" with their healthcare provider about whether treatment is still appropriate for them.'

WHERE'S THE CATCH?

In spite of all the evidence that HT was so great for women, when I started writing the first edition of this book, I felt a bit sceptical. I knew that the information that I was gathering from the women I spoke to was anecdotal, but I couldn't understand why so many battled on HT. They felt bloated and overweight, suffered from painful and hypersensitive breasts, had breast tissue that was so dense that it was hard to do effective mammograms, had bad headaches, adult acne and raised cholesterol levels, and struggled with insulin resistance, sugar cravings and depression. I also knew that I wasn't alone in these doubts and that many women's rights activists were complaining about the fact that menopause was seen as a disease and that doctors' attitudes undermined women and manipulated them to be on HT.

In addition to these critics, there were the 'natural progesterone' gurus like Dr John Lee, who Leslie Kenton praised in *Passage to Power*, or those, like Dr Jonathan Wright, who extolled the virtues of bioidentical hormones in a combination called triple estrogen, which contained estradiol, estrone and estriol, and emphasised the theory, **contrary** to medical opinion, that estrogen should never be taken without progesterone, **even** if a woman does **not** have a uterus.

Although some of the findings of these natural progesterone gurus may have seemed reasonable to women with no medical background, on closer examination there were aspects of their thinking that concerned me. I didn't understand why they didn't put their theories to the gold standard of medical tests, the double-blind randomised controlled trial. Some of them refused to debate with other healthcare professionals in the public, academic arena and once again I was wary of the claim that any hormone, bioidentical or not, was an anti-ageing 'magic bullet'.

In addition, while it is essential to take a progestogen with estrogen if you have a womb, it is not recommended if you do not have one. I couldn't understand why so many women thought that 'natural' progesterone was the Holy Grail. I felt claims that 'natural' progesterone could cure everything from depression to porphyria were somewhat exaggerated.

RESEARCH AND HT

This is probably a good place to explain the complications associated with the research findings on HT. Most women, even those who have discovered the joys of surfing the Internet, don't have the medical expertise to read and interpret statistics. So they hear reports on the radio or television, read sensationalist articles in magazines, or listen to a number of statistics given by their doctor during their 15-minute appointment, which make sense to them at the time, but which are incomprehensible later. I am not suggesting you should take a course in statistics or read complicated medical articles, but when you see an article or read something on the Internet, you should have some tools to help you evaluate whether it makes medical sense and whether you can use the information in it to make an informed decision.

Points to remember when researching HT via the Internet

The Internet has become the quickest, easiest way to access health-related information. But because there is such a vast amount of conflicting material (the last time I googled the words 'menopause information' there were over 15 700 000 results), you need to be on high alert and very critical of what you read to make sure you're not getting dangerous misinformation. There are many really excellent menopause-related sites but others don't have your best interests at heart. Information you read on the Internet is not necessarily true.

Midlife women are an extremely lucrative and profitable target market and the main aim of many of the sites is to sell them something. Many of these women are desperate to find help and information for menopause-related problems, which can make them very gullible. Remember that medical information on the Internet is completely unregulated and it is often extremely difficult to know whether the information you are reading is true or not.

Here is a checklist to use as a guide to see whether the site you are using is reputable.

- **You should be able to see who posted the site:** who is responsible for it and for the information on it, for example major medical centres (such as the Mayo Clinic), universities (such as Harvard Health Publications), foundations and societies (such as the International Menopause Society), government agencies (such as the National Institutes of Health), and medical sites (such as netdoctor.co.uk). **The name of the writer of the text should also be available** and **their credentials should be clearly stated**. You should be able to contact the organisation involved without a problem.

- You should be able to **identify the sources of information** and see if the research has been verified or published by academic journals. An independent panel of medical experts has usually reviewed the information in these journals.

- **Check out the date of the site** to see when new material is posted or when it was last updated. Scroll down and the date will usually be found at the bottom of the page. If a site has medical information, it should be updated regularly; a trustworthy site will typically include the latest research.

- It should be very easy to see whether the site is for healthcare practitioners or for consumers. **Look out for featured or advertised products**. If products are shown or there are things to buy, it is highly likely that the company or person managing the site has a strong vested interest in marketing that product to you.

- **Language is a red flag** when surfing certain menopause sites. Be alert for words like 'anti-ageing', 'guaranteed to work', 'miracle cure' and 'new discovery'. If this new discovery was so miraculous, it would be widely reported in the mainstream and scientific media, and your healthcare practitioners would be informed about it and would recommend it. Watch out for pseudo-scientific jargon using words like 'detoxify' and 'energise', which are often used to sell a product. These words may have some elements of truth but are often used to cover lack of scientific evidence. Buzzwords like 'conspiracy' and 'poison' are also red flags.

- Use your common sense; if the claims made about a product seem too good to be true, then they probably are. **Information on a website should be clear, factual and objective**, not emotional or exaggerated. Try to distinguish between facts and opinion. Your antennae should be twitching if the product claims to treat a wide range of symptoms or prevent a number of diseases. **Ask yourself whether the information you have read is credible.** Search for and verify evidence to back up the claims made on reputable medical sites.
- Testimonials from patients signed with a signature like *John S.* are probably not real. In these cases **cynicism and scepticism are your allies**. True medical professionals are not afraid to sign their full names and designation when they write about something.
- Always ask your doctor or a trusted healthcare professional before following any medical advice from the Internet. A good litmus test would be to check whether it has been certified by a non-profit organisation called **Health on the Net (www.HON.ch)**. This was founded in 1995 by a group of academics, researchers and clinicians from the World Health Organisation (WHO) wanting to help the public find reliable and credible medical information on the Internet. If a site meets the HON criteria they are awarded a logo and credentials, which are verifiable. All websites that have this credential are included on the HON search engine, which is called MedHunt. Make sure the logo is there and click on it to see if it takes you to a page on the HON website to prove it has not been copied. If the logo is not there, you can search for the site on MedHunt and if it is reputable, you will find it there.

How to recognise good research

What makes a good study, one that doctors are prepared to accept when deciding whether or not to recommend a treatment? Many doctors believe that long years of medical experience, during which they have had many opportunities to observe the effects of HT, qualify them to recommend a treatment, but as medicine has become more and more scientific, and it has become possible to test different medicines and understand the risks and benefits better, we can make decisions that are more informed. Medicine that is based on good research is forcing doctors to look differently at the treatments they prescribe. They are now beginning to see that many of the trials on which they had based their opinions were not properly controlled and so the results, which they were using as gospel truth, were incorrect.

As a rule of thumb, a good study should be carefully controlled, using a large sample group, which is divided into two groups. One of the groups, the control group, is on a **placebo treatment** (a harmless substance that has no therapeutic effect), so it can act as a basis of comparison with the group actually taking

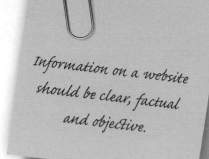

Information on a website should be clear, factual and objective.

the treatment. The words '**double-blind**' mean that neither the people conducting the experiment nor the subjects taking part in it know who is receiving the actual treatment until the research has been completed, so that their information is unbiased.

A **randomised controlled trial** (RCT) is a trial in which people with similar characteristics (e.g. all with low bone density or all with hot flushes) are investigated. The people taking part in the trial (**the sample group**) are randomly assigned to two or more groups. They cannot choose which group they will be in and neither can the person running the trial (**the investigator**); they have a random chance of being assigned to either group. One of the groups (**the intervention group**) will receive the intervention that is being tested and the other group (**the control group**) will receive a different intervention or a placebo. The Women's Health Initiative (WHI) discussed below was an RCT.

It may also help to know the difference between an RCT and an observational study. Unlike an RCT, in **an observational study** conclusions are drawn about the possible effects of a treatment, and though an investigator observes, records and interprets the data in the study, he or she has no control over the treatment being used by the groups of people studied. There are different types of observational studies, including *cohort studies* where a defined group of people (women using HT compared with those who do not use it, for example) are studied over a period of time to see the results; *case control studies*, where people who have a health risk or an illness (heart disease or breast cancer, for example) are compared with a similar group of women who do not have that disease, or *cross-sectional studies*, which are 'snapshots in time' observing the effect/s of an intervention on a representative population group (postmenopausal women taking HT as compared with those not taking HT) and certain factors that may affect their health (do they have raised levels of LDL – bad cholesterol?). The latter are often used to apply public health policy.

The next time you read some information on HT or look at a pamphlet telling you how good the results of a study were, see if it has the following criteria:

- A large sample number
- A control group
- Is it a double-blind study?
- Is it an RCT?
- Has it been carried out over a reasonable period of time to show some significant results?
- Have the researchers declared their interests? The manufacturer of the drug under review may be funding them. Dr Robert Wilson's research was heavily funded by several pharmaceutical companies, including Ayerst, which we know today as Wyeth Ayerst and which was the sole manufacturer of Premarin.
- Read the research with a healthy dose of scepticism: just because something is in print doesn't mean that it's correct. Remember that no study can cover all the different types, age groups, different hormone treatments and regimens. So what might suit you may not suit another woman. Don't take the printed word as an absolute truth.
- Ask your healthcare practitioner whether the research is rated. Studies are usually rated Level I, Level I-1, Level II-2, Level II-3, Level III. If it is Level I it is a properly randomised controlled trial; as the levels drop the study becomes less and less good until it is rated Level III, which means it is based on anecdotal opinions, descriptive reports and experiences of respected clinicians; in other words, it is not evidence-based medicine.

So, what was one of the main things that went wrong with the early research on HT? In many of the earlier studies, the researchers didn't take into account the kind of woman who wanted the 'benefits' of HT. She wasn't just any menopausal woman. She was probably someone who worried about her figure, so she would eat properly and exercise, which would be good for her cholesterol and for her general health.

She would also be the sort of person who would visit her doctor regularly, so her practitioner could pick up any pending problems or medical conditions before they became too severe. She was the kind of patient that doctors call compliant; she takes her medicine and listens to instructions. So when researchers showed how healthy women taking HT were, they were ignoring a very important factor in the research: that the kind of woman taking HT would probably be healthy anyway.

Another problem was that while doctors were saying that HT was good for women's hearts, they were basing their research on studies that had used only men! Or they were basing it on observational data that seemed to suggest that women got coronary heart disease much later than men and only when they become menopausal. So it seemed logical to their doctors that estrogen was protecting them.

As with other aspects of HT and its presumed benefits for women, there had been a plethora of research data showing the benefits of HT in the cardiovascular system of women, but I wondered why, if HT was so good for their heart health, so many women who were on HT were also taking cholesterol-lowering drugs (*statins*). And inevitably, in the late 1990s, a conflict between these hopeful results and other newer results surfaced. By 2000 there was clear evidence that there was an increased risk of blood clots (*venous thromboembolic disease*), as well as stroke. The Heart and Estrogen/ progestin Replacement Study (HERS) found the opposite of what doctors had expected: estrogen and progestin did not appear to further reduce the overall risk of heart disease in women who already had heart problems. In fact, there seemed to be an increase of coronary incidents in the first year of taking HT. So, where women had been told for many years that it was practically their duty to take HT to prevent heart disease, other results seemed to disprove these claims.

THE WOMEN'S HEALTH INITIATIVE (WHI)

These rumblings came to a head in May 2002, when all the previously accepted wisdom about HT was shattered by the results of a very large, well-constructed study, the Women's Health Initiative (WHI). The WHI was a 15-year multimillion-dollar research programme established in 1991 by the National Institute of Health to address the most common causes of death, disability and poor quality of life in postmenopausal women – cardiovascular disease, cancer and osteoporosis.

It was not primarily a study of menopause; the intention was to investigate the risks and benefits of HT to postmenopausal women of 50 and over who were not experiencing perimenopausal symptoms and who were taking either a combination of estrogen and progestin, or estrogen alone. So the results of the WHI would not necessarily be relevant to younger women who had premature menopause and took HT at an early age. The WHI wanted to see the differences between those taking the treatment and those who were on the placebo. The medical profession awaited the results with interest, although generally they believed that their faith in the benefits of HT would be justified.

They were destined for a shock. The results were so alarming that the accepted attitudes of the medical fraternity towards HT were forced to change. The first disturbing fact was that although the study was scheduled to last until 2005, the Data Safety Monitoring Board (DSMB) involved, which had set down certain guidelines relating to the safety of the study, recommended that it be stopped in July 2002 because it appeared that in relation to stroke, the risks of HT outweighed the benefits. A DSMB is an independent committee composed of community representatives and clinical research experts who review data while a clinical trial is in progress to ensure that participants are not exposed to undue risk. It may recommend that a trial be stopped if there are safety concerns or if the trial objectives have been achieved.

The trial of estrogen alone continued, since many doctors felt that it was the progestin that had caused the problem and that the continuing trial would confirm their belief. This was not to be. In February 2004 this trial was also terminated early because of the increased risk of stroke and the fact that there appeared to be no benefit in relation to heart disease. In this case it was the National Institute of Health in America that decided it would be unethical to continue the study.

This termination produced a torrent of outrage. It was as though the ideals dearest and closest to the hearts of most doctors and gynaecologists had been assaulted. And indeed they had. These doctors had spent much of their professional lives recommending HT and swearing by its benefits; to have their beliefs challenged by such a significant study was shocking. The fallout from the termination of both arms of the study was enormous. When the first arm was terminated terrible rows broke out between the different menopause societies in different countries. Dr Jacques Rousseau, who headed the research at the National Institute of Health (NIH), became a pariah in the eyes of many gynaecologists, and the publications that came out of the WHI data were attacked from all sides.

What did the WHI say?

The study shocked doctors because the initial results of the estrogen/progestin part of it showed that for every 10 000 women taking HT there would be eight more cases of breast cancer than among those on the placebo treatment, seven more cases of cardiac events, 23 more cases of dementia, 18 more cases of blood clots (*venous thromboembolism*) and eight more strokes.

On the upside there would be six fewer cases of colon cancer and five fewer hip fractures.

The estrogen-only part, which was halted in February 2004, showed an increased risk of stroke; eight more women out of 10 000 would be at risk for stroke and it seemed that there was no effect, either good or bad, on heart disease. The NIH decided that the risks outweighed the benefits, in spite of the fact that after an average of seven years into the study the women involved appeared to be at no increased risk for breast cancer.

Looking at these numbers you might say to yourself, 'Well, eight more cases of women per 10 000 women a year doesn't sound so bad.' The factor that halted the trials was not the absolute but the relative risk. On the downside, this relative risk showed that there was a 29 per cent increased risk of heart attack (a significant figure), a 26 per cent increased risk of invasive breast cancer and a 41 per cent greater risk for stroke. But on the upside, the risk of hip fracture decreased by 39 per cent.

Although the next paragraph may seem complicated, it is vital that you understand this complex concept because, in medicine, information about absolute and relative risk is essential to any decision you might make about whether or not to take hormones. It is also a very complex concept, which took me a long time to grasp and I will try to explain it as clearly as possible.

Absolute and relative risk

You might go to your doctor and say, 'I read in the WHI study that there was an increased risk of my getting breast cancer or having a stroke.' Your doctor might reply that the absolute risk is still small, about eight more cases of stroke per year per 10 000 women taking HT. This doesn't sound too bad, except of course, if you happen to be one of those eight, but still, in the greater scheme of things, why should those figures have caused such concern? The answer is relative risk. In the WHI study, the NIH decided that the continuing relative risk for stroke was not acceptable in a prevention trial for healthy women, given that HT appeared to offer no benefit to offset the risks — it did not protect women against heart disease.

So what exactly is relative risk? If we do a study of middle-aged women at risk for heart disease and we find that it occurs frequently — for example, 20 middle-aged women in every 100 have a heart attack — but when we give them certain medication, like a cholesterol-lowering drug, which reduces the number of those women who have heart attacks to 10 out of 100, the absolute number reduction would be 10 women per 100 (a relative risk decrease of 50 per cent, which is meaningful). However, if the event happens only rarely, for example, 20 middle-aged women in every 100 000 have heart attacks, and giving them the medication reduces the number to 10 in 100 000, the absolute risk reduction is only 10 per 100 000, but the relative risk reduction is still 50 per cent.

This is why relative risk is the big problem for many doctors, who feel that it is a tool for people who 'play' with statistics. They feel that sometimes the relative risk is widely overstated, causing a panicky reaction from the media and, subsequently, from their patients. In other words, what opponents of the WHI are saying is that although the statistics in the WHI show a significant relative risk, the absolute risk is small. However, despite this small absolute risk, because so many women worldwide were, until recently, on HT, the number of women who were at increased risk for a stroke or breast cancer was large. If the events occurring are rare, relative risk makes these rare events look much more dramatic, so it would be more sensible to look carefully at the absolute risk revealed by the study.

Why all the fuss?

Given these facts, why was there such a panicked reaction to the WHI study? Well, firstly the media picked up on the increased relative risk as a result of HT, didn't understand it properly and had a field day. Then, many women felt that if they were one of the eight women in 10 000 who might be at increased risk for stroke and became one of those statistics, when it might have been prevented by not taking HT, that would be one woman too many. Although the absolute results from the WHI looked reassuring, with only eight more cases of breast cancer per 10 000 women, if we do some simple maths and take these figures to their quite startling conclusion, the scenario would be very worrying. For every one million women on HT there would be 800 more incidences of breast cancer, so that in countries like America for example, where millions of women are on HT, it could mean that if 25 million women were taking HT there would be 25 000 more cases of breast cancer. So, if you play with these numbers they look quite meaningful. If there are 100 million women on HT worldwide, we are looking at 80 000 more women with breast cancer because they took HT, and this number in any terms is huge!

Finally, with myriad treatments and interventions on the market today, the WHI showed that old-fashioned, observational medicine was no longer good enough. *Evidence-based medicine* had now become the order of the day. Evidence-based medicine means that in evaluating a clinical decision, doctors should make use of the best available evidence from the most current, academically sound research. Many women today are more aware of their rights and are better educated, and the Internet has given them new, though often suspect, sources of information. These liberated women feel more comfortable about asking their doctors questions and demanding answers.

Good research will have factored in all sorts of issues: family history, weight, nutrition, alcohol intake, smoking, amount of exercise and general health. Drugs and interventions must be tested and doctors and patients must have access to the results of the tests in order to decide whether the risks outweigh the benefits. Conscientious doctors will use the research to help women decide whether it will be good or bad for their specific health profile in the long run to take the hormones.

But even when citing evidence-based medicine in their clinical practice, healthcare practitioners should exercise caution because evidence-based medicine suggests that specific recommendations from a study be limited to the women for whom the study is relevant. This means that if a study examines the effect of HT on women aged 45–50 it may not be relevant for all postmenopausal women whose ages may ranges from 40-60. For example, the WHI used only one type of estrogen, conjugated estrogen (CE), either alone or with one type of progestin (MPA). As I explain in Chapter 4, many kinds of estrogen can be used in HT and may have different effects. There can never be enough randomised controlled trials, which are the gold standard for evidence-based medicine, to cover all the different factors that make up diverse populations of women or the different treatments available.

Where is the WHI today?

In the original Women's Health Initiative (WHI) study 161 800 postmenopausal women were enrolled. In 2004 when the first phase of the study was over, the women in the original group were asked if they wanted to join the WHI extension study for another five years. Researchers would look at the long-term effects of the original interventions, in this case the use of HT on postmenopausal women, to see whether original participants had changed the way they used HT and to ask and get information about a wide range of scientific questions relating to menopause and ageing over a significant length of time. In total 115 400 women signed up and by 2010 had helped to provide a wealth of information on postmenopausal women's health. In the 15 years that women have participated in the WHI studies, hundreds of articles relating to the information that was collected have been published in scientific journals.

Because of its size and the length of follow-up time, the WHI is unique in medical research on ageing women, despite the criticism that has been levelled at it since the data were first published. Although there are many observational trials dealing with similar issues, certain trials within the WHI are still the only large ran-

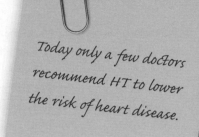

Today only a few doctors recommend HT to lower the risk of heart disease.

domised controlled trials analysing data about HT and its risks and benefits, and generating multiple reports about ageing women and lifestyle. So, in spite of the limitations of the WHI, the findings are taken very seriously indeed by academics and clinicians. By December 2010, over 500 papers had been published concerning the data collected in the WHI and the WHI extension study, and hundreds more are in the pipeline.

The debate about the WHI data persists, and analysis and reanalysis continue, as clinicians and researchers try to reach consensus about the risks and benefits of HT. The WHI continues to uncover misconceptions, raise vital questions and underline how incredibly complex the role of interaction of estrogen is in the ageing female body. It has highlighted the fact that doctors must look at the risk/benefit profiles of their individual patients when they discuss the options of HT during the peri- and postmenopause.

The impact of the WHI continues to be far reaching. By 2007, research describing how gynaecologists felt about prescribing HT after the WHI showed that older male gynaecologists were more sceptical than younger practitioners, both male and particularly female, about the results of the WHI. The reason for this discrepancy is probably that the younger group were trained differently to understand and respect evidence-based medicine and so may have had less of a problem changing their preconceptions. It is comforting, though, to note that today research shows that in spite of doubts on the part of the older clinicians, overall the way they prescribe HT has definitely changed and only a few recommend HT to lower the risk of heart disease or for disease prevention in general.

Interestingly, research shows that in France, where the most common kind of HT used is transdermal estradiol and micronised progesterone, the manner of prescribing HT did not change after the WHI (I will discuss this type of HT in Chapter 4). Many thought that important and conclusive answers were produced about the risks and benefits of HT as far as women who had generally been menopausal for at least 10 years were concerned. However, other clinicians believe that the WHI did not provide definitive answers about whether the use of HT among younger menopausal women (between the ages of 50 and 59) was harmful, because of information (data) emerging from certain **subgroup studies**. (A subgroup study is one where a smaller group of subjects from the main study are chosen by different characteristics such as age or gender to see whether these characteristics would change the overall results shown in the main group.) The main objections were that the results from the data of the WHI indiscriminately included all age groups, only one HT regimen was used, and issues such as timing and duration of the treatment, types of HT and bioidentical hormones were not analysed. In addition, there appeared to be a difference in the risk profile of women who are on estrogen-only therapy (ET) and estrogen plus progestin therapy (EPT).

One of the most relevant sub-studies emerging from the data from one of the WHI subgroup studies was called the *timing hypothesis* – this refers to the time when you start taking HT, in other words the length of time after menopause that you start HT. This research suggested that younger menopausal women would benefit from ET. It showed that the possible benefits of ET, especially in relation to heart disease, may be related to the time that estrogen is given to postmenopausal women – that is, whether it is given at the onset of menopause or later. The WHI-Coronary Artery Calcium Study (WHI-CACS) came out strongly saying the earlier younger women are given ET, the greater the long-term benefits (see Chapter 7). This finding continues to be debated, and although some studies show there appears to be almost no risk for heart disease when HT is given to young, healthy, menopausal women, and may even protect against it in the long run, others disagree, saying this theory has not been adequately substantiated.

A publication written by a group of top academics who further analysed the results from the original WHI said that the results did not support the theory that in relation to the potential risks of estrogen plus progestin therapy, women who started HT soon after menopause had a lower risk of heart disease and greater health benefits in relation to the potential risks. The results of the Kronos Early Estrogen Prevention Study (KEEPs), discussed in Chapter 7, should help to clarify this issue. However, there needs to be urgent ongoing research to provide a more balanced perspective about the risks and benefits of HT.

The latest results from the WHI

And, finally, more support for the timing hypothesis. In April 2011, in the prestigious *Journal of the American Medical Association (JAMA)*, some final results were published for the first time about the WHI estrogen-only randomised trial. This study examined health results in 10 739 women **with hysterectomy** who took ET for approximately six years, as compared with those on placebo, and who were then followed up for over 10 years. The findings showed that using ET, in this case conjugated equine estrogen, was **not** related to either increase or decrease in the risk of heart disease, stroke, blood clots, hip fractures or colon cancer mortality. Estrogen-only therapy was associated with a decreased risk of breast cancer. Age group differences were important; in younger women (50-59) there was a lower risk of invasive breast cancer and a better risk profile for disease and for the general death rate, as opposed to older women. Please note that these results apply to women who had a hysterectomy only!

The findings of this study really highlight the differences between taking estrogen only (which you can do if you don't have a womb) as opposed to estrogen plus progestin, as far as breast cancer risk and other diseases are concerned. There may also be other results if different estrogens, such as 17-beta estradiol, are used. The age at which you take HT also makes a big difference. So it is vital for doctors to thoroughly discuss HT with women, explaining how their age and whether or not they have had a hysterectomy may affect them. Remember the study showed that in older women taking ET, the risks of heart disease, colon cancer, chronic disease and general death rate were greater in the follow-up period, and the risks and benefits of using ET for longer than five to six years cannot be generalised from the results of the study for women in **any** age group and as far as breast cancer risk is concerned. Another very recent large study suggests, as I describe in Chapter 7, that breast cancer risk increases with the length of time HT is used, although it agrees that the risk is greater with EPT than ET, and stresses that the type and route of administration of HT do not make a difference. So, as you will see in Chapter 4, caution in taking HT is advised at all times.

A wake-up call

In spite of the criticisms about the study, the Women's Health Initiative gave doctors throughout the Western world a wake-up call. It showed that HT appeared to have no effect on reducing heart disease in postmenopausal women. It showed that in some cases, whether or not there was consensus about the way the statistics had been interpreted, the risks of HT might outweigh the benefits. It showed that much of the previously accepted research and conventional wisdom about menopause and HT was incorrect. It showed doctors that HT should be prescribed with care and caution and that it was not a universal panacea for all menopausal ills, and it changed the way that HT had been prescribed for several generations. The WHI study showed that the risks of HT as well as the benefits need to be clearly explained. It showed that HT did not necessarily represent the fountain of youth for middle-aged women, and that all the alleged benefits may not have been founded on solid research. It showed that much of the previous data might have been skewed or based on incorrect, observational evidence. It showed that we didn't know as much about HT as we thought we did, and that there were other treatments and interventions that needed to be properly tested. It showed that equine estrogen in combination with synthetic progestin may cause problems. In fact, some research suggests that progestin may be the 'elephant in the room' as far as risk for breast cancer is concerned.

So, even though there are some problems with the study design and the way some of the data from the WHI research was interpreted, the study was a catalyst which sounded a warning both to women and their healthcare practitioners and changed the way HT was viewed.

EMPOWER YOURSELF

- **Don't let the statistics overwhelm you:** When your doctor quotes a bunch of statistics to show you the benefits of a hormone treatment, don't be overwhelmed. Ask him or her to explain the statistics to you. Ask whether the risk is relative or absolute. Ask about the research, check out the sample numbers and find out whether the research is recent and whether it has been published in a prestigious journal such as the *New England Journal of Medicine, The Lancet* or the *Journal of the American Medical Association.*
- **Search the Internet with caution:** Use the guidelines above to decide whether a site is reputable.
- **Don't be afraid to ask your doctor about new research** and be able to understand for yourself whether the study was a randomised controlled trial (RCT) or an observational study.

4

What now? Hormone therapy explained

THREE TREATMENT TALES

Louisa is an attractive, intelligent woman of 54. She explained that she felt fine on the hormones she was taking – a combined oral contraceptive and an estrogen supplement every day – but wanted to know more about them.

I asked her why she was taking both the contraceptive and the hormone therapy (HT).

'Because of my age, my doctor tested me while I was on the contraceptive; he wanted to know if I was perimenopausal,' she said. 'He found that my hormones were a bit low, so he told me to add some hormone therapy to the oral contraceptive. Six months later I went back for my check-up and he told me that at my age I must be menopausal and tested my E2 (estradiol), which was a bit low, so he said it was time to go on to proper HT and gave me combined HT. I felt terrible on it and got night sweats for the first time ever. So I asked him if I could go back onto the previous combination for another six months.'

I was a little perplexed by this story. Her gynaecologist had tested her hormone levels while she was still on the oral contraceptive, which meant that the results would be inaccurate. As a woman of 54, it was almost impossible that she would still be fertile, so why was she still on birth control tablets?

Furthermore, her levels were a bit low because she was either peri- or postmenopausal. It was not clear why her doctor supplemented her hormone levels. He should have taken her off the contraceptive, waited for it to clear from her system and done a proper hormone level test before he prescribed HT, which may or may not have been necessary.

Colleen had had a total hysterectomy when she was 33 and had been put onto conjugated equine estrogens (CEE) (unopposed estrogen; no progestogen, because she no longer had a womb). Today, some 24 years later, she is still taking it. On Mondays, Wednesdays and Fridays she takes 1.250 mg; on Tuesdays and Thursdays she halves the dose and takes 0.625 mg.

She is very unhappy about her weight but is terrified to come off the estrogen because she is worried that she will instantly shrivel up, look old and feel miserable. A few years ago, when she had been on CEE for nearly 20 years, she stopped it cold turkey and felt so dreadful that she immediately went back on it.

Again, I was perplexed. Why should Colleen be taking the stronger dose at all? Since the Women's Health Initiative (WHI) study most doctors, and indeed the manufacturers, were recommending a much lower dose of estrogen for a shorter period of time and in the form of a gel or a patch, not a pill.

Even more worrying was that Colleen had not been monitored and had not had her levels tested for more than three years. Whenever she mentioned her concerns to her healthcare practitioner, he was very non-committal; his attitude was: 'If you're okay don't worry', and because she'd had a total hysterectomy he didn't feel there was any problem with her continuing this dose. He did not bother to explain to her any of the risks associated with taking high doses of estrogen in the long term, which include increased risk for breast cancer, heart disease and strokes.

The reason she felt so awful when she stopped the estrogen cold turkey was that no one had explained to her that her body would have become used to the hormone and it might have been better for her to lower her dose of estrogen or taper off the estrogen gradually and see how she felt, allowing her body to adapt to the new situation. She had asked her pharmacist and he knew so little that she started scouring magazines and newspapers for answers, but came away feeling more confused than ever.

Rosie hated the idea of HT but had, for a while, used a trans-dermal estradiol patch and bioavailable progesterone to maintain her womb's healthy lining. 'I felt good on it,' she said. 'I didn't have any hot flushes, I had more energy and I didn't feel so down, but because of all the media hullabaloo about the dangers, I got anxious and came off all the hormones.

'After a while I started having hot flushes again and I didn't feel great, so I thought I would try the natural route and went to see one of the local alternative medicine gurus. Everyone was singing his praises. He was very eager for me to try all sorts of exotic treatments but I wasn't too keen, so I said no.

'This doctor then referred me to a homeopath, who told me that my estrogen levels were low but my progesterone levels were not, so I was given an estrogen cream.'

The cream was in a squat white plastic jar. It had a label with very little information on it: 'Melilotus-homaccord. Ignatia Homaccord apply ¼ tsp to skin daily for three weeks, estradiol 0.5 mg, estriol 2 mg'.

What is interesting about this story is that while Rosie's estradiol level was low, it was less than 37 pmol/ml (<10 pg/ml), her progesterone level was very high – 12 pmol/ml (3.7 pg/ml), which is the same level as in an ovulating woman.

I didn't understand how a fully menopausal woman could have a progesterone level that high if she wasn't taking additional progesterone. In fact, on further questioning, it transpired that Rosie was using a body cream which contained progesterone, although it wasn't on the list of ingredients.

The homeopath, however, hadn't bothered to find this out, even though it was hormonally impossible that Rosie would have such high levels of progesterone naturally when her estrogen levels were so low. Although the homeopath recommended the estrogen cream, which contained a high amount (2 mg) of estriol, which is meant to be a less powerful estrogen, the cream also included 0.5 mg of estradiol, which is a powerful and active estrogen. In fact many manufacturers are suggesting that women may want to use even lower levels of estradiol since they are able to find symptom relief with this dosage.

When you read the above stories are you surprised that women are so confused? For each of those tales there are a hundred others. Each story shows how women were subjected to different hormone regimens and in each one the women were not given the requisite information by their doctors to allow them to make sensible choices. They were not properly tested, family histories and health histories were not carefully taken and the doctors ignored the most recent medical research, doing what they thought was best, without much regard for the consequences of their actions and often paying no attention to the wishes of their patients.

As we saw in Chapter 3, the problem is that we know a bit about HT but not enough. Research is costly and lengthy, and it is difficult to set up credible studies. What research there is may be flawed because there is often bias, conflicting financial interests and skewed data. There is also a flood of data being released that is full of contradictory information. Because the situation is so confusing, it is very hard for women, even those who are well informed, to know what to do.

Doctors may also be confused and sometimes anxious about prescribing something that may be harmful to their patients; a product that might look okay today may prove to be a health risk tomorrow. Of course, there are also doctors who prefer to rely on their own clinical experience, don't believe in evidence-based medical research and continue to give their patients large doses of estrogen.

This chapter should help you clarify your options and make some sensible choices that are appropriate for you and your individual menopause.

POSITION STATEMENTS OF MENOPAUSE SOCIETIES WORLDWIDE

When the estrogen/progestin arm of the Women's Health Initiative (WHI) trial was terminated, followed by the estrogen-only arm, menopause societies throughout the world convened boards of experts to help their confused members and to give them some guidelines about prescribing HT.

These guidelines are reviewed on an ongoing basis. The experts are some of the best and most experienced in the field of menopausal medicine and they examine a wide body of literature on the subject. They debate among themselves, consider the options carefully and, where the research data seems clear, use their clinical opinions and expert knowledge to write up comprehensive position statements on HT that they hope will clarify the confusing research and make sense of the hype in the media.

These position statements are too lengthy to be included in this chapter. Because they are so extensive and written in medical language, I have summarised and simplified the positions of five of the most powerful and influential menopause societies in the Western world on my website for readers who want more information. You can read the position statements at **www. nicolejaff.com**. Basically, they all agree, regardless of their stance on HT, that **hormone treatment should be specific to each woman, taking**

into account all her health risks and the possible benefits of the treatment. Doctors may agree or disagree with these position statements; you can draw your own conclusions. When I discuss specific risks and benefits of HT throughout the book, I pay close attention to these statements. It is also important to understand the terminology that is used when discussing HT and it is suggested that these terms are used consistently.

THE TERMINOLOGY OF HT AND HT REGIMENS

There is a plethora of data and different opinions the debate rages on and is not likely to abate. Read carefully, make use of the information that is available to you, and keep an open mind about the risks and benefits of HT.

ET	Estrogen therapy (also known as Estrogen-only therapy)
EPT	Estrogen-progestogen therapy combined
HT	Hormone therapy (includes both ET or EPT)
Progestogen	Includes both progesterone and progestin
Systemic ET/EPT	Preparations that work throughout your body, not just on your vagina
Local therapy	ET preparations that work mainly in your vaginal area and are not absorbed in clinically significant amounts throughout your body
Timing of HT initiation	The length of time after your menopause when you start HT

WEIGHING UP YOUR OPTIONS

I am not a medical doctor, but I have been consulting with menopausal women for many years and during this time I have followed as much of the available research on menopause as possible. I have read as widely as I could on this subject and spoken and listened to the opinions of many different experts in the field. I have sat in conferences and workshops, trying to weigh up carefully and logically what I have heard. I have looked at the financial interests of those who were passing out the information. What I write may well be proved wrong by future research and if so I will change my suggestions, but at present the following is my opinion.

Before you even consider taking HT...

You should make an appointment with your healthcare practitioner and spend some time discussing the risks and benefits of HT and whether it is suitable for you. If necessary, when making the appointment, you can tell the receptionist that you may need more time than usual or a longer consultation. Some menopause practitioners make the appointments later in the day and set aside time for these discussions.

Choosing the right doctor

Patricia was very upset when she spoke to me. She had had a total hysterectomy when she was 48. Though happily married, she had no sexual desire and her vagina was painfully dry. Her gynaecologist had prescribed a transdermal estradiol gel and a local vaginal estriol cream. However, neither of them seemed to work. When she tried to discuss these issues with her doctor, she felt unheard and dismissed. She said that he has a very busy practice and when she goes there he is very distracted and she feels she is just part of a 'fast processed sausage machine'. When she arrived for her annual check-up, the waiting room was full of young, pregnant women and she waited for over an hour while he dealt with an emergency. Although the receptionist had her contact details, she hadn't bothered to call Patricia to warn her that there would be a wait.

When her doctor finally saw her, she sensed he was disinterested in her problems and was distracted. He rushed through the consultation, didn't bother to give her an internal examination and only gave her mammogram results a cursory glance. He didn't do a Pap smear, and she assumed that it was because she no longer had a cervix. She had made the appointment because she wanted to discuss her menopausal status with him and to reassess her current HT regimen, neither of which he did, allocating her barely 10 minutes of his time. She felt she deserved better service given the very high fee that she was paying for her annual examination, but he obviously didn't have the time and couldn't have cared less about her menopause problems.

Patricia would probably do better with a gynaecologist who specialises in menopause. Her doctor had delivered her two children and she felt loyal to him, as he had been the right healthcare practitioner for her during those years. The problem may have arisen because women who are having babies have very different concerns from women who are moving into the menopause transition and her doctor was obviously not particularly interested in menopause and so may not have been the best person to deal with the complex issues that often arise at the time in a woman's life. Patricia needs a doctor who is both sympathetic and knowledgeable and prepared to spend some time explaining what is going on with her body in menopause. Midlife women want a clinician who has in-depth knowledge about menopause to help guide them through the decisions they may need to make about HT, lifestyle choices and their health, both reproductive and general as they age.

Patricia's doctor should have listened to her when she complained that the HT regimen he recommended wasn't working and spent some time discussing another solution. Vaginal dryness can be a huge problem for many women and must be addressed. There are many local vaginal estrogen preparations as well as different types of estrogen and Patricia needed to find those that worked for her. He also should have explained why he didn't do a Pap smear and an internal examination. It's still important to do an internal (pelvic) examination even when the cervix and womb have been removed, and there are different criteria as to when a Pap smear is necessary (see Chapter 6).

In order for you to get the best healthcare in midlife, you need a sympathetic and well-informed gynaecologist, a good general practitioner (GP) who will monitor your health throughout the year, and a physician who will give you an annual check-up. I have spoken to many women who are seeing a variety of different specialists; they often do not liaise with each other, and these women end up taking a wide variety of prescription medications, which can have different side effects and interactions. If you have a range of health problems, your physician can act like the conductor of an orchestra, discussing the treatments with both you and your other doctors, and ultimately take responsibility for your overall health.

A checklist to help you find the right healthcare practitioner in menopause

- The receptionist and the office staff often reflect the doctor's attitude. They should be polite and friendly. Their attitude when you call to make an appointment may be an indication of what might happen during your consultation.

- When you phone in with a question about your health, your call should be answered promptly; either by the doctor or in some cases the nurse practitioner. Don't be fobbed off with an answer from the receptionist – it's the healthcare professionals and not the receptionist who should answer medical questions.
- Your healthcare practitioner should be interested in menopause and affiliated to the appropriate societies.
- Your specialists should attend conferences and workshops so they know about and understand the latest medical information. For example, members of NAMS (North American Menopause Society) throughout the world can write a special exam, which will earn them a certificate as a certified menopause practitioner and entitle them to the initials NCMP (NAMS Certified Menopause Practitioner) after their name and titles. Your doctor and/or specialists should be up to date with the available research and focused on their particular area of expertise.
- Because the field of menopause is changing so rapidly and because there are so many complex issues attached to it, it makes sense to speak to a specialist who has a serious interest in this area of reproductive medicine.
- You should be easily able to see your doctor's degrees and qualifications. Depending on the country you live in, your doctor will be registered with a professional body, like the Health Professionals Council of South Africa (HPCSA), General Medical Council (GMC) in the UK or if they are in the USA, they should have passed a special licensing exam such as the United States Medical Licensing Exam (USMLE), which is sponsored by the Federation of State Medical Boards (FSMB) and the National Board of Medical Examiners (NBME). If your doctor is a specialist, they will have a higher degree from a specific medical board certifying them to practise as a specialist in their area of choice. Some of these specialities require recertification after a time.
- Your doctor should always be respectful, listen attentively and give you a reasonable amount of time. He or she should be confident enough to admit when a problem falls outside their area of expertise, and should be happy to refer you to an appropriate medical specialist when necessary.
- Your healthcare practitioner should monitor your health by giving you a series of tests, listed at the end of this book (pages 306–307). They should explain the results simply and in an understandable manner.
- Your doctor should be prepared to discuss the risks and benefits of HT and any prescribed medication or medical issues, and never make you feel stupid when you ask a question or need further information. His or

her attitude to HT is very important in discussing whether it is indicated for you. Read pages 57–59 to understand when and when not HT should be prescribed. He or she should explain any matters under discussion in simple English. You should not feel overwhelmed by medical terminology that is incomprehensible to you. There is a glossary of many of these terms at the end of this book to help you understand what they are saying. Good communication is intrinsic for your partnership with your healthcare practitioner.

- Healthcare practitioners should enquire about the medications and supplements you take and if they do not enquire, you need to inform them.

What should happen at your annual gynaecological examination?

You already know that before you decide to take HT you should have a thorough medical examination. This can be time-consuming and expensive, but it is worth it. Commit to caring for yourself; don't go blindly into treatment.

Your doctor should ask you about your family history, paying special attention to whether you had a mother, or maternal or paternal grandmother, who had breast or any other cancer and whether other close family members died of cancer, heart disease or a stroke, or whether they had osteoporosis. Your doctor should discuss the relevance of this information with you. Specific tests should be performed to see if you are at risk for blood clots. Your doctor should make a record of the medication or supplements you are taking and whether you had a thrombosis or risk of one when you were pregnant. If this is so then you might need specialised testing, called a thrombotic screen, which involves a number of tests and includes a clotting profile. This should be done if your doctor feels that you are at risk for blood clots.

Your doctor should also be aware of whether you smoke, whether you drink and if so, how much you drink daily. In my opinion, if you are a very heavy drinker or you smoke, it is too risky to be on estrogen. Your weight must be checked. Overweight women are at greater risk for heart disease, and this may be increased when they take estrogen. A body mass index of 25 to 30 or greater than 30 should be a warning flag. Your blood pressure should be checked.

Any medical problems should be noted and you should tell your doctor if you suffer from migraines. If he or she doesn't ask you any of these things, bring them up yourself. Levels of cholesterol, fasting glucose and your thyroid should be checked.

Before you decide to start taking HT you should have a mammogram, a transvaginal endometrial and ovarian scan and a bone density scan. You may want to have your hormone levels tested, but be sure the measurements that are being taken are accurate. One of the most glaring errors that occur in

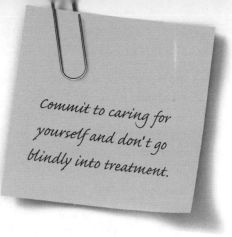

Commit to caring for yourself and don't go blindly into treatment.

the care of menopausal women is the confusion that arises when doctors measure hormone levels. It is accepted that you can't measure the estrogen of women on oral contraceptives or non-bioavailable hormones. The serum estradiol levels you measure can only be from bioavailable hormones. So what often happens is that a doctor tests the hormone levels of a woman who is on conjugated equine estrogens (CEE) but because he or she is only measuring one type of estrogen, and the CEE has not been converted into that estrogen, it looks as though the woman's estradiol levels are low and so the dose of her hormone therapy is increased. This is why women on HT often have the symptoms of excess estrogen.

Take time to discuss all your concerns with your doctor during this appointment. Ask him or her about recent research and discuss the possible risks and benefits. Depending on your health status, your doctor will explain why she or he thinks it may or may not be beneficial for you to start taking HT. Your doctor should only make this assessment based on your individual risk profile. It is important to remember that the benefits and risks of HT will not be the same for you as for others. Your age should be noted, since research – as described earlier in Chapter 3 – now seems to show that there is a relationship between your age and when you start HT after menopause, which might affect your long-term health either positively or negatively.

SHOULD YOU TAKE HT?

I think it is important to stress here that women who, because of natural or induced causes, are plunged into premature menopause (before age 40) or early menopause (between 40 and 45), which is before their natural menopause is due, should have hormone therapy, subject to their doctor's consent and **if HT is NOT contraindicated**. Here is why.

Because the results of the Women's Health Initiative (WHI) were applied to all postmenopausal women, it happened that a very different group – namely young women who suffered premature menopause or early menopause for various reasons, either natural or induced – may have suffered unnecessarily, and had some unintended consequences. Ongoing research, mostly observational studies, seems to show that while these women are at lower risk for breast cancer, ironically they are at greater risk for earlier heart disease, osteoporosis, Parkinson's disease and possibly greater cognitive decline as they age. Research has shown that women who had their ovaries removed when they were very young are at greater risk of death from heart disease, but that HT given to these women may reduce this risk. This information encourages clinicians to review each individual case before recommending the removal of ovaries in young women and when prescribing HT. It is clear from other research that HT may have smaller risks and important benefits in these young women. Each woman's case should be considered individually and rigorously as to the length of time they should take the hormones, and the type of hormones that will be most effective and offer the highest benefits and lowest risks.

Once you have had all the appropriate tests, it is my opinion that you should take HT if hot flushes are affecting your quality of life. If you get a hot flush once in a while or only a couple of hot flushes or temperature changes during a day and are coping well with these, there is no need to take HT. You may want to try non-hormonal or alternative remedies or just live with this small, transient change in your life.

But … it is time to take HT if you wake up during the night drenched in sweat; if night sweats are disturbing your sleep patterns with the result that you feel ratty, weepy and depressed the next day. It is sensible to take HT if, during the day, you are immobilised by hot flushes and if you find that summer has become unbearable. If the accompanying symptoms of the hot flushes are nausea, giddiness, a ringing in your ears, a pounding heart, intense heat, and/or a very red face, and if all or any of these symptoms are affecting the way you live your life and the way you feel emotionally, it would be a good idea to take some form of HT.

Another reason to take HT would be if your vagina is so dry that sex is miserable, or that your dry vagina is causing urinary infections and problems. But if you are experiencing these symptoms and are not plagued with hot flushes, I would suggest that you take HT in the form of a local vaginal estrogen product.

Some doctors feel that women who are at risk for osteoporosis in the first years of menopause should take HT to prevent fractures, but if these women don't have severe menopausal symptoms there are other products on the market which may be a better choice, and I will discuss these options in Chapter 9.

When not to take HT

You are not a candidate for HT if you are older than 60, very overweight, have high blood pressure and are at risk for stroke, heart disease or blood clots. Smokers or heavy drinkers should not take HT. Neither should women who may be at risk for breast cancer or have had or currently have breast cancer. If you have liver disease or have any known or suspected estrogen receptor and/or progesterone receptor-positive malignant tumours, HT is not a wise idea.

Be careful if you have any genital bleeding. The cause should be diagnosed before you begin any HT regimen. If you suffer from severe migraines, unless it has been clearly indicated that they are not due to fluctuations in your hormone levels, you should be careful when you take HT. If you have a skin disease known as *porphyria cutanea tarda* you should also not take HT.

WHAT KIND OF HORMONES SHOULD YOU TAKE?

Estrogen

There is no need to suffer from hot flushes and a dry vagina when we know that estrogen helps these symptoms. Choose the type of estrogen carefully. You have probably heard a lot about bioidentical hormones and 'natural' progesterone. There's nothing really natural about them. Bioidentical is not really even a scientific term. It was invented to describe hormones that were similar in biochemistry to the hormones produced in your body or your ovaries. Amongst these hormones are DHEA, estradiol, estrone, estriol, progesterone, cortisol and testosterone. The word 'natural' used in this sense means that they are biochemically similar or identical to the hormones produced by your ovaries and body. But the word natural refers in fact to the source of the hormones. Women use the word natural because they think that these hormones come from plant substances and have not been chemically altered. In fact they are extracted from plants like wild yam and soy and must be chemically altered to become the bioidentical hormones mentioned above. But whether they are bioidentical or not, they have been manufactured (*synthesised*) in a laboratory.

It is important to note that the term 'bioidentical' is also used for many brand name, well-tested HT products containing hormones that are chemically the same (*identical*) to hormones produced in a woman's body (like 17-beta estradiol or progesterone). These products have been approved by medicine control boards.

There are many different hormones available containing estrogen. They have names such as estradiol hemihydrate, estradiol valerate, ethinyl estradiol, estropipate, sodium estrone sulfate, conjugated equine estrogens (CEE), estriol, estradiol and 17β-estradiol. The last three are the same as the estrogens found in your body. The others may be very similar but they are not identical.

You know from Chapter 3 that one of the estrogens in CEE is equilin. Although it has a similar effect to human estrogen, this equine estrogen is stronger than your main circulating estrogen, which is called estradiol and is bioavailable, and it doesn't have the same molecular structure as estradiol. So when your body breaks CEE down (*metabolises* it), it may not do it in the same way as it would a bioidentical estrogen and the estrogen stays in your system for longer.

So it seems to make more sense to me, on a gut level, to use a bioidentical product that closely resembles your own endogenous hormones (those that are produced by your body). There are thousands of women using bioidentical hormones in different forms – patches, creams, rings and gels – many of which have been approved by medical control councils, but as yet there are no large randomised controlled trials (RCTs), like the Women's Health Initiative, on the risks and benefits of these hormones, so much of the information about them is observational.

Healthcare practitioners have to generalise about the effects of one HT product used in a clinical trial and apply it to all the others. However, the experts agree that it makes sense to accept that there are probably differences between all these different estrogens and progestogens and the effects they have according to the way they are administered: How potent are they? What is their bioavailability – meaning what concentration of that product is found in your body and for how long does it remain there? What are their androgenic effects and their glucocorticoid effects (how do they affect cortisol levels and glucose metabolism)?

There is a lot of discussion about bioidentical products, which are meant to have the same composition as the estrogen in your body (*endogenous estrogen*). In other words, they are made up of estriol, estradiol and estrone, and/or estriol and estradiol respectively. I discussed these three main estrogens in Chapter 2. The theory is that if you are going to balance your hormones, why not use a mix identical to the one that is in your own body? But there are a few issues here that concern me.

By the time we reach menopause the estrogen composition in our bodies has changed. The main estrogen is no longer estradiol but estrone. Research into breast cancer indicates that concentrations of estrone, estradiol and estrone sulfate are high in women with breast cancer, despite low levels of circulating estrogens. So I am concerned about adding more estrone in a hormone cream where estradiol and progesterone in peri- and postmenopausal women are

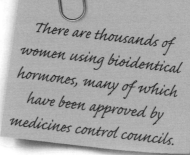

There are thousands of women using bioidentical hormones, many of which have been approved by medicines control councils.

more likely to convert into more estrone anyway. However, like everything else in the field of HT, there needs to be a lot more research to find out the precise role that estrone and estrone sulfate play in breast cancer in peri- and postmenopausal women who are taking HT. Also, although the advocates of these combination creams would have you believe that estriol has the same effects as the stronger estrogens without the risks, one would wonder why estradiol and estrone need to be added, given the risks we know they involve.

The claims for estriol are that it is much less potent than estradiol and it may have fewer of the risks commonly associated with estrogens. But this has not been proved definitively in clinical trials. Although it can never be given in the same doses as estradiol, estriol still carries certain risks – it may cause the lining of the womb to thicken and it may stimulate certain breast cancer cells. It has not been shown to prevent bone loss. On the upside, when used locally in a vaginal cream, it may help alleviate dryness in the vagina and is often prescribed for women who have breast cancer and suffer from vaginal dryness. We need longer and better research to show that estriol, when used over a long time in the higher doses that seem to be necessary for it to work, will not produce the same risks as estradiol. Take the emotion out of the equation and examine the facts.

Progesterone

Here is the big question: what about progesterone – to add or not to add? The terminology relating to this hormone is often very confusing for women. So for the sake of clarity, look at the diagram on the next page.

The word progesterone is usually used to describe the hormone in your body or bioidentical micronised progesterone, which is the same as your own endogenous progesterone (the progesterone that your body produces). Progestins, on the other hand, are synthetic products and not biochemically the same as the progesterone in your body. Both progesterone and progestins have the same effect on the lining of your womb, causing it to be shed when it is ready. In this book when I write about progesterone, I mean the hormone that is identical to your own progesterone, and when I refer to progestogens I am referring to the wide range of hormones that have the same characteristics as your sex steroid hormone progesterone and progestins.

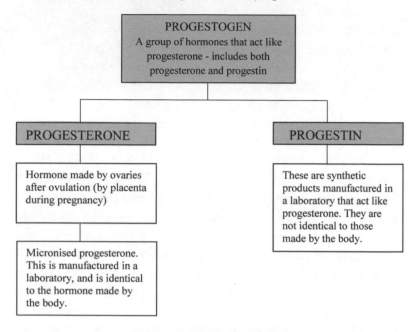

Understanding progestogen

Here are some facts that may help when you read the medical information leaflet that comes with your HT. Some progestins are more similar in chemical structure to progesterone and testosterone and these are called *19-nortestosterone derivatives*. The WHI and other recent research studies seem to show that the addition of MPA (*medroxyprogesterone acetate*) and other more androgenic progestins (which are divided into two groups, *pregnane derivatives* and *19-norpregnane derivatives*), to hormone therapy may increase the risk for cancer, stroke and heart disease. There may also be other effects, like bloating and water retention, although some new-type progestins like *drospirenone*, which is derived from *17-spirolactone* and not from 19-nortestosterone, *dydrogesterone* and micronised progesterone can dampen the effect of *aldosterone*, a hormone that controls the levels of fluid in your body and which, when combined with estrogen, may prevent water retention and may be a better choice. However, a very recent observational study suggested that oral contraceptives containing the progestin drosperinone are associated with increased risk of blood clots as opposed to those containing levenogesterol.

There is also research showing that synthetic progestogens can contribute to depression in women, while micronised progesterone may be helpful in combating depression and maintaining sleep patterns. Some research suggests that medically regulated bioidentical progesterone does not appear to have the damaging effect of synthetic progestogens on the thin, flat cells called the *endothelium* that line the inside of the blood vessels of the entire circulatory system. When the endothelium is damaged it can lead to heart disease and stroke. More research is required in this area but recently in a well-designed trial, the results showed that different types of progestogens when combined with transdermal estrogen might have different effects on clotting risks in women taking estrogen. When transdermal estradiol was combined with a micronised progesterone, the risk seemed lower than the risk in those women who took progestins that were norpregnane derivatives.

So once again, the question comes down to what type of progestogen would be safest and best when taking it to protect your womb while taking estrogen.

A lot has been written about 'natural' progesterone, which I want to emphasise once again is not natural but is synthesised in a laboratory like all the other progestins. The big difference between this and progestin is that it is chemically identical to your own body's progesterone. I don't believe that slathering on progesterone cream indiscriminately is a good idea. 'Natural' or not, it is still a powerful hormone and overdosing with it can cause a lot of bad side effects.

If you are keen to use a 'natural' progesterone make sure that it is one that has been passed by a medicines regulatory body. There are good micronised progesterones available, although to control bleeding you may need higher doses, which may then cause other side effects. Micronised refers to the procedure where the progesterone is broken down into minute particles to allow it to be absorbed more easily, and natural refers to the plant source from which it is derived. Many of the brands of so-called natural progesterone have not been tested and the doses they contain are not standardised, so even progesterone packaged with the same brand name may differ in quality and in the amount of bioavailable progesterone it contains. It may also not control bleeding or the thickness of the lining of the womb. So be careful if you are using this cream in conjunction with estrogen therapy.

Some healthcare practitioners recommend 'natural' progesterone to alleviate menopausal symptoms. Their rationale is that there are progesterone receptors throughout your body and progesterone is a precursor or building block hormone for estrogen and testosterone, as discussed in Chapter 2. They suggest that if you take progesterone, it may give you high enough levels of those hormones to maintain a healthy hormonal balance, but there is just not enough hard research on this method of HT to be sure it does not carry too many risks and undesirable side effects.

In 2009, a double-blind controlled trial compared whether using only a natural progesterone cream was helpful for menopausal women complaining of symptoms. It found that it made no real difference (researchers call this a **statistically significant difference**). In addition, some of these creams contain wild yam, which is useless, because human beings do not have the necessary cofactors to convert this into anything useful. It is also not disclosed that these creams sometimes contain progesterone, which may be a safety issue, especially if a woman is at risk for or has had breast cancer.

Remember Rosie from the cautionary tale at the start of this chapter? She complained that she was sleepy all the time and felt listless and depressed. When I questioned her closely I found she was happily applying a body lotion that contained large amounts of progesterone. She had absolutely no idea how much she was taking; she bought the cream from a health food store as a recommended product for the symptoms of menopause. When she had a blood test she found that her progesterone levels were constantly as high as the levels in an ovulating woman, and remember that level only peaks in a normally menstruating woman; it doesn't remain as high on an ongoing basis.

Some studies suggest that certain progestins may cause problems in the long run. But once again, more research is needed to give definitive answers. So if you haven't got a womb, you should not take a progestogen. If you have a womb, you will definitely need to take a progestogen because if you do not, you could be at risk for cancer of the lining of your womb. Some small studies suggest it may be safe not to take a progestogen or to only take it intermittently if you are taking low-dose or ultra-low-dose estrogen, but the problem is that although this very low dose of estrogen appears to help prevent osteoporosis, it may not alleviate menopausal symptoms. More studies are needed to establish whether taking a progestogen intermittently is safe in the long term and whether it is preferable to taking a continuous combined dose. If you and your doctor decide to go this route, you must understand the risks and be closely monitored by a transvaginal ultrasound scanner.

The big discussion is when you should have your progestogen: only in what would have been the second part of your cycle when you were a menstruating woman (the luteal phase), or a small dose daily? Some people believe that if you still have your womb you should give your body a break at the time your period would have happened in your cycle when you were still menstruating normally. Others believe that women should take a progestogen continuously with their estrogen.

An alternative to an oral progestogen is a loop (an intrauterine device) containing a progestogen (Mirena). This type of loop, containing 20 mcg of a progestogen called *levenogesterol*, is derived from 19-nortestosterone and appears to control bleeding and prevent the lining of the womb from thickening. It may also not have the suggested adverse effects of an oral progestogen because it is local, so the amount of progestogen that enters your system is lower, although a fair amount of this progestogen is still absorbed. More research is needed to establish whether its effects on the breast or heart differ from those of other available progestogens. There have been cases of postmenopausal women who use this device experiencing spotting or breakthrough bleeding. NAMS does not recommend its use in its most recent position statement.

There is also the option of taking a progestogen after a few months of estrogen-only treatment to ensure a bleed. You have to see which regimen suits you best and if you decide to go a different route from standard EPT, the lining of your womb must be very carefully and regularly checked. Discuss your options with your doctor and make sure that you have the lining of your womb monitored regularly to see that it isn't getting too thick. Don't forget too, that if you have had an endometrial ablation (see Chapter 6) you will still need a progestogen if you are taking estrogen because small pockets of the endometrium (lining of the womb) may remain. The dose of progestogen that you need if you still have your womb will depend on the type of progestogen you use and the amount of estrogen you take.

Remember you **cannot** take estrogen alone if you have a womb but since progestogen may cause many undesirable side effects and there are questions about the risks of adding progestogen to an HT regimen, some fascinating studies are under way to see whether an estrogen (CE) combined with an estrogen agonist/antagonist may be the answer for some women and will prevent the need for a progestogen when taking ET. The problem is not as easy as it sounds; just as there are various types of selective estrogen receptor modulators (SERMs) which react in the different ways to the receptors, there are also many different types of estrogen, administered in different ways, so the researchers will have to work out how all these other factors will affect women.

Bioidentical hormones – what you should know

Elaine's husband had recently been transferred and because she had a long and happy marriage, she agreed to give up her thriving practice as an educational psychologist and move to another country with him. She was nearly 60 at the time and was already menopausal. She is an attractive woman and gregarious, but she found the move very difficult. She didn't feel well and though she had always been highly competent, felt unable to cope. After a few months she felt so below par that she asked her new friends if any of them could recommend a doctor. One of them raved about an anti-ageing specialist, saying he was fabulous and would be a huge help. Although she was usually sceptical, Elaine felt so despairing that she made an appointment to see him.

The doctor was very good looking and very compassionate. She told him that she was suffering from stress, insomnia, high blood pressure and exhaustion. The doctor nodded understandingly, though he didn't take her blood pressure and didn't examine her at all. He said that he was an expert in the field of anti-ageing and hormone imbalances and told her she was suffering from hormone depletion, suggesting that she have a battery of blood tests, which would identify this. He also recommended that she buy a wide range of supplements from him, which he said would help with her stress and insomnia. These products were very expensive but she was glad to pay the price as she felt so awful.

After having the blood tests, she returned to the doctor who told her that her hormones were dangerously low and sold her what he called a bioidentical hormone replacement cream, containing estrogen and testosterone. He explained that she should apply this cream daily to the tops of her legs and/or to her inner upper arms. He still had not examined her, and at no point did he discuss the risks and benefits of the cream with her or explain that there are greater risks for heart disease in women older than 60 who take HT.

The cocktail of supplements she had bought from him did not help her stress and she found a helpful GP who told her to stop taking these products and gave her commercial medication to help with her anxiety and insomnia. She felt better but continued to use the bioidentical HT. A few months later Elaine was surprised to see a thick growth of long dark hairs on the top of her thighs, where she had applied the cream daily. She was very upset, as she is blonde and never had any hair growth like this before. She tried to contact the doctor, who did not return her call. When he finally got back to her he did not suggest that the cream might be causing the problem. After a few more weeks when the hair growth intensified, Elaine contacted him again. His receptionist was not keen to let her speak to him but after several more calls, she eventually got hold of him.

This time he said she should repeat the blood tests and suggested that to be safe Elaine should apply the cream to areas of her body where there were no hair follicles, such as the soles of her feet. Elaine waited another six weeks, becoming more and more frustrated that he had not bothered to give her the results of the tests though he knew she was very anxious about the unwanted hair and also any other possible long-term side effects. She finally managed to speak to him and he explained in a long-suffering tone that her testosterone levels were now very high and she was obviously very sensitive to the hormone cream he had prescribed. He suggested that she use an alternative cream that contained no testosterone. Elaine, by now angry and upset, asked him what other side effects could result from high testosterone levels. She was very relieved when she heard that acne, which is a side effect, had not happened to her, and she stopped using the cream. He had no other suggestions about how to alleviate the embarrassing unwanted hair on her legs, though a dermatologist subsequently told her that the only option for the permanent removal of this hair would be laser treatment.

She is now seeing a gynaecologist who specialises in menopause and feels much better.

The term 'bioidentical' is used to refer to many well-tested hormones that have been approved by the various medical control councils; you can take these and know exactly the dose you are putting into your body. They are not the complex mixture of three estrogens that I mentioned earlier, but since estradiol can convert into both estrone and estriol, and progesterone can convert into estrogen and testosterone, you will probably have some of these hormones in your body anyway if you only take estradiol. Both compounded and manufactured bioidentical hormones are available on the market, but many have not been approved. However, some doctors do prescribe them and this chapter should give you enough information to make an informed decision.

In the aftermath of the Women's Health Initiative (WHI) study, with heightened awareness and fears about the risks of HT, women began to investigate alternatives to commercially produced hormone products. Searching for relief from menopausal symptoms, many became aware of bioidentical hormones, which are marketed as safer and more effective according to information that is often based on old research and quasi-scientific evidence. I recently read a PowerPoint presentation given by a well-known 'anti-ageing expert' saying that synthetic hormones have 'been proved to be unsafe in HRT' and 'bioidentical hormones are the only safe option for effective ovarian hormone supplementation'. (Remember that these bioidentical hormones are synthesised in a laboratory exactly the same as commercially produced hormones.) However, although there is an increasing tendency to use compounded, bioidentical hormones for individual hormone therapy, the term *bioidentical therapy*, which was coined by marketers, has no efficacy meaning and is neither defined nor standardised. The term *bioidentical* means that these hormones are structurally identical to the hormones produced by a woman's ovaries. Bioidentical hormones can be both manufactured and compounded. Women are told that these products are 'natural', which, as I indicated above, is simply not true.

If you are told that the bioidentical hormones you are using are compounded, this means that a doctor has asked a pharmacist to combine, mix or alter certain ingredients to create a medication that has been customised for you. These hormones are made from plant derivatives and are then prepared, mixed, assembled, packaged, or labelled as drugs.

The whole point of compounded, bioidentical hormones is that they should be specific to the person for whom they were prescribed. Unlike commercially manufactured hormone therapy, many of these bioidentical hormones claim to replace hormones rather than treat specific menopausal symptoms. There is a great deal of hype about returning hormone levels to 'normal', so proponents of bioidentical hormones say that they are actually 'replacing' hormones, while traditional HT is used to treat transitional menopausal symptoms.

In fact, it has not been established what the 'best' or most 'normal' hormone levels in postmenopausal women are and a woman's physical comfort may not even be related to her hormone levels – you often simply need a small amount of HT to help your symptoms rather than a whole regimen to replace your hormones. So, with the aim of 'replacing' your hormones, these products usually include estradiol, estriol, estrone, progesterone and testosterone. Many bioidentical hormone products have not undergone rigorous clinical testing for safety or efficacy, and issues regarding purity, potency and quality are a concern.

In addition, some bioidentical hormone products on the market are not compounded but still believed by many women to be safer than so-called artificial hormones. But don't be fooled. Patients often receive incomplete or incorrect information about these products. Bioidentical hormones are not necessarily safer than the so-called artificial or synthetic hormones. A hormone **is** a hormone, though different types have different levels of potency, so there are the same safety issues with compounded bioidentical hormone products as there are with hormone therapy medications that have been approved for use by various regulatory bodies. There is no scientific evidence to support claims of increased efficacy or safety for individualised estrogen or progesterone regimens. It is clear that all hormone regimens, whether bioidentical or commercially manufactured, should be subject to the same stringent controls.

Unlike manufactured hormone products, bioidentical hormones generally have no warning label because they have not been regulated by a medicines control board and no package insert describing their risks and benefits, and have not been approved through rigorous testing or Level I research.

Information is found on the Internet and the people who sell these products, often celebrities, laypeople or healthcare practitioners who are affiliated with the product and have a vested interest, quote all sorts of research and also do what I discuss in Chapter 5, which is to pick sentences out of research, edit them and use them out of context. I recently saw a site which listed literally hundreds of articles 'supporting' the use of bioidentical hormone therapy – their own make, not regulated ones – and to my surprise saw that many of the articles critically examining and dismissing these claims were listed. An article criticising bioidentical hormone use may actually be quoted as supporting it, using the edited quote next to the source on the assumption that most women don't have the time or knowledge to read and analyse the actual article.

There are no randomised controlled trials (RCTs) comparing bioidentical hormone therapy with commercially regulated bioidentical products and it doesn't seem likely that there will be in the future. Many of the studies of bioidentical hormones are short term, carried out on animals, are not placebo-controlled or use very small sample numbers. Most do not meet the criteria set out on page 38 for Level I evidence, which is the gold standard of research. As one doctor said to me: 'If a menopausal rat walked into my consulting room, I'd know exactly what to treat it with!' The trouble is we're not rats, we are menopausal women, and should demand that anyone recommending bioidentical hormones should produce adequate evidence.

Studies done on bioidentical hormones have revealed that fewer than half the samples contained the ingredients claimed or the amount of active hormone they promised. Because the amount of estrogen or progesterone in many of the products is not clearly indicated, it is easy to take more estrogen than is necessary. Just because the estrogen in a product is bioidentical doesn't mean it is safer. The risks and benefits of taking these products should be very clearly described to women by the practitioner prescribing them.

Remember that hormones that have been passed by a regulatory body must be consistent in their quality, purity, potency, efficacy and safety. The products from compounding pharmacies are not regulated in the same way and their quality can vary. As I said earlier, a hormone is a hormone, and in my opinion, it is highly irresponsible for health food shops and people who are not experienced in reproductive endocrinology or in the field of menopause to sell creams or gels containing these very potent hormones to unsuspecting women. They are **not harmless** because they are bioidentical! The women who buy these hormones, often at much greater cost than the commercial hormones, are vulnerable because they do not have the medical background to evaluate the research, and their worst fears about breast cancer risks, heart disease and ageing are exploited. In any case, as you read earlier, before you begin an HT regimen you need to have a thorough medical examination. It is unlikely that someone serving in a health food store has the medical expertise to carry this out. This may also apply to healthcare practitioners who sell these products but who have not specialised in reproductive medicine and do not have the requisite equipment to carry out the necessary examinations. Ask yourself when your doctor sells you these products whether you have had a full check-up first.

If you are keen to take bioidentical HT that has not been passed by a regulatory control board, do it sensibly: enlist the help of your general practitioner, gynaecologist or physician. Find out exactly how much of the particular hormone you are taking in each dose and be sure that it is the correct amount. If you have a womb, make sure you have an annual endometrial scan to see that the lining is not becoming dangerously thick. Have an annual mammogram and have your hormone levels monitored to check the potency of the unregulated product. I must stress the point though that if you decide to use these hormones, it is a case of 'buyer beware'. Don't forget that compounding pharmacies also promote their products and are well aware of their market, and remember that bioidentical hormone products that have been passed by regulatory boards are widely available in many different forms.

Hormone therapy is not anti-ageing medicine

The trend for celebrities, self-appointed experts and laypeople to promote these products has grown. Suzanne Somers of the television sitcom *Three's Company* is one of these anti-ageing gurus. She has an enthusiastic website and has written several books lauding the benefits of anti-ageing medicine and bioidentical hormones, including *The Sexy Years* and her latest book, *Sexy Forever*, making claims that are not supported by strong scientific or medical evidence. Somers herself takes higher levels of estrogen than the experts recommend.

There is a tendency among some of the proponents of HT and those who advocate bioidentical hormone therapy to tell women that they must take hormone therapy because it will keep them young. This is, in my opinion, an extremely dangerous stance. Beware of the healthcare practitioner who is in love with this idea and overenthusiastic about the perceived benefits of HT! Estrogen is not the elixir of life; there are many other medications for disease prevention, which may not carry as many risks. There is **no** robust evidence at this time to show that HT should be used for anything other than the alleviation of menopausal symptoms and the data indicates that it should be taken in the lowest possible dose for the time appropriate to an individual woman's risk profile.

The jury is still out as to whether estrogen therapy (ET) protects against heart disease and two long-term studies, KEEPS and ELITE, address this. I discuss this issue in Chapter 7. There is no evidence that ET improves your mental ability or protects against dementia. In fact, a recent study showed that once the effect of general ageing is taken into account, there is no association between blood serum estrogen levels and mental function. There is an urgent need for more research in this area but ageing is genetically programmed into our bodies. You will get older but the way in which you age is **your** responsibility. There is no magic bullet to keep you young and long-term or high-dose HT or bioidentical therapies may carry all sorts of risks that will outweigh the benefits. HT has not yet been proven to prevent disease or retard ageing, though there may be health benefits if treatment is begun at the start of menopause. It is vital to eat sensibly, exercise religiously, deal with your stress and watch your weight. These are the things that will keep you looking younger and feeling better. At this time research suggests that HT should not be used for disease prevention or as anti-ageing medicine.

Testosterone

Currently a lot is being written about women in menopause and their decreased desire for sex. I have my own ideas on this subject, which I will deal with in the section on sex and menopause, but since some doctors recommend testosterone when prescribing HT to perimenopausal women, I will try to give you the low-down on it.

Some doctors have been using testosterone implants for years but this testosterone is not bioidentical, it is usually *methyltestosterone* – a synthetic type – and is often given in quite a high dose that may well upset your delicate hormonal balance and create unpleasant side effects like aggressiveness, greasy skin, unwanted facial hair, adult acne and weight gain. It may also impact badly on your cholesterol levels because it is an androgen and can drive up your LDL (bad cholesterol).

Some women really battle with low sexual desire and have had blood tests showing that their levels of testosterone are very low indeed. But this in itself is a problem because serum testosterone levels reflect only a tiny amount of the total testosterone available in your body, so measuring total and free testosterone may only give a limited picture of a woman's testosterone levels.

Interestingly, new research has shown that testosterone continues to be produced by the cells in the ovaries (*stroma*) for some time after the onset of natural menopause, so low levels of testosterone in menopause may not be a cause of low libido.

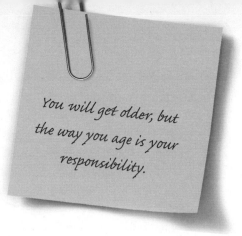

You will get older, but the way you age is your responsibility.

On the other hand, women who have had surgical menopause often find that the dramatic removal of their ovaries causes a sharp drop in sexual desire even if they are taking estrogen. Newer research has shown that these women had improved sex lives when using a transdermal testosterone patch, which gave them a daily dose of 300 mcg of testosterone in conjunction with transdermal ET. Other studies into a low-dose testosterone patch showed that after four weeks of use there was a marked rise in sexual desire and after six months all the women using the patch were very satisfied with their sexual encounters, though the long-term effects of testosterone, including on breast tissue, are still not clear. The good thing about this patch was that there were very few of the usual side effects – a slight increase in facial hair and some very minor cases of acne, and all agreed that the sexual satisfaction far outweighed these disadvantages. If you are very keen to use some testosterone, I would suggest you stick to the rule of using one that is bioidentical and has been passed by a medicines control council. As with all hormone therapy, testosterone therapy should be individualised and all the risks and benefits should be considered.

DHEA

Because DHEA (*dehydroepiandrosterone*) is the main building block hormone for so many of the steroid hormones, including estrogen, progesterone and testosterone, certain healthcare practitioners like to prescribe a bioavailable DHEA. It was banned by America's Food and Drug Administration (FDA) in 1985 as a medical treatment but is now available in the USA and many other countries as a dietary supplement.

There are many products that are called DHEA, one of which is a pharmaceutical product that is biochemically similar to your own DHEA. Take care, as there are many other preparations, found mainly in health shops, which are labelled DHEA and may contain some of this bioidentical DHEA, but may also include many different kinds of additives and hormones that could be harmful. You should read product labels and discuss doses with a qualified healthcare practitioner before starting therapy.

Healthcare practitioners specialising in complementary medicine have touted DHEA as a miracle hormone with myriad helpful effects, including burning fat, building muscle, strengthening your immune system, boosting your libido, energising you, preventing memory loss and helping to diminish stress. Well-researched scientific studies are more cautious, but agree that DHEA does play a role in the health of menopausal women, as described in Chapter 2. Research into DHEA is ongoing but has not yet verified all these claims, especially as far as oral DHEA is concerned, but on the upside some research showed that vaginal DHEA may improve vaginal dryness, leading to better sexual functioning.

As you read in Chapter 2 women have different levels of DHEA, so when offering women DHEA therapy, scientists are not sure how women with low levels will react to DHEA medication as opposed to those who have levels over seven times higher. The recent research about DHEA is compelling and offers another option for the relief of menopausal symptoms, but make no mistake, like all other hormones DHEA is very potent and if you decide to take it you should be aware of the problems that may be caused by overdosing. These include: sleep pattern interference; increased masculine characteristics like hair growth on your body and face while your hairline recedes; a greasy, porous skin; an increased risk of heart disease because DHEA lowers the level of good cholesterol (HDL) and raises that of bad cholesterol (LDL); and weight gain, because it increases insulin resistance. (The two types of cholesterol are described fully in Chapter 7.)

Just because DHEA is one of the main building block hormones doesn't mean that adding it to your system will solve your perimenopausal woes and metabolise in such a way that your hormone levels will be the same as when you were in your twenties. I would suggest that you only add DHEA to your HT regimen if you are under the care of a very experienced endocrinologist or specialist who has the expertise to monitor you and to understand the correct dosage.

HOW SHOULD YOU TAKE YOUR HORMONES?

Although there is no clear research about whether it is better to take HT orally, through your skin or by an intrauterine device, I think the best way to take it is through your skin (*transdermally*). The reason is that when you take HT in the form of a pill it must first pass through your liver (*hepatic first pass*) in order to be absorbed by your body. This is believed to interfere with a very important hormone called *insulin-like growth factor 1* (IGF1), which has a good effect on your bones and helps to maintain bone density. IGF1 also has an insulin-like effect.

When you take oral estrogen it may interfere with the delicate production process of IGF1, resulting in raised levels of insulin, which means that your metabolism slows down, your blood sugar drops and you crave sweet things and carbohydrates. On the other hand, when you apply estrogen to your skin it is absorbed and, like the estrogen that is manufactured in your own body (*endogenous estrogen*), it is carried to your heart and from there, as I explained in Chapter 2, it is distributed to the estrogen receptor sites before it gets to the liver. When you take estrogen orally, a higher dose than occurs naturally may be delivered to your body in one go and reaches the liver within a few hours, which means that your body has to deal with metabolising this rapidly instead of in its normal steady way.

In Chapter 2, I likened the complex and subtle way the hormones in our body are programmed to the instruments playing in harmony in an orchestra. If one member is out of tune the whole melody is discordant. Logically, it seems to me, this is what happens when you take estrogen orally.

When you take the estrogen through your skin, especially through a slow-release patch or by applying measured doses of the cream or gel, your body is getting its estrogen in a way that is almost identical to the way it received it when your own body was producing enough estrogen, allowing for very stable, continuous hormone levels. It seems that this may be a safer way for your body to receive HT.

Recent research has also shown that unlike oral estrogen, transdermal estrogen had no effect on IGF1 levels or those of C-*reactive protein* (CRP), a protein that is produced by the liver only when your body is experiencing severe inflammation. This is important because once again it shows that transdermal HT does not appear to interfere with the way the liver works. Research has shown that although CRP levels may be raised when you have a heart attack, it is not clear what role it plays in heart disease; whether it is just a marker of this disease or whether raised levels may be a risk factor in heart disease. Other research showed that with transdermal estrogen there was no meaningful rise in triglycerides (a type of fat found in your body that is used for energy, though high levels of these can be dangerous) and suggested they had very little effect on blood pressure.

Women taking transdermal estrogen had lower levels of estrone sulfate than those taking their HT orally, and the estrone sulfate levels in those using the patch were similar to the levels found in menstruating women. This is important because it is thought that increased estrone sulfate levels may be implicated in breast cancers. Researchers also found that women prone to migraines suffered far more when taking oral HT, while there was no increase in the frequency and severity of migraines in women using the patch. Data from the ESTHER (EStrogen and THromboEmbolism Risk) study showed that there might also be a lower risk of blood clotting with transdermal estrogen, micronised progesterone and less androgenic progestogens. New research shows that though this way of taking estrogen may lower the risk of clots, the type of progestogen it is combined with may also affect your risk. A recent extremely large long-term observational study showed that low-dose, transdermal patches were related to a lower risk of stroke. But as always, there needs to be further gold standard research to get more definitive answers.

There are also more and more products containing 17β estradiol that you can take through your skin. Some women who don't have wombs are very happy with a 20 mg estradiol implant, which appears not to affect cholesterol levels or to add to the risk of stroke, and slowly releases estradiol throughout the day without causing the problems that may occur when you take one dose at a time. Once again though, you need to discuss all the pros and cons of this implant with your doctor. I personally prefer being able to change the dose at a moment's notice if I have to.

WHAT IS THE SAFEST AND BEST DOSE OF HORMONES?

In their position statements NAMS (North American Menopause Society) and SAMS (South African Menopause Society) recommend that women take the smallest amount of estrogen possible to alleviate the symptoms of hot flushes and dry vaginas. So I would suggest that you begin with the lowest dose available and increase it if you find it isn't making a difference.

It is interesting to note that as soon as the results of the Women's Health Initiative (WHI) study were published and the media were having a fine time panicking the public, hundreds of thousands of women stopped taking their HT 'cold turkey' and profits of companies like Wyeth (who manufacture Premarin) plummeted by 30 per cent in one year. Suddenly all the big companies started advertising hormones with very low doses of estrogen and progestins.

In the following comparison I have selected the most relevant points and highlighted important words and numbers in italics.

In *Menopause* in 1997 Prempro advertised like this:

- Simplicity of a single tablet
- One prescription for you, one tablet for your patients
- The most prescribed HRT regimen in America
- Proven endometrial protection with a *low* dose of only *70 mg* of progestin over four weeks of therapy. One PREMPRO tablet contains *0.625 mg* of the conjugated estrogens found in Premarin® tablets and *2.5 mg* of medroxyprogesterone acetate.

In *Menopause* in 2004 things had changed somewhat:

- Today, menopausal symptom relief starts here *0.3/1.5.* The *lowest effective* dose. Proven efficacy with the *lowest* starting dose
- 52 per cent less estrogen, 40 per cent less progestin
- Manage patients at the lowest effective dose. Women should be started at *0.3 mg/1.5 mg daily*
- Wyeth – our commitment to women's health continues
- '*Go low* with Prempro.'

Suddenly there is a plethora of low-dose estrogen products on the market, all of them paying attention to guidelines which suggest that much lower doses of estrogen and progestogen are as effective and much safer. In your doctor's waiting room you will notice a series of pamphlets advertising these new 'low-dose' products. So you can be sure that no matter how much the manufacturers of hormones argued against the results of the WHI, they took notice of the Food and Drug Administration (FDA) recommendations and of the fact that women had woken up to the risks of large doses of HT, and reacted by lowering the amount of estrogen in their products.

Many very low-dose estrogen patches and creams are already available and more will be coming on to the market, so keep your eyes open for them and ask your pharmacist to let you know as soon as they become available. Start with the lowest dose you can – you can always increase it if it isn't effective. Research has shown that women using products with doses as low as 0.025 mg no longer battle with hot flushes. But, as a rule of thumb, acceptable lower daily doses are 0.3 mg of the CEE tablet, a dose of oral micronised 17β-estradiol of 0.50 mg and ranging from 0.014 mg to 0.025 mg for transdermal estrogen (the patch, creams or gels). Remember, if you have a womb you must take a progestogen if you are taking estrogen.

I am a great believer in the mantra 'less is more', as you will realise when you read the chapter on vitamins and supplements. Be moderate with your hormone therapy. Another important point is how you take your HT. Because bioidentical hormones metabolise quickly, I think that it may be sensible to take your daily portion in divided doses even if the manufacturer suggests only one application daily. Rub the cream or gel on in the morning and the evening for the best results. Try to mimic your body's rhythm. If you are using the patch you need to split up your week exactly. So apply it on Tuesday morning and then replace it with a new patch on Friday evening.

LOW-DOSE COMBINATION CONTRACEPTIVES (ESTROGEN AND PROGESTIN) AS HT

As I explained in Chapter 1, there are women in early perimenopause who start having irregular periods and menopausal symptoms like hot flushes, but can become pregnant because they are still ovulating. They are not yet ready to use menopausal hormone therapy, but they may be struggling with these symptoms, so a low-dose combination birth control pill during this time may be the answer. This is because it helps to reduce symptoms and protects you against becoming pregnant at the same time until you reach menopause. It can also regulate irregular periods, help acne (which affects some women as they transition into menopause), and helps decrease the risk of cancer of the ovaries and the lining of the womb. These low-dose oral contraceptives do not seem to increase the risk of heart disease, stroke or breast cancer if they are used for a longer length of time.

Some women prefer to use a combination contraceptive in the form of a patch or ring depending whether a medicines control board in your country has approved it. Sometimes using oral contraceptives can hide the fact that you are perimenopausal, so depending on your age you may want to stop them for a while and use non-hormonal contraception, like condoms, until you are sure.

The same warnings about HT apply if you want to try this form of HT: you should be healthy, have no additional risks such as heart disease, blood clots and breast cancer and you should not smoke. You should have the same monitoring as a woman on HT. Some side effects include breakthrough bleeding for a while when you start this regimen and breast tenderness. When you stop these low-dose oral contraceptives you will have some bleeding, even if you are menopausal and your periods have stopped.

When Myra became menopausal at the age of 51 her kindly, small town gynaecologist insisted that she start HT, though other than an occasional hot flush she had no problems with symptoms. She made no objection, because she knew it was standard practice at the time and all her friends were on it. Her doctor was very accommodating, changing her HT regimens several times until she found a product that suited her. Her gynaecologist saw her only every couple of years thereafter, did not insist on annual examinations to monitor her progress, and from his enthusiasm about HT, Myra felt he was doing her a favour by renewing the prescription year after year.

Myra did not really enjoy being on HT because she had looked forward to the end of her periods, which now continued for the next 10 years thanks to the monthly bleeds caused by her combined EPT. In 2002, when the first WHI study results were widely reported, she felt worried about the negative effects of HT, decided to stop the treatment and felt fine. In 2006, she had moved and realising she had not had a check-up for over six years, went to see a new gynaecologist. She was now 66. He sent her for a bone scan and told her to have her cholesterol tested. When she returned to hear the results, he laid into her angrily. 'He made me feel that by stopping HT I had ruined my health,' Myra recalled. 'He told me that a section of my spine was weakened and that I could suffer a fracture at any time.'

Feeling dreadful, guilty and thoroughly scared, Myra took the story to her GP, who recommended a specialist physician. Appropriate medication has improved her bone density, she changed her lifestyle, including a better diet and exercise, and her cholesterol levels are back to normal. She says that at 70 she feels as fit as a fiddle.

Several interesting points are highlighted in Myra's story. HT is recommended for women with moderate to severe hot flushes and related symptoms that affect quality of life; she had none of them. Her doctor did not insist on an annual physical examination or mammogram to monitor her. She took herself off HT because she had read the exaggerated media reports about it, but never discussed this with her doctor. Like many woman who feel healthy, she did not bother to get an annual check-up, which is vital if you want to take responsibility for your health. The new gynaecologist, who should have known better by 2006, subscribed to the concept that being on HT is vital for women's health, believing that it protects against heart disease, when research shows that it actually increases heart disease risk in older women. Being on HT for more than three to five years may increase breast cancer risk. Although estrogen does protect against bone loss, as soon as you stop it there is often a dramatic loss of bone and the positive effects of HT are rapidly lost. In addition, the risks of long-term HT in older women clearly outweigh the benefits. It is quite normal for a woman in her sixties to have some bone loss in her lumbar spine but bone density alone cannot put you at fracture risk. There are several other factors that can contribute to this (see Chapter 9).

Most doctors now cautiously believe that women can safely stay on HT for up to five years. This may also depend on the timing hypothesis: at what age you started HT as you transitioned into menopause, and when you were fully menopausal. If you are taking HT for that length of time, the rule about having regular check-ups and being carefully monitored by your doctor applies even more strictly. Today the consensus is that if you still have bad menopausal symptoms after five years, have tried to stop HT but can't because these symptoms are making you miserable and you are not at risk, or if you cannot take the appropriate medication for bone density loss for one reason or another, you can continue HT as long as you are very carefully monitored and understand all the risks and benefits. The aspect of individuality is vital in making decisions about the length of time you take HT. Remember, the benefits outweigh the risks in some women, while there are many risks for others.

I would suggest that you re-evaluate how you feel after a year. If you don't have hot flushes and the other symptoms have disappeared, you could slowly taper off the HT. There is no definitive research about whether tapering off is better than stopping abruptly, though a recent study shows that women who tapered off HT seemed to do better than those who stopped abruptly, but many women seem to prefer coming off their HT regimen slowly. What often happens though is that the flushes have stopped but your vagina still doesn't feel great. This is when I would suggest you try vaginal estrogen, which has a local rather than a *systemic* effect. Systemic means that the HT is absorbed in your bloodstream and has a clinically significant effect (the treatment has obvious results, i.e. your hot flushes are fewer and not as severe).

Local vaginal estrogen

Some healthcare practitioners prefer vaginal estrogen creams, tablets or pessaries (small oval-shaped pills that you can put into your vagina). An estriol cream can be very helpful and doesn't have any side effects. It can be applied three times a week and seems to work, though some women don't like the mushy feeling of the cream.

The method I think is most convenient and least invasive is an estradiol-releasing vaginal ring. A low-dose estrogen thin rubber ring, similar to a diaphragm, is placed in the vagina and tucked securely behind your cervix, where you don't feel it, alleviating the problems of a dry vagina by releasing small amounts of estradiol in a consistent way over a period of three months. It mostly has a local effect on your vagina; some estrogen may enter your blood but the circulating amounts are very small (20-30 pmol/l per day or 5.4-8.2 pg/ml).

> Eleanor's sex life had been put on hold because, as she told her GP, sex had become so painful that she found it almost unbearable to make love to her husband and they were both, understandably, feeling very frustrated. Her doctor recommended the estradiol-releasing ring and Eleanor started using it. Within two weeks she found that her vagina had stopped feeling dry and painful and that sex was normal again. But when she went to her gynaecologist for her annual check-up he told her to stop using it. When she asked him why, he replied that he didn't like it, but gave her no further explanation.

Many doctors only prescribe the estradiol-releasing ring for much older women who are suffering from some of the urinary tract problems, like urinary incontinence and urinary tract infections, which often accompany a dry vagina, rather than to alleviate the problem of a dry vagina that comes with menopause, but it seems to me to be a safe and uncomplicated way to beat this problem too. As Eleanor's story illustrates, some doctors do not like it, but many women have found that their vaginal problem improves markedly with the use of the vaginal ring. The ring can remain in place for three months and should be changed after that, which means that four rings should be used each year.

It is thought that the ring can be used indefinitely, even if a woman has a uterus, and up to now it has been believed that the effects are almost entirely local, which means that the estrogen that is released is confined to the vaginal area and doesn't circulate throughout the body. However, some of the latest research has shown that the vaginal ring not only relieves vaginal dryness but may alleviate hot flushes. This means that some of the estrogen released from the ring circulates throughout your body, which is known as a systemic effect, rather than just a local effect. So although much less estrogen is absorbed systemically with both the ring (and the tablet), some research has shown that there are changes in the cholesterol levels of some women who are using these, which means that specialists have still not decided whether the amount of estrogen absorbed systemically from the ring is safe for cancer survivors.

More research is needed to find the lowest, most effective dose of vaginal estrogen that would only work locally. So if you are at risk for breast cancer or any other estrogen receptor-positive cancer and decide to use the ring, you must discuss all the risks and benefits with your healthcare practitioner and continue to be carefully monitored. Other local vaginal estrogen preparations such as an estriol cream, which have been found to be effective, might be safer in this case. This debate aside, research on the ring shows that it generally has no adverse side effects and even women who no longer have a cervix find it comfortable and easy to use.

DESIGNER HORMONES

Some hormones used in HT have been specifically manufactured to try to overcome some of the problems found in regular estrogen and progestogen products. There has been a lot of research into these products but more is needed, especially using larger sample groups to try to understand their risks and benefits more fully.

Tibolone

Tibolone, a designer preparation, has a combination of weak estrogenic, androgenic and progestogenic effects on your body. It is not available in the USA, but is used in the UK, Australia and Europe. It reduces hot flushes and is recommended for women with osteoporosis because it increases bone mineral density. It also has several additional positive effects, including the fact that it does not appear to lead to thickening of the lining of the womb and the estrogen in it is tissue-selective, which means that it has a beneficial estrogenic effect on certain tissues, including those in the vagina and bone, but not on breast tissue or the lining of the womb. It does, however, have some unpleasant side effects, which include breakthrough bleeding if you still have a womb, weight gain, bloating and water retention and, more worrying, it seems to cause an increase in LDL, the bad cholesterol, and a reduction in the level of good cholesterol. Tibolone does not appear to increase the risk of clots in women and seems to improve sexual functioning in women with low sexual desire.

In 2006 a trial to determine the effect of tibolone on new vertebral fractures in elderly women – Long-Term Intervention on Fractures with Tibolone (LIFT) – was stopped prematurely as the Data Safety Monitoring Board (DSMB) found that there was an increased risk of stroke in the group taking tibolone as opposed to the control group. However, the authors of the Endocrine Society Position Statement point out this was in a group of older women and tibolone does not appear to increase this risk in younger postmenopausal women, and there also appeared to be a lower risk for breast cancer after three years of use. In May 2007 another randomised placebo-controlled clinical trial, LIBERATE, designed to assess the safety and efficacy of tibolone, when used for the relief of menopausal symptoms in patients with a history of breast cancer, was discontinued ahead of schedule because the DSMB found that there were more breast cancer recurrences in the group of women who were randomised to receive tibolone.

The consensus in 2009 was that tibolone is a useful treatment option for healthy women who have just started menopause and have their wombs. However, medical scientists agreed that it should not be prescribed to any woman who had, has had or who may be at risk for breast cancer. It appears to double the risk of stroke in women older than 65. It seems that differences in the results of breast cancer risk in the two trials were because the one group of women had osteoporosis, were thinner and were not taking tamoxifen, while the other group in the LIBERATE trial were much younger (averaging 52 years old), were fatter and most of them were taking tamoxifen. Once again, my personal preference is for bioidentical hormones, which metabolise as nature intended them to, though many doctors in countries where it has been approved by the medicines control boards are happy to prescribe tibolone, and their patients feel good on it.

SERMs or estrogen agonists/antagonists

Selective estrogen receptor-modulators (SERMs) are designer hormones. They are also called estrogen agonists/antagonists (Eaa). These medications are designed to have an estrogenic effect on certain areas of your body that will benefit your brain and bone, but block the action of estrogen in other tissues, such as those in the breast and womb where long-term use of estrogen could be risky. They have been prescribed for several years now for specific medical conditions such as the control of breast cancer, low bone density and osteoporosis.

The best-known SERMs are *tamoxifen* and the second-generation SERM *raloxifene*. Although tamoxifen has been used for nearly 30 years to treat women with estrogen receptor-positive breast cancer and millions of women have done well on it, it does have some unpleasant side effects. One of the most serious of these is that it doesn't relieve hot flushes; it sometimes aggravates them. It is thought that this happens because tamoxifen blocks the effects of certain estrogen receptors in the body, including in the brain. Research has shown that after more than five years on tamoxifen there is increased risk of endometrial cancer and stroke (Chapter 8).

Raloxifene was developed to help prevent osteoporosis in women and has been very effective in this area. Like its predecessor, it has an anti-estrogenic effect on breast tissue and it doesn't stimulate the lining of the womb. It appears to lower the bad cholesterol and triglycerides, although it doesn't raise the levels of good cholesterol. Like tamoxifen, it doesn't alleviate hot flushes and may make them worse. The most serious side effect of this SERM is blood clots and so it is felt that women at high risk for blood clots, heart disease and stroke should not use raloxifene. Benefits and risks of both raloxifene and tamoxifen have been extensively studied and I will discuss them further in Chapter 8.

What's new? Estrogen agonists/antagonists in combination with estrogen

There are now some third-generation SERMs, including *bazedoxifene*, which are showing some very promising results in trials, are FDA approved, and researchers are looking at innovative new ways to use them in combination with ET. The scientists hope that this combination will help menopausal symptoms and improve bone density without causing the lining of the womb to thicken or to have adverse effects on breast tissue.

DIFFERENT KINDS OF HT REGIMENS

As discussed above, there are different ways to take HT and it's important for you to decide which regimen is best suited to your lifestyle and body chemistry. Some women loathe the patch; they may be allergic to the adhesives on it or find that it peels off when they are exercising and, of course, it's useless for those women who do daily water aerobics. Others like it and feel really good on it especially if they don't like the problem of remembering to take hormones daily. They may find after a discussion with their doctor that they can find a dose that is ideal for them if they cut the patch in half or if they don't like the problem of remembering to take hormones daily. Other women are more comfortable with a gel or cream.

If you have a womb you need to decide, with your doctor, whether you want to take progestogen daily in conjunction with your estrogen or only sequentially, and there are also different options here. You can take it every two weeks. If you are taking a very low-dose estrogen you may find that the lining of your womb doesn't thicken and you may only need progestogen intermittently, but in this case you must understand the risks and be closely monitored by a doctor who is skilled in the use of transvaginal ultrasound.

How to find out what's best for you

Sometimes it's hard to know which HT regimen is best for you. But it's here that you have to take responsibility for yourself. You will know if you feel good on something. You will know when your hot flushes have stopped, you are sleeping better and sex is no longer uncomfortable. It's okay to start an HT regimen and then stop it if you start experiencing uncomfortable symptoms.

Whatever you choose, it may not work immediately. In fact, with most products it is at least two weeks before you feel a difference, but if after you have started a new hormone you feel bloated or nauseous, your breasts are tender, you feel symptoms of PMS or become very moody or irritable, the product you are trying is not for you or you may need to try an even lower dose or a different combination. Work with your healthcare practitioner; ask your doctor for all the options and decide what is best for you. It's your right to feel as good as possible and you may need several attempts before you find the hormone therapy and hormone regimen that really suits you.

As I write this there are several very low, transdermal estrogen products in the pipeline, so keep your eyes open and ask your doctor or pharmacist to let you know when they arrive on the shelves. When you are deciding on a hormone treatment read the product insert carefully. There are many viable products, but in my opinion those that are closest biochemically to the hormones in your body, are low dose and are taken transdermally, are preferable.

- **Other medication:** When you are having a check-up before you go on HT or when you return to your gynaecologist for your annual check-up, make a point of telling him or her if you are on any new medication or if you have had any illnesses or medical incidents during the year. For example, you can't expect your doctor to be psychic and know intuitively that a cardiologist has put you on a blood thinner or that since your last appointment you have been diagnosed with high blood pressure. It's not up to you to decide what is and is not relevant about your medical history. Let the expert decide. If you don't impart the information you can't blame your doctor for making a bad decision. Everything that relates to your medical history during the intervening months is important if you are to have a successful partnership and not put yourself at unnecessary risk if you are on HT.

- **Use your judgement:** Think for yourself and use your own judgement. The fact that your doctor's wife is on 0.625 mg of CEE doesn't mean that it's okay for you.

- **Stopping HT:** When you decide to stop your HT, though there is no definitive medical evidence, you may want to wean yourself off it slowly. The way in which you do it depends on the type of HT you are taking. Discuss this with your doctor. I believe that it is better for your body to become accustomed to having low levels of estrogen. If you stop it abruptly you may experience the same sort of symptoms that come from fluctuating levels of estrogen in perimenopause.

- **HT pointers:**
  - Follow a sensible lifestyle
  - Have a full check-up
  - HT should only be taken to alleviate moderate to severe hot flushes, night sweats and a dry vagina
  - Hormones should be biochemically similar to your own hormones
  - HT should be applied transdermally – the dose should be as low as possible
  - HT should be taken for the shortest possible length of time
  - Your age at menopause and the time after menopause when you decide to start HT may have important health implications
  - If your only remaining symptom is a dry vagina, try a local vaginal estrogen product
  - If you are on HT you should have regular check-ups, including an annual transvaginal examination and a mammogram.

5
If I shake you, will you rattle? Vitamins and minerals in menopause

Laurie is an attractive 58-year-old brunette who came to see me because she felt terrible: 'I'm nauseous and my head aches. I feel very tired and I can't remember things. It's strange, because although I feel exhausted, at the same time I feel nuts, like I'm wired. And if that's not bad enough, I recently lost a lot of weight and now I've put it on again. I can't seem to keep it off no matter what I do.'

Laurie's symptoms fitted right in with those of perimenopause, but they seemed to be unusually bad. She explained that she was very aware of her health and was taking several vitamins and supplements daily. She was also drinking three to four litres of water a day because she had been told it was healthy. She could not understand why, when she took such care of herself, she should feel so awful. She told me that she was nervous about taking HT and was a great believer in alternative medicine, which she thought would help her through menopause.

I asked Laurie to show me all the supplements she was taking and was horrified to discover that she was swallowing a daily dose of 16 different vitamins, supplements and homeopathic tinctures. In addition, she was taking at least six painkillers daily because she had such bad headaches. From a purely logical point of view, given the number of supplements Laurie was taking, it seemed to me that her liver was working overtime.

She was obviously having rebound headaches from the painkillers and drinking far too much water, so she was flushing large amounts of the supplements down the drain and putting a lot of stress on her kidneys. In addition, it didn't seem that the products she was taking were alleviating her perimenopausal symptoms; they were making them worse!

Many peri- and postmenopausal women are firm believers that vast quantities of vitamin and mineral supplements will not only get them through menopause but will also keep them healthy and eternally young. This is a very thorny topic. In fact, as I read the extraordinarily wide selection of literature and media advice on the subject, I felt very confused. For all the passionate outpourings from the conventional medicine industry denouncing supplements, there were equally passionate refutations, claims and denials from the producers and proponents of supplements in the complementary and alternative medicine industry.

Once again, we women are caught in the crossfire. We buy into the idea that by not taking specific vitamins and minerals we are abdicating responsibility for our own health and well-being and compromising our chances of a healthy life and old age, yet we are worried by reports that not only may we be wasting our money on these supplements, but they may actually be harmful.

A friend who arrived from America carrying plastic bags brimming with different vitamins, knowing that I was sceptical about their efficacy, brought me eight different newsletters and glossy magazines on the subject. While I was reading them I suddenly realised why women are conned into believing that supplements are vital to their future health. The articles in these publications are sometimes written by medical doctors; they use medical terminology and speak with consummate authority on the subject. They recommend various supplements in self-assured, breezy, consumer-friendly language.

They offer hope and certainty that we can prevent ageing and ill health; once again, they offer a quick fix. Just as the pharmaceutical companies played on women's fears about ageing when they sold us that magic bullet HT, the producers of supplements are hooking into the same anxieties and we are buying into the hype.

The problem is that some of the people who write these articles, although they are often pictured in white lab coats with stethoscopes draped casually round their necks, may not be licensed and may have degrees that are not recognised by conventional medical authorities. Many of them are sponsored by the producers of vitamins and mineral supplements and, just as I warned you to be wary of research articles on HT that did not declare their interests, I am warning you to pay attention to the hidden interests behind the information you read about supplements. Most of the 'practitioners' are selling the supplements about which they write so glowingly, so their advice is not impartial!

I know that medical science is not perfect and I know that 'there are more things in heaven and earth than are dreamed of ', and that there is still enormous research to be done into this subject, but in order to remain true to my belief that knowledge is power and that women's fears should not make them vulnerable to voracious commercial interests, I am going to nail my colours to the mast and tell you how you might be able to negotiate the supplement dilemma.

A GIANT INDUSTRY

Let's begin with some facts. The alternative medicine and vitamin and mineral supplement industry is a giant one. A recent survey in America showed that there were more than 29 000 different supplements available. Women, in a desperate quest for health and youth, spend billions annually on products that have usually not been subjected to the rigorous research and development that conventional medicines must undergo.

Most conventional medicines take at least 12 years to develop before the controlling bodies of their respective countries allow them to be manufactured. Their efficacy has to be proved and their side effects stated before they appear on the market. Supplements can be sold as soon as the manufacturer has produced them. There is no onus on manufacturers to give any information on the label other than the ingredients, no need for them to clarify the efficacy and safety of the products or make any reference to the side effects that these products may cause.

Supplement manufacturers are also allowed to make structure-function claims. In other words, they can't say that calcium cures osteoporosis but they can say: 'Calcium makes bones strong'. Because these products are not carefully controlled they may be contaminated with toxic heavy metals like lead, mercury and arsenic, and the amount of the ingredients stated on the label may be misrepresented, so that you may be taking more or less of a supplement than you believe, or even taking something that has not been listed. The doses suggested on the label may not be correct and may have bad effects; for example, many supplements are said to slow down the rate at which something in your body decays or breaks down because of its interaction with oxygen (*antioxidant*), but certain vitamins in the wrong amounts may actually speed up the decay (an *oxidant* effect).

Some of these products may very well be effective. It is just that as yet there is not enough rigorous scientific data available that shows clearly that they really do what they claim. In the past, government bodies like the Food and Drug Administration (FDA) in the USA, the Medicine and Healthcare Products Regulatory Agency (MHRA) in the UK and the Medicines Control

Council (MCC) in South Africa classified supplements as foods, so anyone could put a supplement onto the market.

There was no difference between the memories of those who took the ginkgo and the control group who didn't.

The producers of these unregulated supplements could then make extravagant, perhaps unjustified claims about the efficacy of the product, not bother to supply data about its safety, and label it in such a way that you could not rely on the ingredient information but would get hooked by phrases like 'younger skin at your fingertips', or statements using complicated medical language that gives an impression of superior knowledge. For example: 'The cell protective effects of Indole-3-carbinol help to maintain proper function of estrogen receptor sites on cell membranes, help maintain p21 suppressor gene function, help detoxify pesticides and other environmental pollutants including dioxin, aid in the conversion of 16α-hydroxyestrone to 2-hydroxyesterone, promote the health of prostate and breast tissue.'

When these statements appear on labels or in advertisements for American products they must also carry a box (which is often in minuscule print) saying: 'These statements have not been evaluated by the Food and Drug Administration. This product is not intended to diagnose, treat, cure or prevent any disease.' This is all well and good but very few of us read the tiny print, and the claims made, when taken at face value, sound very impressive. Furthermore, the onus is on the FDA to prove them wrong. In the circumstances, there is absolutely no need for the manufacturers to subject their products to rigorous, well-designed scientific studies.

Another problem with the information we receive on supplements is that the claims are not substantiated. The trials that are cited have small sample numbers, are not properly controlled, and are often of short-term duration; usually not more than six months. They may often be based on anecdotal information or testimonials (letters that say: 'Since taking supplement X I have lost 15 kg and feel younger and healthier than ever').

Many of the people who sell supplements may not have been properly trained in the field and may not understand the complicated biochemical processes whereby food is digested and our bodies obtain the vitamins and minerals essential for our health and well-being. They also may not understand the complicated interactions that can occur between so-called natural substances and conventional medication.

When someone in a health food store or pharmacy offers me ginkgo biloba, telling me authoritatively that by taking it I will improve my memory, I feel like shouting: 'Who says?' I would be delighted if careful scientific research proved this to be true. Which of us menopausal women has not sat with a blank look on our faces, trying to retrieve some information or bemoaning the loss of our memories to our friends? It would be great to get some help in this area, but a recent rigorous study of more than 200 healthy adults taking recommended doses of ginkgo showed there was absolutely no difference between the memories of those who took the ginkgo and the control group who didn't.

So why do we, when we are peri- and postmenopausal, think that we need to take vitamin and mineral supplements and *nutraceuticals* (products taken from foods and said to have proven medical benefits, especially in the prevention of heart disease)? I think it is because we want to be responsible for ourselves and our health, and that in some sense we have bought into a concept that has become the rallying cry of complementary and alternative medicine in the twenty-first century – anti-ageing and preventative medicine.

While I believe that it is very important that women take responsibility for their own wellness and live the kind of lifestyle that helps to prevent illness and disease, I think that we get too hooked into a mindset that promises eternal youth and immortality. Ultimately, most of the anti-ageing claims that the complementary and alternative medicine industry make have not been proved in well-designed, scientifically proven clinical trials. What we do know is this: we will age and we will die.

The best we can hope for and take responsibility for is that to the best of our ability, we will try to live a balanced, sensible life that will ensure a happy and healthy old age. However, we are bombarded with advertisements, information and hype from the media, entreating and beseeching us to take more of this or that supplement.

It is true that we live in a world where our crops are fertilised with all kinds of chemicals and pesticides, that we eat eggs and chickens that are produced in inhumane batteries and that our meat may be pumped full of hormones and antibiotics. Much of the food we eat has food colourants and preservatives and some of us are hooked on fast foods that are high in sodium and saturated fats.

But here's the good news: most of us generally eat enough good quality foods to ensure that we get most of the nutrients we need. In fact, the vitamins that you get from foods probably act more efficiently than a single dose of a particular supplement. Our bodies have been synthesising foods for thousands of years and are very efficient. If our diet is well balanced there is no reason to believe that we won't be getting enough of the right vitamins and minerals. In Chapter 10 you will see some recommendations for a really healthy and nutritional food plan. However, I sometimes recommend certain supplements that may be taken in moderation and within prescribed limits, and I list these on pages 114–115.

In spite of this knowledge, many healthcare practitioners are eager to prescribe large doses of supplements. I have read of menopause experts who unashamedly suggest that women can easily take 10 or more capsules and tablets every day. I personally think that's an awful lot of supplements to remember to take daily, especially since stress is one of the conditions that add to our vitamin depletion. In my opinion, once we feel we should be taking those supplements, it is just another thing to remember and to feel bad about if we don't.

However, I must make a confession. For several years before I really woke up and started looking at the available research, I was a great advocate of supplements. I bought into all the propaganda and, looking back to my client files of 10 years ago, I see that I generally suggested at least seven or more supplements daily. Today I am convinced that less is more and nothing is better for middle-aged women than taking responsibility for a healthy lifestyle.

Another problem with taking a wide variety of supplements is that many of them contain small amounts of other supplements in addition to the main ingredient. So you may think you're only supplementing with glucosamine because that is the main product listed on the front label, but what you are taking may also contain vitamins C, E, B1, B2, B6, B12, nicotinic acid, pantothenic acid, zinc, selenium, boron, silicon and manganese. So you have the additional responsibility (and stress) of being aware of the amounts of the different vitamins in each of the supplements you are taking in order to keep your dosage within the safe upper limits suggested.

DEFINITION OF VITAMIN AND MINERAL SUPPLEMENTS

Vitamins are organic substances that the human body needs, in varying but usually small quantities, in order to grow. They help to break down and use (*metabolise*) the food we eat in the most efficient way, ensuring that our bodies grow and develop, and that we have healthy, functioning cells. Because the body cannot produce all its own vitamins, these organic substances work together with other substances called enzymes, which are special proteins that help the chemical processes in the body, so that the vitamins are used in the most appropriate way. Each vitamin has a number of specific functions in the human body and a deficiency of one or more can result in illness. For example, in the old days, sailors on long sea voyages who didn't have access to fresh vegetables developed scurvy from a lack of vitamin C.

There are two groups of vitamins: those that are water soluble (vitamin C and the B-complex vitamins) and those that are fat soluble (vitamins A, D, E and K). The former are found throughout the body's tissues, where they interact with enzymes to ensure that your body functions in a healthy and life-enhancing way.

Excess amounts of water-soluble vitamins are eliminated from your body in your urine, but make no mistake, too much vitamin C or too many B vitamins can be toxic, so pay careful attention to the amounts you are taking. Remember, if you are taking several supplements daily you may be getting extra amounts of any one vitamin. Two of the fat-soluble vitamins, A and D, can be very toxic but even too much of vitamins E and K is not wise. Your body, as we discussed in previous chapters, is a finely tuned machine, and moderation is everything. Just as too much of a particular hormone can upset the body's delicate balance, too much of any one vitamin can cause problems. In the case of supplements, more may **not** be better.

Like vitamins, supplements can contain amino acids, which are the building blocks of proteins, herbs and/or botanicals, which are any of the parts of a plant that can be synthesised and used in the product in a variety of ways; and enzymes.

I keep talking about the importance of a healthy diet but many women are not sure what this means, so I have included a list on pages 95–100 describing the function of each vitamin, in which foods it is found and, most importantly, what amounts of it are generally safe to take. Most of the antioxidants the supplement manufacturers are promoting are found naturally in these foods. If we can obtain our vitamins and minerals from foods they are cheaper, truly natural and are better absorbed, since the body, developed over thousands of years of evolution, will know how to synthesise them.

The vitamins that come from foods come combined with other vitamins and minerals, and interact in the body in an intricate way, providing the healthiest, most effective results. If you do decide to take mega doses of supplements, you should be aware that many of the trials done on these substances have not been long term and the long-term poisonous effect (*toxicity*) of the products may not be properly known or understood. Many of these products may also interact powerfully with any conventional medicines that you may be taking. Remember, just because a supplement is said to be natural doesn't mean that it's harmless.

The lists below are intended as a guideline to show you that many of the supplements we are told to take are present in a sensible and varied diet. You should only need to supplement your diet if you don't get enough of a particular vitamin or mineral; have been ill or chronically stressed; have an eating disorder; or eat fast food morning, noon and night. There are healthcare practitioners, like registered dieticians, who have been properly trained and can assess your diet to see whether you might be deficient in one or more of the vitamins and minerals listed below.

Approach supplementation with caution and never go above the Safe Upper Limit (SUL). The SUL, or tolerable Upper Intake Level (UL), means the maximum daily amount of a nutrient that should not cause harmful health effects in most people in the general population. It is set to protect the most sensitive individuals in the healthy general population and applies to chronic daily use. These are important reference values if you'd like to understand what is in the vitamins and supplements you are taking and should be written on the information labels.

Another reference value is the Recommended Dietary Allowance (RDA), which is the average daily intake level of a particular vitamin or mineral that meets the nutrient requirements of most healthy people, in all gender and age groups. If there is not enough evidence to suggest an RDA, an Adequate Intake (AI) is set. Dietary Reference Intakes (DRIs) is the term used for the reference values that have been used to plan and assess what the nutrient intake should be in healthy people and have been developed by the the Food and Nutrition Board (FNB) in the USA under the aegis of the Institute of Medicine (IOM).

If you eat a really varied diet containing lots of fruit, vegetables, whole-grains, the right kinds of protein, nuts and dairy products, you should get more than adequate amounts of vitamins and minerals for healthy living. The suggested amount of fruit and vegetables is at least five to nine servings daily.

VITAMINS

Guidelines for the daily dose are for women 31–70 years old, unless I indicate differently. The suggested daily dose is called the **Recommended Dietary Allowance (RDA)** and I use **Average Intake (AI)** when there isn't enough evidence to be definitive. The **SUL** is the **Safe Upper Limit**, the highest amount you can take safely daily. **IU** stands for **International Units**, which are the measurements usually used on food and supplement labels. Also note that **mg** means **milligrams** and **mcg** means **micrograms**. Different manufacturers use different units of measurement and where two types are used, I note it.

Vitamin A (also known as retinol)

Function: Vital for healthy skin, teeth, bones, tissues and vision.
Food source: Liver, egg yolk, butter, cream, fish-liver oils.
Guidelines for daily dose: RDA = 700 mcg (2 333 IU); SUL = 3 000 mcg (10 000 IU).

Beta-carotene

Beta-carotene is a precursor of vitamin A (the body can make vitamin A from this vitamin)
Function: It is an antioxidant. It is converted to retinol, which is essential for vision, and then to retinoic acid, which is involved in growth and cell differentiation.
Food source: Dark leafy greens, yellow and orange vegetables and fruits.
Guidelines for daily dose: 3–6 mg. This dose has not really been established but this amount is estimated to be safe.

Carotenoids

(Including lycopene, zeaxanthin lutein, alpha-carotene, cryptoxanthin)
Function: Powerful antioxidants; also help with healthy vision, skin and lining of blood vessels and help to protect the skin from sun damage and cancer.
Food source: Yellow and orange vegetables, dark leafy vegetables, avocado and red and pink fruits like tomatoes, watermelon and pink grapefruit.

Thiamine (B1)

Function: Vital for the maintenance of healthy nerve cells and the central nervous system; important for growth and digestive functioning; helps in the body's conversion of carbohydrates to energy.
Food source: Wholegrain products, seeds, wheatgerm, meat products, dairy products, legumes, eggs and some fruits.
Guidelines for daily dose: RDA = 1.1 mcg; no SUL established.

Riboflavine (B2)

Function: Maintains the growth of cells and is involved in red blood cell production; important for the metabolism of carbohydrates, proteins and fats; maintains the mucous membranes of the skin, eyes and nervous system; involved in the production of adrenaline by the adrenal glands.
Food source: Milk, eggs, enriched cereals, grain, ice cream (the real kind), liver, some lean meats and vegetables.
Guidelines for daily dose: RDA = 1.1 mcg; no SUL established.

Folic acid

Function: Plays a vital role in the production of DNA; can prevent birth defects like spina bifida; involved in the formation of white and red blood cells, and may reduce homocysteine levels.

Food source: Green leafy vegetables, beans, orange juice, liver, yeast extract, some fruits.

Guidelines for daily dose: RDA = 400 mcg; SUL = 1 000 mcg.

Niacin (B3)

(Nicotinic acid and nicotinamide are the active forms)

Function: Maintains healthy skin and nerves; maintains lowered cholesterol levels; converts food to energy; oxidises fats and proteins.

Food source: Beef, pork, eggs and cow's milk, peanuts, chicken, fish and yeast.

Guidelines for daily dose: RDA = 14 mg; SUL = 35 mg.

Pyridoxine (B6)

Function: Helps with the synthesis of protein in the body; formation of red blood cells and normal brain functioning, and aids the digestive system; involved in the formation of antibodies and boosts the immune system; involved in regulating moods and relieving depression.

Food source: Fish, pork, eggs, milk, wheatgerm, brewer's yeast, brown rice, soybeans, oats, wholegrains, peanuts and walnuts.

Guidelines for daily dose: RDA = 1.5 mg; SUL = 100 mg.

Vitamin B12

Function: Vital for the red blood cells and central nervous system; important for the normal metabolism of all cells, especially in the gastrointestinal tract, bone marrow and nervous tissue.

Food source: Eggs, dairy products, animal proteins, liver and kidneys.

Guidelines for daily dose: RDA = 2.4 mcg; no SUL established.

Pantothenic acid

Function: Food metabolism, involved in the manufacture of hormones and cholesterol.

Food source: Chicken, beef, cereals, liver, egg yolk, kidney, yeast, broccoli, wholegrains, mushrooms, avocado, milk, sweet potato, salmon.

Guidelines for daily dose: RDA = 5 mg; no SUL established.

Biotin

Function: Metabolises protein, fat and carbohydrates; regulates insulin hormones and cholesterol (cholesterol is the building block for most hormones and functioning of cell membranes, especially in the brain).
Food source: Liver, egg yolk, kidney, muscle and organ meats, most leafy vegetables, some fruit, milk and the bacteria in your gut.
Guidelines for daily dose: AI = 30 mcg; no SUL established.

Vitamin C

Function: Healthy teeth and gums; promotes healing; involved in the body's absorption of iron; is a powerful antioxidant.
Food source: Ripe fruit, especially citrus fruit; vegetables, especially red peppers.
Guidelines for daily dose: RDA = 75 mg; SUL = 2 000 mg.

Vitamin D

Function: The body manufactures this after exposure to sunlight. Promotes absorption of calcium, so is vital to the development and maintenance of healthy bones and teeth; regulates the body's levels of calcium and phosphorus.
Source: Exposure to sunlight; also found in fatty fish, fish-liver oils, liver, eggs, butter, cream.
Guidelines for daily dose: RDA =15 mcg (600 IU); SUL = 100 mcg (4 000 IU).

Vitamin E

Tocopherol (d-alpha-, beta-, gamma- and delta-tocopherol are excellent, but beware of synthetic vitamin E).
Function: Powerful antioxidant; protects red blood cells from being destroyed in too large numbers and keeps membranes healthy.
Food source: Nuts and seeds, wheatgerm, leafy vegetables, legumes, egg yolk.
Guidelines for daily dose: RDA = 15 mg (22.4 IU); SUL = 1 000 mg (1 500 IU).

Vitamin K

Function: Vital to blood clotting; also involved in brain functioning and may help to maintain strong bones in the elderly.
Food source: Broccoli and leafy green vegetables, vegetable oils, small amounts found in eggs, dairy products and meat.
Guidelines for daily dose: AI = 90 mcg; no SUL established.

MINERALS

A mineral is a natural inorganic substance with a specific chemical make-up that is vital for healthy body functioning. The minerals I have listed below are those that are most important for a healthy diet. You may know of others. If your eating plan is sensible, you will be getting traces of all of them, which should be enough to maintain general good health.

Guidelines for the daily dose are for women 31–70 years old. Sources for the vitamin and mineral guidelines are given in the Reference and Resource List on pages 323–327.

Calcium

Function: Essential for bone formation and for cardiovascular, nerve and muscle functioning; maintains cell structures.
Food source: Milk and milk products, especially cheese; sardines with bones; dark leafy greens like kale and broccoli; sesame seeds and oranges; soybean products. Low-fat milk and plain low-fat or fat-free yoghurt.
Guidelines for daily dose: RDA = 500–1 200 mg; SUL = 2 000 mg.

Iron

Function: Iron in red blood cells carries oxygen, which is necessary for the production of energy, the functioning of the immune system and cognitive performance. Iron is an important component of some enzymes.
Food source: Red meats, liver, fish and poultry; dark leafy vegetables, cocoa, molasses, wholegrains, oysters, lentils and dried beans, prunes, raisins and some fruit.
Guidelines for daily dose: RDA = 18 mg (19–50 years) 8 mg (51 and older); SUL = 45 mg.

Magnesium

Function: Magnesium is essential to maintain both the acid-alkaline balance in the body and healthy functioning of nerves and muscles (including the heart), as well as to activate enzymes to metabolise blood sugars, proteins and carbohydrates. It is essential for metabolising vitamin D.
Food source: Seeds, unrefined grains, beans and leafy vegetables.
Guidelines for daily dose: RDA = 320 mg; SUL = 350 mg.

Potassium

Function: Together with sodium it maintains normal cell functioning, water balance, acid-base balance, muscular and neural functioning, and is important for cellular growth. Muscle mass and glycogen storage are related to the potassium content of the muscles and it works with various enzymes in helping the pancreas to secrete insulin.

Food source: Most fruits, root vegetables like potatoes, milk, beef, liver, chicken, soy, turkey, shellfish and dark leafy greens.

Guidelines for daily dose: 4 700 mg; no SUL established.

Selenium

Function: Works in conjunction with vitamin E to provide a powerful anti-oxidant.

Food source: Seafood, eggs, liver, kidneys, red meat and chicken. Depending on oil content: wholegrains, brazil nuts.

Guidelines for daily dose: RDA = 55 mcg; SUL = 400 mcg.

Zinc

Function: Supports the health of the immune system; helps to synthesise protein, lipids and carbohydrates, and maintains the health of reproductive organs and cell division. Zinc is a component of insulin.

Food source: Meats, fish, beans, wholegrains, pumpkin seeds, mushrooms and brewer's yeast, oysters, shellfish and herring.

Guidelines for daily dose: RDA = 8 mg; SUL = 40 mg.

TRACE MINERALS

Chromium

Function: Involved in the metabolism of carbohydrates, fat and protein; involved with insulin action; may benefit triglyceride levels.

Food source: Brewer's yeast, oysters, liver, seafood, wholegrains, meat, broccoli.

Guidelines for daily dose: AI = 25 mcg (31–50 years), 20 mcg (50 and older); no SUL established.

Copper

Function: Involved in maintaining the immune system, healthy red and white blood cells, brain development, cholesterol and glucose metabolism.

Food source: Wholegrains, nuts, shellfish, liver and dark green leafy vegetables.
Guidelines for daily dose: RDA = 900 mcg; SUL = 10 000 mcg.

Manganese

Function: Important in activating different enzymes to help healthy body functioning; crucial in healthy thyroid functioning, digestion and central nervous system functioning, as well as for the formation of connective and skeletal tissue, growth and development, reproduction, and carbohydrate and fat metabolism.
Food source: Grains and cereal products, nuts, green vegetables, tea, legumes, blueberries.
Guidelines for daily dose: AI = 1.8 mg; SUL = 11 mg.

Molybdenum

Function: Helps to regulate iron stores in the body and interacts with different enzymes to metabolise carbohydrates, oxidise fats; helps keep teeth healthy.
Food source: Meats, fish, legumes, wholegrains, pumpkin seeds, leafy vegetables, cauliflower, mushrooms and brewer's yeast.
Guidelines for daily dose: RDA = 45 mcg; SUL = 2 000 mcg.

Vanadium

Function: Ultra-trace element on which much more research needs to be done. It may be helpful in lowering cholesterol levels.
Food source: Wholegrains, meats and dairy products, seafood, spinach, parsley, mushrooms, oysters.
Guidelines for daily dose: 1.8 mg estimated requirement since the daily requirement is undefined.

SUPPLEMENTS FREQUENTLY PRESCRIBED FOR PERI- AND POSTMENOPAUSAL WOMEN

I met Sherry and Val, both in their mid-fifties, at a workshop, where they were having an animated conversation about the huge amount of money they spent on vitamins and supplements. Both of them were health conscious and Sherry, especially, was an avid reader of everything she could lay her hands on about health in menopause.

'I'm not keen on taking hormone therapy, but I have such awful night sweats, I must have bought every alternative medicine available to help me deal with my hot flushes. Honestly, I've spent a fortune at my local health shop hoping for a miracle cure.'

'I know exactly what you mean,' exclaimed Val. 'I don't want to take HT because I've always been keener on going the natural route, but I'm really battling with hot flushes so I bought a whole slew of products. I take so many vitamins and supplements that I don't know if I'm overdosing on them or if they're safe because they're natural.'

'I am just as confused as you are,' complained Sherry. 'I feel I'm bombarded with advertisements exhorting me to buy this miracle vitamin or that essential supplement and I'm ever hopeful that I will actually find something that will help, though nothing has worked yet. At this moment I have at least a dozen different types of these products in my cupboard, which I take faithfully but still have hot flushes throughout the day and really bad night sweats, which wake me several times a night.'

'I have the same problem,' said Val. 'In fact, I felt so desperate after six months that I went to see a healthcare practitioner who specialises in "natural" remedies, which cost me another fortune as I had to have a whole series of blood tests. He then made me throw out all my previous vitamins and supplements and gave me a whole new lot. I came home loaded with pills and now have a dozen, if not more, bottles of vitamins and other menopausal tablets and still have these debilitating flushes and night sweats. I'm also taking a flower essence for anxiety, which doesn't seem to work.'

Neither of them had discussed these products with their gynaecologists or GPs and both admitted that they hadn't been reading the fine print on the labels, so they had no idea how much or little of a particular vitamin or product they were actually taking and whether these levels were safe and effective or not. They had both, with the exception of Val's visit to the specialist in natural medicines, relied on the advice of the assistants at their local healthcare shops. Both of them told me that they wished they had a clearer idea of what they should and shouldn't be taking.

Peri- and postmenopausal women are offered many supplements, mainly by complementary and alternative healthcare practitioners. Unfortunately, there have not been enough rigorous, efficacy trials on these supplements for me to say with absolute certainty that they will be beneficial to you or will help to improve your symptoms. But although there isn't definitive evidence about the efficacy, benefits and risks of these alternative menopause remedies, women continue to be hugely interested in complementary and alternative medicine, possibly because we have been 'burnt' by conventional medicine and are alarmed at what we read about the risks of conventional medications. The Women's Health Initiative (WHI) report and the subsequent scare about HT further encouraged us to look to complementary and alternative medicines as a solution to our problems. Even before the WHI scare, we were uneasy with the side effects that many of us experienced with conventional hormone therapy.

Women are particularly susceptible to the lure of complementary and alternative medicines because we tend to look at things laterally, trust our instincts, be less suspicious of difference and more prepared to accept that life is complex. We think there may be solutions other than conventional ones to problems. We also long for the eternal youth that complementary and alternative medicines promise us. What we don't realise is that we may also be 'burnt' by these products and, because we are susceptible to the lure of promises that we can prevent ourselves from ageing, we need to have a very clear idea of the risks and benefits of the different supplements that are available to us.

The Web is very useful for accessing information – there are literally thousands of sites devoted to this subject – but remember to apply the same critical approach to these sites that I suggested in Chapter 3 when you are accessing information about hormones.

Just to refresh your memory, when reading about 'natural' remedies for peri- and postmenopausal women remember the following:
- **Check who runs the site.** Is it a reputable government, medical or academic institution? And are the writers qualified – a string of letters or some technical-sounding name doesn't mean that they are bona fide; the degrees may come from bogus institutions.
- **Is the purpose of the site to sell you something?** Does it have advertisements and sponsors, and are there all sorts of links that lead you to products that are for sale?
- **Check that there are sound references.** Much of the information on dietary supplements uses the trick of selecting a line of information from

a study and repeating it out of context, or using a phrase from a study without citing the study or its reference anywhere in the publication.

- **Watch out for overly scientific language** categorically stating the effects of a product without citing the study or the reference from which it comes.
- **Check the date of the information** on the site. Improved research may mean that something that was a breakthrough in the 1990s has changed radically in the intervening decade. For example, see the changes that have happened concerning vitamin E and vitamin D dosing recommendations in the past few years.

You should apply the same stringent criteria to articles on the subject. I recently read a newsletter written by one of the so-called gurus of complementary medicine, which says the following (*the italics are my comments*):

Vitamin A deficiency reduces immune function by diminishing the function neutrophils, macrophages and natural killer cells [*says who?*]. Normally I suggest 10 000 to 25 000 IU. But if you're working on an infection, such as influenza, I recommend a loading dose [*what does this mean? How will your liver cope with it?*] for three days at 300 000 units daily. Then drop to 25 000 units daily thereafter [*see above for guidance on vitamin A: 3 000 mcg or 10 000 IU*]. If you're worried about toxicity – don't be (unless you're pregnant). The Merck manual says that you must take 100 000 units for several weeks to months before you reach toxicity with vitamin A.

Whitaker, J. 'Other Supplements to Boost Resistance'. *Health and Healing*, December 2004, Vol 14, No 12, p 3.

All the reading and research I had done had led me to believe that a supplemental daily dose of no more than 2 333 IU would be safe. So practising what I preach, I looked up the Merck manual, which says: '*Chronic toxicity* in older children and adults usually develops after doses of >3 000 mcg (10 000 IU)/day have been taken for months' (my emphasis), but on the same page concludes with the following: 'Prolonged daily administration of large doses *must be avoided* because toxicity may result' (my emphasis).

Then I logged onto the Natural Medicines Comprehensive Database, http://www.naturaldatabase.com/, which is updated regularly and is the closest I have found to a physicians' reference book (it lists all the information, side effects, benefits and so on of the conventional medicine you take). It says that vitamin A is safe in adults when used in doses of less than 10 000 IU per day and gives the following reference: Food and Nutrition Board, Institute of Medicine, *Dietary Reference Intakes for Vitamin A, Vitamin K, Arsenic, Boron, Chromium, Copper, Iodine, Iron, Manganese, Molybdenum, Nickel, Silicon, Vanadium, and Zinc.* Washington, DC: National Academy Press, 2002. Available at: www.nap.edu/books/0309072794/html/.

The above serves to illustrate my point. Be very careful what you read and who you believe; eat and live as healthily as possible and don't go wild with huge doses of any one supplement. There is, as yet, no clear scientific evidence that more is better.

There are hundreds of different supplements in the marketplace but those I list below are the ones most commonly prescribed for peri- and postmenopausal women. I have tried to give you an overview of each of them: their risks, efficacy and benefits. In some cases I have given the scientific name with the herbal supplements, so that if a homeopath prescribes a tincture for you, you will know what you are taking. Remember that many over-the-counter remedies aren't well controlled and the quantities of active ingredients they contain could be toxic in some cases.

The first four supplements are thought to act like the hormone estrogen. Much research has been done into these but there are still not enough long-term, double-blind randomised controlled trials. However, because of the interest in these supplements, good trials are under way and it may not be too long before we can say with much more certainty that they do what they claim to do and are safe, as well as beneficial.

Because of the huge interest in complementary and alternative medicine, your healthcare practitioner should be aware of the growing number of products that have been tested and that may be safe and effective in relieving symptoms. Your doctor is well trained and qualified enough to understand the research documents so don't be afraid to show him or her information or ask his or her opinion so that you can have an informed discussion. Your doctor should always ask you if you are taking any complementary or alternative medicines and this should be included in your medical history. Many women swear that a particular supplement has helped reduce hot flushes, but this is often the result of what is called the 'placebo effect', the situation in which those in the control group believe so strongly that the substance they are taking is going be good for them that they actually exhibit the same physical changes as the experimental group.

The point above about the 'placebo effect' is so important that although I wrote about it in Chapter 3, I'm going to repeat it. In a good double-blind, randomised controlled trial (RCT) there are two groups: an **experimental**

group, which is taking the product being tested, and a **control group**, which is taking a harmless but ineffective substance called a placebo. The people in the control group believe that what they are taking is the substance that is being tested. Neither of the groups knows whether they are the control group or the experimental group. Much of the research that has been done into plant estrogens up to now has not been of long enough duration to eliminate the placebo reaction, but it does show how powerful the mind can be in controlling symptoms like hot flushes. According to a very well-known professor of complementary medicine, of the alternative treatments (including acupuncture, homeopathy, herbal supplements and reflexology) that he analysed with his colleagues over many years, about 95 per cent were not statistically different to placebo. But our minds are very powerful and if we expect that something will help us, it often does.

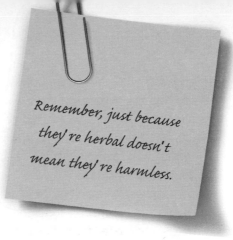

Remember, just because they're herbal doesn't mean they're harmless.

PLANT ESTROGENS

A word of warning here: because so little is known about the way these plant estrogens interact, be careful of taking two or more in combination. One of them may be fine for you, but some of the supplements that health food shops recommend to peri- and postmenopausal women contain all or some of these. **Remember, just because they're herbal doesn't mean they're harmless**. If you are taking these, you should be monitored as closely as you would be on HT.

Soy isoflavones

Soy protein, which comes from soybeans, is a very important dietary supplement because soybeans are rich in calcium, iron, potassium, amino acids, vitamins and fibre, and soy also contains all the essential amino acids necessary in a healthy human being. This last point makes it an excellent source of replacement protein for vegetarians.

Most peri- and postmenopausal women know about soy because it contains plant estrogens, which are called phytoestrogens, and in soy are known as soy isoflavones. The best known of these are genistein and daidzein. It is thought that soy has a hormonal action in women because daidzein is metabolised to an estrogenic compound known as equol. The flora in your gut help this process and this is why some women convert daidzein better than others, because we all have different levels of gut flora. Some women are not able to metabolise daidzein to equol at all, which is why there are women who complain that the soy isoflavone supplements don't help their menopausal symptoms.

Another problem is that the amount of soy isoflavones may differ from soy supplement to soy supplement. The type of soy isoflavone may be significant; recent research has shown that a daily dose of 15 mg of genistein significantly reduces hot flushes in some postmenopausal women.

There has been an enormous amount of research into and discussion of the role that soy plays in helping to alleviate menopausal symptoms, as well as about the many benefits claimed by healthcare practitioners. Different practitioners recommend different doses, but it appears that a daily dose of between 35 mg and 110 mg of soy isoflavones is safe for up to six months and may slightly decrease hot flush frequency and severity. Long-term trials are under way to provide better information about the safety and efficacy of soy isoflavone supplements.

One of the worries about soy is that because it appears to act like estrogen in helping to reduce hot flushes, some researchers think that in the long term it might act like estrogen on breast tissue and on the lining of the womb, but a recent one-year study of women taking genistein found that it had no apparent effect on the lining of the womb. However, women who are at risk for estrogen-related cancers (breast, ovarian and uterine) and are sensitive to estrogen should be very aware of any estrogen-like symptoms when taking this supplement, if they decide to risk taking it at all. Because the research in this area is still fairly new, some information suggests that soy isoflavones may protect breast tissue from estrogens, while other evidence shows that they may stimulate it. Because of its estrogenic properties, soy may interfere with tamoxifen. There is mixed evidence about whether dietary soy supplements will cause thickening of the lining of the womb and its long-term safety in this regard has not yet been established.

Soy also seems to be helpful in reducing bad cholesterol, but research has shown that it is better to take actual soy protein, like lecithin powder, for this purpose rather than capsules or tablets. Other research shows that soy may have a very strong antioxidant action. There is ongoing research to determine whether soy isoflavones are helpful in maintaining or building bone density; some double-blind randomised controlled trials have shown that soy isoflavones are effective in maintaining the bone mineral content in women who are in late menopause, while other double-blind research shows that they do not protect against bone loss in women with early menopause. These contradictory results are because of the different study designs, the levels of estrogen in a woman's body and the type and way each soy supplement is metabolised. But scientists still need to establish definitively the effects of soy isoflavones on bone density and fracture risk, and their long-term safety.

Black cohosh (Actaea racemosa, Cimicifuga racemosa)

Many of my clients have been given this in tincture or tablet form by alternative and complementary healthcare practitioners to alleviate the symptoms of menopause. The best known brand product is Remifemin, which is manufactured in Germany, where it has been available for more than 50 years and has been carefully regulated. Trials have shown that a daily dose of 40 to 60 mg can be used safely for about six months but longer-term studies are still needed. Some producers recommend a dose of 20 mg twice daily.

There has been some non-conclusive evidence that the substance may have some adverse effects on the liver. Of even more concern is the possible long-term effect of black cohosh on breast tissue and lungs. Although several trials have already shown that it does not really have significant estrogenic effects, in fact it acts like the selective estrogen receptor-modulators (SERMs) I wrote about in Chapter 4, except that black cohosh is a plant (*phyto*) SERM. This is precisely why there is a need for well-designed, long-term, controlled clinical trials of this product, with substantial sample numbers. However some recent trials show that black cohosh is significantly less effective than estrogen in reducing hot flushes and night sweats, and sometimes even worked less well than the placebo used in these trials.

There are ongoing randomised controlled trials under way at prestigious academic institutions that hope to determine whether black cohosh acts in the long term like estrogen on breast tissue and the lining of the womb, and whether it has beneficial effects on heart health or bone formation. One of these recently completed trials, showed similar results as those above – when compared with the placebo treatment, black cohosh did not reduce hot flushes and night sweats. But of greater interest was the fact that a chemically and biologically standardised daily dose appeared to be safe and did not seem to affect breast tissue or the lining of the womb, or cause liver toxicity. There is always a caveat because supplements containing black cohosh are not regulated, so if you take it you should be aware if you develop any signs of liver problems, such as dark urine, pain in your abdomen or jaundice, you should immediately consult your healthcare practitioner.

Red clover (Trifolium pratense)

A safe dose of red clover appears to be 40–160 mg daily and the best-known brand is Promensil, an Australian product containing isoflavones. Red clover isoflavones contain four isoflavones: *biochanin A*, *formononetin*, *genistein* and *daidzein*. Promensil's website promises that the product will do the following: relieve the symptoms of menopause, hot flushes and night sweats; help improve general well-being; and maintain bone health and cholesterol. However, in some double-blind, randomised placebo-controlled trials of menopausal women, red clover has not been shown to be clinically effective in reducing hot flushes over a period of 12 weeks and much more evidence is needed to support all those claims. Newer research suggests that in some small, randomised control trials, a small benefit has been shown with red clover when compared with placebo. The studies also do not show that red clover helps improve bone density.

So, given the results of several trials and reviews of the literature where red clover was taken in varying doses for varying times from 12 weeks to a year, it is unlikely that red clover will reduce your menopausal symptoms, but as in the case of black cohosh, large well-controlled clinical trials are currently underway and once they are completed we may be better able to rate the efficacy of red clover and establish definitively whether it has an anti-estrogenic effect on breast tissue and on the lining of the womb, and is beneficial to heart health and bone formation. As with the randomised controlled study of black cohosh, commercially available products of red clover with a standardised dose of red clover was found to be safe if taken over a period of 12 months and did not prevent blood from clotting. It was also shown to reduce the symptom of anxiety over a period of time.

Other research has shown that red clover may have an anti-inflammatory effect on the arteries, so a lot of work needs to be done there as well. Some women may want to use either red clover isoflavones or black cohosh to alleviate their menopausal symptoms and if either of these supplements works for you, there is no harm in trying it for a while, but be alert for sensitive, tender breasts, have a scan of the lining of your womb annually and be aware of any changes in your body.

Until more research has been done I would suggest that you avoid taking products that combine these two herbal supplements because we don't know how they react together. I also wouldn't recommend other products containing one or either of the above supplements in combination with other herbal supplements, because we cannot be sure of the dosage, quality or efficacy of these products. There are some medical scientists who recommend that the dosage of these products be standardised, since they vary so widely and in one study many of the products analysed contained less than 25 per cent of the isoflavone content described on the label. A well-known English menopause expert has described a four-point quality safety code, SAFE when using complementary medicines. **S**tandardised levels of the active ingredient, **A**bsence of drug interactions and contaminants, **F**ound to be an effective and safe product, **E**ffective levels of active ingredient. This may be a good way of assessing the complementary therapy you decide to take.

If you're interested in checking out the clinical trials. the Natural Medicines Comprehensive Database is available (http://www.naturaldatabase.com) and, although you need to pay a small subscription, if you are really concerned about what you are taking and if your own healthcare practitioner doesn't have this information, I would highly recommend that you suggest they subscribe to it or do so yourself. This database uses objective, evidence-based research, explains mechanisms of action and safety concerns and describes the efficacy of the product. This information is kept up to date based on the latest research.

Dong Quai (Angelica sinensis)

Dong Quai is also a plant estrogen and is thought to be safe in 400 mg daily doses in powder form. Complementary and alternative healthcare practitioners are enthusiastic about prescribing it to help with menopausal symptoms, but like the other substances in this group, its safety and efficacy has not yet been adequately proven. It appears to have estrogenic effects, which may be why it seems to alleviate hot flushes in some women. Because it may have estrogenic effects, you shouldn't take Dong Quai if you're sensitive to estrogen or at risk for estrogen-sensitive cancers. Some people find that Dong Quai increases bleeding risk.

Flaxseed or linseed

Flaxseeds contain lignans, a type of plant estrogen, though they are not present in flaxseed oils. Information about flaxseed is covered in detail in the section on omega-3 fatty acids (page 112).

Glucosamine

Glucosamine and chondroitin are compounds are found in nearly every tissue in your body, particularly in the cartilages. This supplement is recommended for the aching joints and arthritis that often plague us as we get older. A dose of 1 500 mg daily seems to be safe, with no bad reactions, and long-term research has shown that this daily dose may relieve symptoms of osteoarthritis. You will find that glucosamine is often combined with a supplement called chondroitin. This may cause problems if you have a shellfish allergy. Once again there is no evidence to show that they work better together than alone. In a recent meta-analysis, when 10 studies of glucosamine, chondroitin and the two in combination were reviewed, it was found that compared with placebo, these did not decrease joint pain or improve joint mobility, although users were generally convinced that these supplements helped them. The study also showed that both glucosamine and chondroitin appeared to be safe to use. There need to be more, better-designed gold standard clinical trials to confirm which formulation is best and to determine overall safety and effectiveness.

As with many products, glucosamine supplements are not carefully regulated so you should try to buy a reputable brand name. Some healthcare practitioners prefer glucosamine sulphate to glucosamine hydrochloride, but as yet there does not appear to be definitive evidence as to which form is more effective. (See the GAIT study in Chapter 9.)

Coenzyme Q10 (CoQ10)

This is a compound similar to a vitamin that is found in your body. It is thought that the amounts of CoQ10 in your body begin to decline as you get older, which is the reason why so many complementary and alternative healthcare practitioners recommend it to middle-aged women. Supplements may be recommended in doses ranging from 30 to 100 mg.

Although small amounts of CoQ10 are obtained from certain foods, particularly seafood and meat, the body produces almost all we need for healthy living. It is fat soluble and is found throughout the body in almost all the cells, with high levels in the major organs of the heart, pancreas, liver and kidneys, but these amounts are not bioavailable to (*metabolised or utilised by*) the body.

Interestingly, the CoQ10 found in soybean oil has been found to be bio-available, which reinforces my belief that soy protein may act as an antioxidant. CoQ10 maintains healthy cell function and plays a vital role in the production of *adenosine triphosphate* (ATP), which is essential to the storage and production of energy in the muscles in a process by which all the energy and nutrients in food are released to ensure that they are assimilated by the body.

Because of the role CoQ10 plays in cell respiration and the release of energy it is thought to be a powerful antioxidant, which may play a protective role in the human body as it begins to age, especially in relation to heart disease. The results of research studies over the past few years seem to bear this out. Trials have also shown that CoQ10 may help to lower blood pressure, reduce insulin levels and LDL (bad) cholesterol, and increase levels of some important vitamins and HDL (good) cholesterol. However, these trials had several design flaws so they should be regarded with caution and it would probably be sensible to wait for larger randomised controlled trials before supplementing with CoQ10. You should also be careful about mixing CoQ10 with other medications because it may have adverse reactions or lower the efficacy of the drugs you are taking.

Ginseng (Panax ginseng, Panax quinquefolius)

Ginseng is called an adaptogen by complementary or alternative healthcare practitioners. This means it is believed to play a specific, beneficial role in the body where, they say, it helps to regulate certain functions before it is harmlessly absorbed or eliminated.

The problem with ginseng is that there are several different kinds, including Siberian, American and Panax. Ginseng has been used for thousands of years in traditional Chinese medicine but because there are varying kinds and varying doses, and because it is extracted in different ways, the supplements you buy may have varying results.

There are all sorts of claims made about ginseng. It is said to improve flagging energy levels, the immune system and the libido. Some practitioners believe that it reduces stress. Since many peri- and postmenopausal women complain of many of these symptoms, it seems logical that they are offered ginseng supplements, but once again, well-designed clinical trials have offered no evidence to back up these claims or show that ginseng is safe in the long term. In fact, it may have some very harmful effects on women who are suffering from high blood pressure, migraines or heart disease. Asian ginseng has been shown to lower levels of glucose in the blood, so it should be used with great caution by those who have diabetes. It has also been known to cause bleeding problems.

Fatty acids

Most of us know by now that the omega-3 and omega-6 fatty acids are absolutely essential to good health. They are vital fats, crucial for the efficient functioning and maintenance of every single cell in our bodies. The main fatty acids that we know about are *linoleic acid*, which is the omega-6 fatty acid, and *alpha-linoleic acid* (ALA), which is the omega-3 fatty acid.

In our twenty-first century diet we probably get more than adequate omega-6 fatty acids from different vegetable oils, nuts and seeds, and from grain-fed meat and poultry, but our diet doesn't usually provide us with enough of the omega-3 fatty acids, so the ratio of the omega-3 to omega-6 fatty acids in our bodies is often unbalanced, leaning heavily on the side of the omega-6 fats. Without going into a confusing description of the body's biochemistry, it is vital for optimum health that the two be balanced. Omega-3 fatty acids appear to be powerful antioxidants, help to prevent inflammation and thrombosis (*antithrombotic*) and they may also help to lower blood pressure. Some research suggests that they may help to lower triglycerides and LDL (bad cholesterol).

In Chapter 10 on weight and diet I write about 'good' and 'bad' fats, but since we are discussing supplements, I would suggest that most middle-aged women should supplement their diets with omega-3 fatty acids, which come from flaxseed oil, fish oil, flaxseeds, hempseeds and purslane; oily cold-water fish like herring, mackerel, salmon and sardines; soybeans, walnuts and walnut oils. If you include any of these in your diet in decent quantities you may be getting enough omega-3 fatty acids, but if you are like most of us and can't be bothered to eat enough oily fish each week, you can supplement using fish oil.

If you are taking a fish oil supplement, be careful of the brand you use; some fish oils may be contaminated by toxic chemicals, so you should be comfortable that the manufacturer is reputable and can back up its quality claims. A downside of fish oil supplements is that they tend to 'repeat' and can cause a fishy taste, but today there are many highly refined fish oil supplements and if you take these with food it shouldn't happen and fish oils are an excellent source of omega-3 fatty acids.

In some cases, vegetarians who don't want to take fish oil or women who have a religious objection can use flaxseed oil. However, alpha-linoleic acid (ALA) in flaxseed must be converted in our bodies to the two important fatty acids: EPA and DHA. There is new research suggesting that only a small amount of ALA in flaxseed is converted to EPA and DHA. This is because ALA is often broken down very quickly in our bodies and because of the high content of omega-6 fatty acids in our typical Western diets. So it is probably better to supplement omega-3 fatty acids in the form of fish oil, where the EPA and DHA are already converted from ALA.

You should have a daily minimum of 1 000 mg of omega-3 in your diet. A 1 000 mg capsule of fish oil provides 180 mg EPA and 120 mg DHA (300 mg together). Two to three of these capsules daily should meet your needs.

There are lignans in flaxseed that are a type of plant estrogen, but these are not present in the flaxseed oil, which contains only the ALA component of flaxseed. Taking flaxseed may help to improve menopausal symptoms and the quality of your hair and skin, so that some flaxseed in the form of oil, seeds or one or two capsules may be a good addition to the diets of peri- and postmenopausal women.

Ginkgo (Ginkgo biloba)

This is mainly prescribed for middle-aged women who find that they are battling a failing memory. Poor memory is a frequent symptom in peri- and postmenopausal women and many of us use or try out this supplement. Although ginkgo is prescribed for a wide variety of ailments, the claim that it can help poor memory is of most interest to menopausal women.

Ginkgo biloba is one of the oldest known plants in the world and has been used in traditional Chinese medicine for thousands of years. A daily dose of 240 mg seems to be safe, but once again there is no consensus on how risky or helpful it is. A five-year study conducted by the National Centre for Complementary and Alternative Medicine (NCCAM) to establish the effectiveness of a daily dose of 240 mg found that it was not effective in lowering or preventing Alzheimer's disease or age-related dementia. Ginkgo is often combined with ginseng in supplements said to improve memory, but once again there is no hard evidence about whether this combination is helpful or safe and a trial sponsored by the National Institute on Aging found that when a group of more than 200 healthy people over the age of 60 took ginkgo for six weeks they did not have improved memory.

Ginkgo is said to increase bleeding but the reason for this is not clear, so it should not be taken if you are on blood-thinning medication.

In fact there are literally hundreds of other over-the-counter remedies and herbal supplements that I have not written about that may prove to be beneficial and risk free. I would advise that you exercise caution when purchasing these and adopt a hefty amount of scepticism. Take the time to research the product on the sites I have suggested, following the guidelines I have given you, and always discuss any supplements you are taking or intend to take with your healthcare practitioner.

SUPPLEMENTS IN MIDLIFE

Now that you have read the vitamin and mineral tables you are probably thinking that your diet and lifestyle are such that you are not getting some or all of the supplements that you think you need. For example, very few middle-aged women get enough calcium from dietary sources and I would think it unlikely that they would be getting enough omega-3 fatty acid.

While I do not advocate huge amounts of supplements, I am definitely a believer in moderate amounts. I think that women who want to take supplements should speak to an expert, someone who is properly trained and registered, and not an assistant in a health food shop or someone who is selling supplements as part of a pyramid scheme.

I have recommended the following supplements over the years:

Multivitamins – If your diet is poor or your lifestyle is unhealthy, I would recommend a good multivitamin supplement. Some practitioners don't like these combination vitamins, while others swear by them, but if you decide to take them I would suggest you lean towards those that come in a food state form (a form that is very similar to the natural form the vitamin in food comes in) because your body will metabolise them more quickly and better.

Calcium – Although you get calcium from your diet, your lower levels of estrogen may mean that you don't absorb it as well, but there have been recent studies suggesting caution when using calcium supplements because too much may increase the calcification in your arteries, putting you at greater risk for heart disease. I discuss this in greater depth in Chapter 9, so briefly, a moderate daily supplement of 500 mg of elemental calcium to make up for any calcium deficit in your diet, should be safe and beneficial. You should always combine this supplement with the correct amount of vitamin D 400–600 IU for maximum absorption.

Vitamin B complex – Many middle-aged women are very anxious or stressed and battle with low energy, and a good vitamin B complex seems to be helpful. On a biased anecdotal note (just what I told you to beware of), a great uncle of mine who was a very well-known physician and way ahead of his time in many of his theories, was a great believer in vitamin B. He lived to a ripe old age and his widow, who lived until her nineties, remaining healthy and exceptionally bright until her death, took a large daily dose of vitamin B supplements for more than 30 years.

Folic acid – If you are taking a multivitamin that has the appropriate amount of folic acid, that's fine. If you are not, 400 mcg daily may lower your risk of heart disease, may improve memory and may protect you against certain cancers.

Flaxseed – in the recommended amount or flaxseed oil capsules in a dose of between 1 000 and 2 000 mg daily. Anecdotally this seems to be good for hair and skin, and may help alleviate menopausal symptoms. A helpful side effect is that it seems to prevent constipation.

I do not personally recommend the following but here is some additional information:

Antioxidants – Many practitioners and some women swear by an antioxidant supplement containing CoQ10 or a supplement containing selenium and vitamin E, or others with beta-carotene vitamin A or C. However, the scientific evidence on the safety and benefits of antioxidants is mixed, so I would suggest that you make sure your diet is rich in antioxidant foods, like wholegrains, fruits and vegetables and omega-3 fatty acids and if you feel there is a need to supplement, discuss the options with your doctor. Research so far is not particularly encouraging and even suggests that some antioxidants, like beta-carotene, may not be safe when taken in the long term.

Alternatives to HT – If you are battling with menopausal symptoms and don't want to take conventional HT, you could try one of the plant estrogens I have mentioned, with soy isoflavones, red clover and and black cohosh probably being the best researched. Remember that there is no definitive long-term research into the risks and benefits of these and they may not be safe if you have, have had or are at risk for breast cancer. Don't combine these supplements as the doses may vary and we have no clear research on their effects or interactions.

EMPOWER YOURSELF

- **Tell your doctor about supplements:** Always tell your healthcare practitioner what supplements you are taking. Many of these supplements have been shown to cause side effects and others may react with medicines that you may be taking, interfering with them or causing unwanted reactions. A good doctor will have taken the trouble to make themselves aware of the latest research on supplements and should be able to advise you. If your practitioner can't help you in this regard, find a certified dietician or a specialist physician who has this knowledge and spend some time discussing your lifestyle, especially your daily diet, with them. They will soon pick up areas where you may be lacking in vital supplements, or be able to tell you that you are on the right track.

- **Do your research:** If you are interested in keeping up with the latest research on complementary and alternative medicine by reading some of the leading medical journals, you may have to subscribe to them, like the Natural Medicines Comprehensive Database (http://www.naturaldatabase.com/), but you can always find the abstracts of the articles on a site like PubMed, which is the U.S.A National Library of Medicine's database. The interest in this field is now so great that you can look for new research on this subject at http://nccam.nih.gov/.
- **Don't be gullible or naive:** Always ask yourself about the self-interest of the person who is trying to sell you the supplements.
- **Buy from a reputable source:** Be sure to buy your supplements from someone who is truly knowledgeable about them. A person who is selling supplements as part of a pyramid group or multilevel marketing just can't be as knowledgeable as an expert, and once again, their advice may be biased by a profit motive.
- **Be wary:** Remember, many herbal treatments can interact with medications and cause toxic effects.
- **Diet:** Eat a healthy, varied diet. You will see from the information in the lists that you will be able to get most of the vital nutritional supplements you need from a sensible, well-balanced meal plan.

6
Hot flushes and hysterectomies

'I'm sitting in the middle of really important presentation,' said Ilana, *'and things are going well. Suddenly I feel a strange feeling; almost out-of-body. I feel sort of disassociated and then I know it's going to happen. I feel this wave of heat travelling up me, growing in a rush. I know that my face is turning blood red and I start to pour with sweat. I feel like I'm in a sauna. My colleagues, mostly men, are looking at me in astonishment and I find myself rushing out of the room to mop up!'*

Nicki smiled sympathetically. *'I know just how you feel. Mine aren't as bad as that, though I feel terribly hot. They seem to come in waves throughout the day and they get worse if I drink my soup or coffee hot. Nowadays everything I drink has to be lukewarm or I find myself reaching boiling point. I also often feel incredibly anxious, sometimes even panicky, when this happens.'*

Chris shook her head. *'That doesn't happen to me at all. I feel a sort of humming in my ears, a tingling feeling like pins and needles in my fingertips, then there's this wave of giddiness. I feel like I'm going to keel over but I'm not much hotter than usual.'*

'Yes,' said Sara. *'It's not that I feel burning hot, it's just that for the past few months I've felt that my whole body temperature is higher. I hardly ever feel chilly now and it seems to me that summers have become much, much warmer than they used to be.'*

'I agree,' nodded Jo. *'But though the days feel warmer, it's the nights that really bother me. I don't even sleep with a duvet any more, even on the coldest winter nights. My husband has had to get his own blanket. Sleep has become a rare commodity. Even if I fall asleep feeling reasonably comfortable, I wake several times during the night drenched in sweat. Sometimes I've had to change my nightdress and put a bath towel underneath me; the sheets are so wet and I don't want to wake my husband up to change the bed.'*

The conversation of this group of middle-aged friends is typical of that of women who are in the throes of perimenopause. They are all experiencing the result of fluctuating levels of estrogen on the hypothalamus in their brains. In other words, they are getting hot flushes. But because they are all biochemically different individuals, the kind of hot flushes they are experiencing varies widely.

Because hot flushes are the red rag of menopause, an enormous amount has been written about them; of all the symptoms of menopause it is hot flushes that women obsess about most. As I wrote earlier, many writers, in a backlash against the old anti-feminist mindset that menopause was a disease, tried to reframe these symptoms by calling them 'power surges'. Leslie Kenton wrote a bestseller called *Passage to Power*, which was one of the first works to suggest that menopausal women were strong and functioning, desirable and desirous, not dried-out old crones. Other feminists had ceremonies where they honoured the menopausal woman as a wise woman or shaman.

I'm not so sure the answer is to rename a hot flush or have a ceremony. I think this puts additional stress on a middle-aged woman by making her feel that she should welcome her hot flushes, believing they are empowering her, when all she longs for is to feel cool again or have a good night's sleep and not wake drenched in sweat. But I do think that the way you handle these flushes has a lot to do with how you perceive them. I believe that knowledge is power. If you know what's happening to you physiologically and you have some handle on how to deal with them, hot flushes will be understood as part of the perimenopausal process; often uncomfortable, terribly disruptive, sometimes unbearable, but ultimately transitional. We know that except in incredibly rare cases, hot flushes do eventually stop.

As I discussed in Chapter 1 there may be a variety of reasons for hot flushes, including early ovarian failure, various medications, a sensitivity to alcohol, thyroid or endocrine problems, and fevers that may be caused by viral or bacterial illness, so if it's unlikely that you're perimenopausal, you should ask your doctor to investigate other reasons.

Hot flushes may begin a couple of years before menopause, and reach their zenith about a year after menopause, but it's still unclear how long they last; guidelines say between two and 14 years, some research has shown they generally last on average for at least five years. But a very recent study suggests, contrary to the previous clinical guidelines, the average duration of hot flushes is about 10 years, depending on the stage of menopause a woman is at when the hot flushes begin. It seems that the earlier your hot flushes begin the longer they will last. So if your hot flushes start as soon as your menopause transition begins, they could last over 11 years, while if you are bothered by them only late into your transition into menopause, they probably won't last longer than three-and-a-half years. However, long-lasting hot flushes may raise a clinical treatment problem for women taking HT for symptom

If your hot flushes start as soon as your menopause transition begins, they could last over 11 years.

relief. This is because there may be greater risks involved in taking HT for a longer time period and for older women who need to continue taking HT.

Some women stop HT after a couple of years only to find that their symptoms recur and sometimes seem to be more severe the second time round. There are those lucky women who never have a hot flush, or whose hot flushes don't last longer than six months, while some less fortunate, especially those who have had an abrupt transition into menopause following removal of their ovaries, have them well into their eighties.

Hot flushes that follow surgically induced menopause are often very severe and more frequent than the flushes of natural menopause. Women who become menopausal as a result of chemotherapy or radiation treatment may battle with hot flushes, as do those who are taking SERMs (selective estrogen receptor modulators) or aromatase inhibitors (see Chapter 8). Hot flushes may start gradually and build in intensity over the months as a woman's levels of estrogen drop. Some women experience a month of hectic hot flushes, which then peter out and recur after a few months. Others have a few unpleasant months and never have another hot flush. Still others suffer only from night sweats or get a hot flush when they are very stressed, while some battle morning, noon and night, and feel that they are constantly on fire. There are also women who find themselves chilled and shivering uncontrollably once the hot flush has passed.

Hot flushes come in many guises and combinations, and it is thought that at least 70 per cent of women who are undergoing natural menopause experience some kind of hot flush. They can last for as little as 30 seconds or build in intensity and then go on for as long as five minutes or more. Women usually experience the hot flush in their upper bodies and it seems to sweep upwards in a wave. Most women say they know when they are about to have a flush, because they experience strange tingling sensations, a growing feeling of warmth or even a strange, disassociated, out-of-body sensation. Hot flushes can sometimes mimic a panic attack. The symptoms of a panic attack often follow this scenario: a brief, unexpected feeling of physical discomfort, often in conjunction with sweating or chills, breathlessness and heart palpitations. This may sound very familiar to a woman describing a hot flush. Permutations of hot flush symptoms seem endless and although we each experience them differently, you will find there are many similar elements when you discuss them with your friends.

In spite of all the research, the way in which hot flushes occur is still not properly understood. What we do know is that all human beings have something known as core body temperature. The normal average body temperature of a healthy person is usually 37 °C. The body is an amazing machine that maintains this temperature by ensuring that the heat it produces balances the heat it loses or gains in its environment. The area that maintains this temperature control and helps your body maintain a normal temperature is in the hypothalamus, which is situated in your brain and which I wrote about in Chapter 2, describing how the hypothalamus sends a message to the pituitary, which initiates the secretion of FSH (follicle stimulating hormone) and LH (luteinising hormone). In addition, your nervous system keeps your hypothalamus in constant touch with what is happening to your body's temperature. It is then the job of your hypothalamus to ensure that your body has the appropriate physical responses that will keep you cool or warm, depending on your environment. So sometimes your blood flow is increased and sometimes it is decreased. Sometimes the way in which you metabolise food is sped up and sometimes it is slowed down; sometimes you start shivering, which makes your muscles contract so that you become warmer, and sometimes it makes you sweat so your body cools down as the sweat evaporates.

Researchers think that a hot flush may be caused by a small, sudden rise in your body's core temperature, which can take place at any point from two minutes to 17 minutes before the actual hot flush. When the hypothalamus detects this sudden rise in the core temperature, it sets into action those physical changes that have been designed to cool the body down by sweating, a change in heart rate and an increased flow of blood to the skin, which happens because the small blood vessels become wider so that the blood can flow through them more quickly.

It is believed that the temperature control area in your hypothalamus responds to the interactions of several of the special chemical messengers (*neurotransmitters*) in the brain, as well as to *endorphins* (substances your body produces when it is stressed) and hormones.

Two of these neurotransmitters are called *serotonin* and *norepinephrine* and are especially important to the way in which hot flushes occur. It seems that both before and after a hot flush the levels of norepinephrine in the blood are higher. We know that norepinephrine is responsible for an increase in our core body temperature and it is also involved in the way our bodies respond to this rise in temperature.

It is thought that appropriate amounts of hormones like estrogen, androgen and testosterone keep the levels of norepinephrine under control. In perimenopause, when the levels of these hormones fluctuate or drop suddenly, the levels of norepinephrine increase and cause a rise in your core body temperature, so the cooling off reactions start up and you begin to sweat, your heart pounds, and you get all the symptoms of a hot flush. It seems that it is not the low levels of estrogen that cause hot flushes but the sudden drops in estrogen levels that occur in perimenopause. In postmenopause, when your estrogen has stopped fluctuating and levelled out, the hot flushes usually stop.

In another twist to this tale, researchers have worked out that the neurotransmitter serotonin seems to be involved. It is thought that when estrogen levels drop, levels of serotonin in the blood drop too, and the serotonin receptors in the hypothalamus increase. This, as you can imagine, is a very complex interaction and when it happens the body usually cools off. Remember that serotonin is the 'feel good' transmitter and special medicines that are called selective serotonin reuptake inhibitors (SSRIs), like venlafaxine, are used to combat depression when serotonin levels drop. The reason I point this out is that when we come to the chapter on menopause and depression in middle-aged women it will give you a head start in understanding what happens when levels of estrogen and serotonin fluctuate or drop in peri- and postmenopause.

Another thing to look at is when hot flushes are most prevalent. The fact that they are linked to your core body temperature means that they are also linked to your body's biological clock. This biological clock is regulated by a structure that is also situated in your hypothalamus, so everything is interconnected. In the early evening, a few hours after your core body temperature reaches its highest point, hot flushes seem to increase in intensity. This is why when perimenopausal women who are suffering from hot flushes travel, they experience a variation in their hot flushes – the biological clock may be upset by time zone differences.

The issue for many women is how to they can best handle their hot flushes. Do they interfere with your quality of life or are they just a minor inconvenience, which you can cope with. Do they interfere with your quality of life or are they just a minor inconvenience, which you can cope with because you know that this stage in your life is transient? As I wrote in Chapter 4, HT is recommended for women with moderate to severe hot flushes – more than eight hot flushes a day. I have seen some women who laugh off the discomfort and others who feel quite desperate about it. There are those who have had mothers or family members with breast cancer, or have even had their own bout with cancer, who are terrified to take HT and really battle, and those who say they don't care, they will take the risk because they refuse to put up with hot flushes. Each woman handles hot flushes in her own way. Here are my thoughts and recommendations on how to deal with them.

DEALING WITH HOT FLUSHES

Lifestyle

There is not much good clinical research available on how lifestyle changes may help your hot flushes, but I think that common sense is the watchword here. I often wonder how our mothers and grandmothers dealt with the problem; perhaps they just suffered in silence. Of course, synthetic fabrics were much less common, which may have made a difference; it may be sensible if you suffer from hot flushes to wear natural fibres and sleep on cotton sheets and use cotton blankets.

As a rule of thumb, choose fabrics that breathe. These may be natural fibres or the new generation of synthetic fabrics that athletes wear to keep the sweat away from the body where it can evaporate more easily. Anything that makes you feel constrained, uncomfortable and hot may precipitate a hot flush. Wear layers during this time and clothes that float rather than those that are tight and clingy, especially tight waistbands or elastic that cuts into your waist. Remember too that most women put on weight during perimenopause so make sure your clothes are loose fitting. Even in winter wear cotton as well as wool and be able to remove layers in a very warm room before your core temperature responds to the heat. At night turn down the heat in your bedroom (but provide your partner with a heating pad or a hot-water bottle and an extra blanket; he shouldn't have to freeze because you're hot). Alternatively, layer the bedclothes at night, so that you can throw off the blanket or duvet on your side of the bed. Other suggestions are to keep a glass of cold water next to you and sip it or, if you're really battling, a novel suggestion from the NAMS e-magazine *Menopause Flashes* is to put a frozen ice pack under your pillow and turn the pillow often so your head is always resting on a cool surface, or wrap it in a towel and place it on your feet!

Some women find that as the warning signs preceding a hot flush start they can pre-empt the hot flush by dabbing cool water on their pulse points: their wrists, the back of their necks and the backs of their knees. I know that some women carry small spray bottles of water in their bags for this purpose. Do you remember seeing old ladies splashing the back of their necks before entering the sea to lower their body temperature? Strange as it might seem, this can help.

Many women find that if they eat spicy or very hot food they precipitate a hot flush, and the same happens when they drink very hot drinks or soup. It may not help, but it can't hurt during this time to have lukewarm drinks and bland food. Too much alcohol may trigger a hot flush, as may a bout of overeating and too much coffee. Very hot baths, hot showers and saunas or hot tubs at this stage of your life may precipitate a hot flush. But because all women are individuals, hot flushes can be triggered by different factors depending on your biochemical make-up.

Smoking and exercise

Stop smoking. Research shows that women who smoke have worse hot flushes than those who don't because smoking interferes with your estrogen production, so that your levels of estrogen will be much lower and you will have less circulating estrogen available in your body. Smoking is also associated with an earlier age at menopause, which means more years of hot flushes! In any case your health will improve exponentially if you stop smoking and, in my view, any woman who smokes is putting her health at risk – period.

On the same track, it may help reduce your hot flushes if you exercise. Even if it doesn't, the benefits of regular exercise, as I will discuss later, are so great that it's worth it. Research shows that women who exercise probably have fewer, less severe hot flushes. This may have something to do with the endorphin levels. Of course, as with everything in menopause, nothing is straightforward and the rise in your core body temperature when you exercise may precipitate a hot flush, but even then those are usually shorter and less severe.

Weight loss

Staying on the subject of health, one benefit of weight loss may be a reduction in hot flushes. It seems that women who carry more weight suffer more. Although women who have higher body mass probably have higher estrogen levels than very thin women, we know that fatter people often battle with temperature, so losing some weight may be helpful; you know it will be healthier in any event.

Stress

There is no research that suggests that stress precipitates hot flushes or makes them worse, so I will just have to rely on anecdotal evidence here. I think that many middle-aged women often get hot and bothered, and when they do they have a hot flush. Whether the 'hot' in the above phrase refers to a rise in your core body temperature, I don't know, but I do know that many women have told me that when they are stressed they have more hot flushes. So on the off-chance that stress is one of the triggers for hot flushes, try to de-stress. When you are stressed these signs may mimic some menopausal symptoms.

Exercise may help you de-stress and other ways to reduce stress are discussed further on in this chapter. If you do experience a hot flush, don't panic, especially if your heart is pounding and there is a ringing in your ears. Breathe in slowly through your nose for a count of seven, hold your breath for four counts and breathe out very slowly through your mouth for eight. Repeat this routine a couple of times. Research has shown that controlled breathing either at specific intervals during the day or when a hot flush begins may be very helpful, and I can say without reservation that this treatment has NO adverse side effects. Some recent research suggests that the relationship between anxiety and hot flushes is very complex and that your doctor should not be too quick to diagnose anxiety when the symptoms you describe may be those of hot flushes, and equally, they should not dismiss the symptoms as belonging to a hot flush rather than anxiety, especially if you are transitioning through menopause. Make sure that your doctor carefully assesses you before coming to any conclusions.

Some other ways of dealing with hot flushes

There are several studies examining ways that women who don't want to take HT for a variety of reasons can cope with hot flushes and also reduce the stress and anxiety that often accompany debilitating hot flushes and night sweats. Later in the book I discuss a stress reduction technique called *mindfulness*. A recent study used this method in conjunction with stretching exercises and after eight weeks these women felt their hot flushes were better, they were no longer so distressed by them, had a better life and sleep quality and weren't as anxious and stressed. In another recent randomised trial, women who completed an intensive mindfulness-based stress reduction programme over a period of eight weeks were less bothered by their hot flushes and night sweats than prior to the course, even three months after they had finished the course. Other experts suggest meditation or yoga as a means to reduce stress and cope with hot flushes.

It may sound a bit off the wall, but here's some evidence-based medicine that offers another option. Several randomised controlled trials suggest that acupuncture, a traditional Chinese treatment that uses tiny stainless steel needles inserted into a point on the body that has been predefined to achieve a particular result, may be helpful in reducing hot flushes. These studies have fairly small sample numbers but they provide some evidence that acupuncture may work, and a recent study showed that it was very effective in breast cancer patients who tried this as compared with venlafaxine. There were no adverse effects in the group of women using acupuncture. This seems to be a safe, effective treatment though not in the long term, as other studies have shown that these good effects were not seen at six and 12 months and further research is needed to understand how acupuncture works in helping these symptoms. The placebo effect I wrote about in Chapter 5 may provide an answer. If women expect something to work, it often does.

Hormone therapy

The most effective help for hot flushes and night sweats is HT, unless it is contraindicated for you. This subject is thoroughly discussed in Chapter 4.

Remember the guidelines: if possible, take estrogen that is chemically identical or similar to the estrogen manufactured by your body, in the lowest, most effective dose. In my view, HT should be taken through the skin (*transdermally*) for the shortest possible time. You need a progestogen if you still have a womb, but whatever you decide as far as HT is concerned, do it with your own individual profile in mind. Many women find they suffer from these symptoms as soon as they stop HT and decide to restart it. Age plays an important part in the decision to restart HT, as do your individual risk factors and potential benefits. These should be thoroughly discussed with your healthcare practitioner before you begin HT again. It's also important to be sure in your own mind how severe or unbearable you feel these symptoms are. You may want to start off with a lower dose than previously and perhaps try a different regimen. Transdermal estrogen may place you at lower risk for blood clots. The very recent research on the timing hypothesis and longer-term use of HT that I discussed in Chapter 3 may be reassuring, depending on your individual health status.

Non-hormonal treatment of hot flushes

Marika called in tears on a Saturday evening. She had been given my name by one of my clients who saw how tearful she was and felt that I might be able to help her. She had a new grandchild and was looking forward to her christening on the Sunday morning. She explained that some months earlier she had had both her ovaries removed because she had tested positive for the BRCA1 gene and her gynaecologist felt she might be at increased risk for breast and ovarian cancer. Even more recently she underwent a double mastectomy as a cancerous lump had been found in her breast. She had had a hysterectomy in her late forties and had been on HT for the past 18 years, but since her last surgery had stopped taking it abruptly. She was experiencing drenching hot flushes and night sweats and felt dreadful.

On the Tuesday before she called me, she had an appointment with her plastic surgeon, where she was discussing a breast reconstruction and complained about these symptoms, telling the doctor that one of her friends had said that clonidine had really helped her. The surgeon gaily wrote a script for the drug. This medication is prescribed to lower blood pressure and is also used off-label (see page 127) to help with hot flushes. Marika immediately started taking the pills. However, by Saturday she could barely stand up – she felt so weak, dizzy and nauseous.

The first question I asked her was whether she was on blood pressure medication. She thought for a minute and said yes, she was on a medication containing telmisartan, which is usually prescribed to lower mild to moderate high blood pressure. Marika had no idea that clonidine was originally approved to treat high blood pressure and this doctor didn't bother to ask whether she was already on anything to lower blood pressure so, with a double dose of blood pressure medication, she was suffering from all the symptoms of extremely low blood pressure. I suggested Marika call her GP or physician immediately and come off the clonidine.

The lesson here is that it's vital for you to know what medications you are on. Even if a new practitioner doesn't request this information before prescribing new medication, you should make sure your doctor has a list of the drugs you are taking. Marika's doctor knew she was at risk for breast cancer, and once Marika mentioned the medicine she thought she was being helpful by giving her a non-hormonal solution. I think if you have several medical conditions, it is essential to have one physician or specialist who acts like the conductor to an orchestra and oversees all the different prescriptions from the other doctors and specialists. Medications can have a wide variety of side effects and potentially dangerous interactions with other drugs, so it is very important that these are carefully monitored. As you can see below, there are other non-hormonal options that might have been more appropriate for Marika.

In certain women, especially those with breast cancer, hormone therapy may not be suitable to help ease severe hot flushes, so other remedies may be suggested. Some of these remedies were not specifically designed to counteract hot flushes, but women using them found coincidentally that they seemed to help. Using these products to treat a symptom or illness that has not been approved of is called *off-label*. This is the legal use of a prescription medicine to treat a disease or condition for which the medicine has not been approved by medicines regulatory boards.

Unfortunately, studies conducted on these products to see if they are effective in alleviating hot flushes are not large enough to establish whether these treatments are safe and effective in the long term. They may be helpful in treating menopausal women who cannot take estrogen therapy but the absence of sufficient information means they are not the treatment of choice for women where HT is the first option. Among these products are the following:

- *Clonidine* – originally used for women with high blood pressure (hypertension). Although research has shown that clonidine in high doses may be effective in reducing the frequency, length and severity of hot flushes, these doses can cause side effects such as insomnia, a dry mouth, constipation, drowsiness, rash, nausea and gastrointestinal disturbances (stomach upsets). So without further and more robust research at this time, it is hard to establish the most effective dosage or for how long this medicine should be given to women battling with hot flushes. It is also not known what the long-term effects associated with this treatment would be.
- *Gabapentin* is used as an anticonvulsant and for treating migraine headaches. There is research showing that postmenopausal women who took a daily dose of 900 mg of gabapentin had reduced hot flushes over a 12-week period. In another study women who took 2 400 mg of gabapentin had a 70 per cent reduction in hot flushes. The latter is a huge dose, which should be slowly increased from a starting dose of 400 mg.

Side effects such as headaches, dizziness, disorientation and sometimes sleepiness and rashes were experienced by some of the women in these studies. The sample numbers in these trials were small and larger long-term studies are needed to determine safety and efficacy. However, the results of a recent trial on a newer-generation anticonvulsant compound called *pregabalin* look promising. It was found that a twice-daily dose of 75 mg seemed to provide significant relief from hot flushes and night sweats. There were side effects such as dizziness, disorientation and some blurred or double vision but in general they appeared to be mild.

- *Vitamin E*, 800 IU/day, which is often referred to as high dose, may be another option, although the clinical evidence is not definitive and the results are mixed. Because vitamin E seems to be non-toxic in low doses, is inexpensive and available without a prescription, it may be an option for women who are struggling. But results, if any, may take weeks to be felt and usually only with higher doses. The concern is that some research indicates that higher doses may cause long-term risks, and women who have heart disease, diabetes or high blood pressure should consult their doctors before taking vitamin E. A recent meta-analysis of current research on vitamin E supplementation showed that there was a greater risk of haemorrhagic stroke, where bleeding in the brain occurs, in some vitamin E users, which resulted in medical scientists advising against using vitamin E indiscriminately. (A meta-analysis is a study where the results of several independent studies are combined and analysed.)

Supplements

Plant estrogen supplements may also be helpful in reducing hot flushes. Look at the detailed information in Chapter 5 and remember that just because something is herbal doesn't mean it's harmless. Soy isoflavones, red clover and black cohosh may be most effective in this area but more research is needed to determine all the risks, benefits and appropriate doses.

Antidepressant medication

Some women who battle terribly with hot flushes and their effects cannot take hormones because of the risks or the adverse side effects. In these cases, antidepressants may work. If you remember, I wrote at the beginning of this chapter about the role of serotonin and norepinephrine in the activity of hot flushes (see my definition of off-label use above). Research has shown that certain antidepressants seem to help reduce hot flushes. The most popular of these is *venlaxafaxine* (Effexor), which interacts with serotonin and norepinephrine, helping to balance their levels in the blood. It seems to be very effective and, of course, for perimenopausal women who suffer from depression, it is doubly useful.

However, as with all antidepressant medicine there are significant side effects like a dry mouth, sleeplessness and decreased appetite, so those women taking venlafaxine need to decide whether the relief they get from reduced hot flushes and less depression is worth the side effects. The decreased appetite may appeal to perimenopausal women who are overweight.

Other antidepressants that seem to work are *paroxetine* (Paxil) and *fluoxetine* (Prozac), which are serotonin reuptake inhibitors. The latter two also have side effects, including loss of sexual desire, which is already a problem for some menopausal women, and weight gain. One of the upsides of using antidepressants to help reduce hot flushes is that the drugs begin to work within a week and it seems that very low doses are effective, which means that the side effects are not too bad.

Other research has shown that *sertraline* (Zoloft), *venlafaxine* (Venlor) and *citalopram* (Cipramil) may help reduce hot flushes in some women. However, individuality plays a part here and some women experience no relief at all with any of the antidepressants. If you decide to embark on a course of antidepressants you should do so with great care and an understanding of the risks and side effects, and you should be under the care of a competent psychiatrist who understands the biochemistry of these medicines and their possible effects on you. In a recent double-blind randomised controlled trial (these trials are discussed in Chapter 3), women taking *escitalopram* (Cipralex) found that the number and severity of their hot flushes were significantly reduced. Although the use of this antidepressant for hot flushes is off-label, the FDA is currently reviewing it to see whether it can be used as a treatment for hot flushes and night sweats. Another medicine called a serotonin and norepinephrine reuptake inhibitor (SNRI) is *desvenlafaxine* (Pristiq), which is also under review by the FDA since a recent study has shown that it works well in reducing the number and severity of hot flushes.

Here is a **strong warning** for women who are taking tamoxifen as a treatment for breast cancer. Recent but conflicting research suggests that certain medications, including some antidepressants, may not be safe if you are taking tamoxifen because they may interfere with the way your body metabolises tamoxifen, so you won't get the full benefit of this medication. Until this concern has been clarified you should probably look for alternative options and not take antidepressants containing: fluoxetine (Prozac), bupropion (Zyban), or duloxetine (Cymbalta). The following may still inhibit the action but less strongly: sertraline (Zoloft), desvenlafaxine (Pristiq), escitalopram (Cipralex), and citalopram (Celexa, Cipramil). You should also avoid quinidine, diphenhydramine (Benadryl), terbinafine (Lamisil) or cimetidine (Tagamet) since these medicines may also interfere with the action of an enzyme in your body called CYP2D6, which has a major role in metabolising tamoxifen. It appears that venlafaxine (Effexor) does not seem to affect it. Remember that different medications may have different names in different countries, so always ask your doctor or check the labels if you decide to take another medicine in conjunction with tamoxifen.

HYSTERECTOMIES

When I was 45 I developed the most excruciating pain during my periods. For a year before the onset of this pain I had been having incredibly heavy periods. Sometimes I thought I was bleeding to death; huge chunks of tissue or blood clots would come away and no matter how often I changed my tampon and even when I wore super-thick pads I would often wake in the night to find myself soaked. I spoke to my GP and she recommended a gynaecologist. This suave gentleman scanned my womb and told me that I had a huge fibroid. He said it made my uterus look as though I was 12 weeks pregnant and that he felt that the only solution was to have a hysterectomy. In any case, I was in my mid-forties, had two children and was not thinking of having any more. He assured me that this was a routine procedure and most women of my age with these problems found that a hysterectomy was the answer. He sounded very convincing, but I have always been reasonably cautious so I spoke to my ex-gynaecologist from America, who had delivered one of my babies and knew me well. He heartily approved the diagnosis, telling me that I would feel like a new woman.

One of my closest friends from America sounded very perturbed when I told her what I planned, but I was so confident that the doctor knew best and I knew so little about hormone therapy and menopause that I was sure that after the six-week recommended recovery period I would feel as good, if not better, than before. I called my gynaecologist again, because my friend's doubts had made me anxious, and voiced my fears. He explained the surgery and spoke to me in reasoned terms. He seemed to have all the time in the world to talk to me. I felt immeasurably reassured, booked my surgery for the week after my 46th birthday and continued quite happily with my life.

At no point during my discussions with this gynaecologist did he explain to me that I was probably perimenopausal; that heavy bleeding and clotting in perimenopause are absolutely normal; that many women's fibroids grow rapidly during this time because of estrogen surges and that as the estrogen levels out, the fibroids stop growing and then shrink. He didn't say: 'Let's wait for a while; there's no immediate danger and urgency. There are no cysts on your ovaries. There are other remedies you can try.' He didn't tell me that smaller fibroids could be removed by a laparoscopy or a hysteroscopy, and larger ones by a myomectomy or treated with embolisation (see the section on fibroids below). He didn't say that because fibroids are sensitive to hormones and tend to grow when they're exposed to estrogen, there were hormonal treatments that could modify the levels of estrogen being produced (see Chapter 4), help the symptoms I was battling with and reduce the size of the fibroid temporarily so that if I became menopausal in the meantime, I may not have to have surgery. Neither did he mention that there were hormones (progestogen, in fact) which I could take to try to stop the bleeding. He didn't say that perhaps we could try an endometrial ablation, which is a laser treatment that destroys the lining of the uterus. It is a procedure suggested for middle-aged women who don't want more children but who are battling with the exceptionally heavy periods that happen in perimenopause.

At no point did this gynaecologist stress that a hysterectomy is major surgery and that there would be no harm in waiting a bit. In fact, the only reason to rush into having a hysterectomy is when there is a risk of cervical or endometrial cancer. He didn't say (perhaps he didn't know) that estrogen therapy might not suit me and could have undesirable side effects, nor did he tell me that I would be plunged into premature menopause with all *its attendant symptoms. He didn't tell me that hot flushes after a surgical menopause were often more sudden and severe. He didn't warn me about what could and would probably happen with sudden onset menopause – I could gain weight, be subject to mood swings, lose my desire for sex and battle with a dry vagina. He didn't tell me that I had the option of keeping my ovaries. None of this came up. He told me blandly that he would put me on HT after the surgery and I would feel great with it. I listened and I didn't question him further. I went into surgery uninformed.*

I woke up feeling deathly sick from the anaesthetic, the pain of my scar and my cut muscles. The gynaecologist arrived in his green operating gear, looking suitably handsome and exhausted. He explained that he had removed my ovaries as they were dark and had endometriosis. Once I could sit up and look around I saw that I had a patch on my thigh. This was my estrogen replacement – 7.8 mg of estradiol hemihydrate to be replaced once a week. It had taken only hours for me to become a fully menopausal woman but it would be a year before I started to feel better.

The ET did not agree with me and I had numerous reactions to it, including wild mood swings, a general feeling of insanity, pounding headaches and skin rashes. I battled with many symptoms of menopause and couldn't find the right combination of HT. The gynaecologist, who had been so readily available pre-surgery, was impatient and abrupt with me as I questioned the treatment, and I felt that I had been utterly unprepared and consequently disempowered and betrayed. I had not expected to feel so bereft at the loss of my womb; the psychological loss and feeling of being less of a woman was as powerful as the physiological symptoms.

In the end I reframed my situation, channelled my anger and taught myself as much as I could about menopause, constantly updating my information. Thanks to a good combination of HT for several years after the hysterectomy and the interest in menopause that my own hysterectomy generated in me, my story has a happy ending.

SOME INFORMATION ABOUT HYSTERECTOMIES

If your doctor tells you that you will have a total hysterectomy this means that the uterus and part of your cervix, or your entire cervix, will be taken out. Many women who have had hysterectomies don't even know whether they have kept their cervix or not, so ask your surgeon to explain exactly what she or he intends to do in your particular case.

Some doctors retain the cervix by *laparoscopy*, which may be a good thing as some women find that they have better sex if the cervix is retained. If you are having a hysterectomy because you have advanced cancer, you may have a radical hysterectomy, which means that your womb, your cervix and part of the upper area of your vagina, as well as your ovaries, are removed.

The surgery to remove your womb can be done in two ways: through a cut in your abdomen, usually just around or on the bikini line, or through your vagina. The latter method is usually a less drastic procedure. If your doctor has recommended that your ovaries should be also be removed (an *oophorectomy*), they and your fallopian tubes will be taken out. Sometimes it is decided that if you are not yet peri- or postmenopausal and you have healthy ovaries, they will be left in. Depending on your particular case one ovary may be left in. But you should always discuss the reason for the removal of your ovaries with your doctor. If you are not menopausal you might not want your ovaries removed as this means that you will usually have a more gradual menopause, though sometimes after the womb is removed your menopause may come earlier because the blood flow to the ovaries changes.

As the medical profession becomes more knowledgeable, more choices are evolving for hysterectomies, such as surgery where much of the womb can be removed by laparoscopy and the remainder through the vagina. In a different technique, the surgeon can do all the preparation for the removal of the womb by dissecting it, using the laparoscope and then pull all the bits out through the vagina. The type of hysterectomy you have depends on the method your surgeon prefers and what she or he believes will be safest for you and enable you to recover quickest.

As I wrote in Chapter 2, your ovaries make more than one of the hormones in your endocrine system, so many women who are not at risk for ovarian cancer, who do not have many or abnormal cysts or endometriosis in their ovaries, may want to think very carefully before allowing healthy ovaries to be removed. For example, it seems as though women with natural menopause continue to produce some testosterone, so the decline in this particular hormone is more gradual.

Research has also shown that those women who have an early surgical menopause may be at greater risk for heart disease because of the abrupt drop in estrogen. The issue of the removal of ovaries is very thorny indeed. There is an extremely serious question here that must be asked about your risk for ovarian cancer. Unlike many other cancers, there are no clear markers or signs of ovarian cancer – it can be silent and is most often fatal, and this is why many surgeons feel that if you are perimenopausal it may be wise to remove the ovaries as a precaution. It is imperative that you take time to ask your doctor about the dangers of getting this deadly disease and elicit his or her professional opinion on whether you should keep your ovaries.

However, as you can see below, there are several good reasons why doctors will recommend a hysterectomy or a hysterectomy in conjunction with bilateral oophorectomy (removal of both ovaries). This is called a bilateral salpingo-oophorectomy (BSO). This surgery may be absolutely necessary and may save your life.

Reasons to have a hysterectomy

- Persistence of severely abnormal cervical cells. It is very important to monitor the cells in your cervix, which is why all women who have a cervix should have an annual Pap smear, as should women who have had a partial hysterectomy and kept their cervix, and those who have had a total hysterectomy for cancer of the cervix.
- Abnormal cells in the lining of your womb, which could lead to endometrial cancer – cancer of the lining of the womb.
- Abnormal ovarian cysts, indicating ovarian cancer.
- If you have a strong family history and if you have the BRCA1 or BRCA2 gene, which increases your risk for breast and ovarian cancer. This risk may be considerably reduced with a bilateral oophorectomy, especially if your childbearing is completed.
- Uncontrolled heavy bleeding that cannot be stopped by other methods.
- A prolapsed uterus (where the uterus drops down into the vagina from its normal position and may even protrude from the vagina). This can occur after childbirth and sometimes if women are seriously overweight. It can even, in some cases, be caused by chronic coughing or excessive strain when lifting heavy objects.
- Very large fibroids that are debilitating, causing pain, interfering with your urinary tract and bladder, and that are too big to shrink.

Nobody decides lightly to have major surgery that involves a general anaesthetic, yet it is amazing how many women opt for hysterectomies without the proper knowledge and preparation. It is true that many women do very well after a hysterectomy but others who have both their ovaries and their wombs

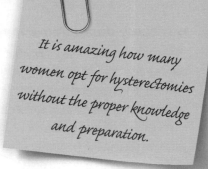

It is amazing how many women opt for hysterectomies without the proper knowledge and preparation.

removed, and find themselves in premature menopause, really battle. Many take at least a year to feel themselves again and spend even more time after that trying to find a hormone therapy that suits them.

As the body of research grows, it is becoming very clear that younger women who are under the age of 50 and have a hysterectomy with oophorectomy are at much greater risk for heart disease and stroke and die at an earlier age. Women who keep their ovaries but have a hysterectomy before the age of 50 may also be at greater risk for heart disease. The thought is that when you have a hysterectomy it may disrupt the blood flow to the ovaries, causing earlier menopause. The point of this research is that unless there is a convincing medical reason, you should be cautious about this kind of surgery. If you have a benign disease you should try at least to retain your ovaries if you are younger than 50, and if you have had your ovaries removed, you should seriously consider your options for estrogen therapy with your doctor **if it is not contraindicated**.

It is not only in women younger than 50 that these risks apply. There are several studies suggesting that since ovaries may play an important role in protecting your heart, removing them unnecessarily even after 50 and before menopause increases the risk of heart disease and lowers the age of death. So unless it is vital for you to have your ovaries removed because you are at high risk for ovarian cancer or they are cancerous, only consider this type of surgery to prevent disease, if you are quite convinced that the benefits will outweigh the risks over time, and not before menopause regardless of your age.

My sense is that if there is not a compelling health reason for having a hysterectomy, it is much easier to cope with menopause when you come to it gradually.

That said, hundreds of thousands of women who have opted for this surgery are now leading happy fulfilled lives. This section is not meant to be prescriptive but to inform you about the surgery so that if and when you decide to have a hysterectomy you feel empowered and confident that in partnership with your doctor, you have made a wise decision.

Is surgery doing you a favour?

The reason I have called this chapter 'hot flushes and hysterectomies' is because hot flushes, which can vary in frequency from one a week to one an hour, are often much worse after a sudden onset menopause caused by surgery during which your womb and ovaries are removed. Sudden onset menopause can also be brought on by certain chemicals and/or some types of radiation used in the treatment of cancer.

For many years gynaecologists believed that they were doing menopausal women a favour by performing hysterectomies as a cure-all for excessive bleeding, fibroids and endometriosis. In fact, they were often plunging perfectly healthy women into premature menopause by removing their ovaries at the same time as they removed their wombs.

As you can see from my story, there are quite a few options your gynaecologist could try before you decide on a hysterectomy and the removal of both your ovaries (*bilateral oophorectomy*). My gynaecologist told me that I needed a hysterectomy because I had such a large fibroid in my uterus. He never suggested surgery simply to remove the fibroid. I had a sense that fibroids were something quite sinister, while in fact they are benign growths of muscle and connective tissue in the walls of the uterus. They may grow more rapidly when your estrogen levels surge in perimenopause or may increase because of hormone therapy. Fibroids generally only need to be treated if they are causing symptoms such as abnormal bleeding and pelvic pressure.

EXCESSIVE BLEEDING

Women in perimenopause often experience excessive bleeding due to the fluctuations of estrogen and the dropping levels of progesterone that I described in Chapters 1 and 2. There are several different hormonal treatments that might help severe bleeding and you should discuss these with your doctor to see whether one of them might suit you. The intrauterine device (loop or coil) containing a progestogen called levonorgestrel has been found to be safe and effective for many women in treating excessive bleeding. There are some side effects and changed bleeding patterns, but it is less expensive and less invasive than surgery.

Another option is a procedure called *endometrial ablation*, where a laser is used to burn the lining of the womb away. Most women who have this procedure never have a period again; some have light bleeding like spotting and in a very small number of women it has no effect at all, in which case a hysterectomy might be the only option.

Current thinking about endometrial ablation is that women who have this procedure may experience a false sense of relief and feel like they no longer have to worry about the lining of their wombs. It is important to note, however, that small pockets of the endometrium (lining of the womb) may be left behind after this procedure, so menopausal women who are using ET should take a progestogen as well to prevent a build-up of the lining in these areas.

ABNORMAL BLEEDING

Although irregular periods and bleeding are a sign of perimenopause, there may be reasons other than your changing ovarian function and fluctuating hormone levels that could cause this. Certain medical conditions can cause abnormal bleeding, so you should see your doctor if you experience any of the following:

- Very heavy bleeding with clotting that you have never had before.
- Periods that continue for more than seven days or are two or three days longer than you usually experience with your menstrual cycle.
- The time between your periods becomes shorter than 21 days, so you find you are having periods more frequently than before.
- You have spotting or bleeding between your periods.
- You bleed after sex.
- Some reasons for abnormal bleeding may include the effect of hormonal contraceptives, a progestogen-containing intrauterine device (IUD) or hormone therapy, fibroids, pregnancy, some medications or herbal preparations, an infection in your pelvis, cervix, womb or vagina, a polyp on your womb or the lining of your womb. More serious reasons include cancer or pre-cancerous changes of the lining of your womb or cervix. However, as I discuss in Chapter 8, it is quite easy to check up on these problems but you should take responsibility for your health and be vigilant for any signs that might indicate a serious problem.

FIBROIDS

As I discussed in Chapter 1, when a gynaecologist examines you a trans-vaginal ultrasound should be an integral part of the examination. Using this, the gynaecologist can determine the position and size of a fibroid. Once an ultrasound is done and it is recommended that your fibroid be removed, you should have an informed discussion to help you understand how the procedure will take place. There are various surgical techniques to remove fibroids. One of these is specifically directed at removing the fibroids alone and is called a *myomectomy*. It is frequently the chosen treatment for premenopausal women who want to bear more children, because it may help to preserve fertility. If you have only a few small fibroids this procedure can be done by means of a *laparoscopy*. The surgeon inserts a small instrument (a laparoscope) through the navel into the abdomen, looks at the problem and then treats the patient.

Another method is *hysteroscopy*, which is a surgical procedure that can be done on women who have a single fibroid protruding into the cavity of the womb and don't wish to have their womb removed. A small camera and appropriate surgical instruments are placed in the cervix and the fibroid is surgically removed. A *laparotomy* is another technique by which the surgeon makes a cut in the abdomen and removes the fibroid. Many women complain that they feel bloated after abdominal surgery. This is because in an abdominal laparoscopy air is blown into the abdominal cavity to improve visibility, and during a laparotomy the abdominal cavity is open and not all the air that enters it during the procedure can be removed.

Finally, your doctor might suggest *embolisation* of the fibroids. This is an advanced X-ray technique where the blood supply to the fibroid is cut off so that it shrinks.

ENDOMETRIOSIS

As I wrote in Chapter 1, the lining of your womb is called the endometrium. Endometriosis occurs when endometrial cells grow outside the uterus instead of inside it, where they can be sloughed off during the usual monthly bleed. The endometrial cells can be found in your ovaries, your fallopian tubes and your pelvic cavity and can cause a great deal of pain. All sorts of other symptoms may be connected with endometriosis, among them constipation or diarrhoea and lower-back pain. An interesting fact about endometriosis is that there may not be any relationship between the amount of endometriosis present and the severity of the pain you are experiencing. Your doctor can diagnose endometriosis by performing a laparoscopy.

A small number of postmenopausal women may continue to experience severe pain from endometriosis. It is thought that this may be caused by the high levels of aromatase which are often present after menopause and the condition may be treated with aromatase inhibitors, which I describe in Chapter 7. Although medicines have been used to alleviate some of the symptoms of endometriosis, they will not ultimately cure the disease, and the treatment of choice is surgery.

HOW TO PREPARE FOR A HYSTERECTOMY

Before you and your doctor decide that you should have this surgery, have an informed discussion with him or her about the best procedure for you. If it is medically appropriate, it seems clear that the least invasive method of surgery, such as a laparoscopy, would be a sensible choice.

Once you have made the decision to have a hysterectomy, plan your time before and after it very carefully. You want to be able to relax when you come out of hospital, so see that you have someone who can help you, cook for you or look after you for at least six weeks when you return home. If you don't have help, enlist your friends and do some serious freezer cooking. Give yourself plenty of recovery time if your surgery is to take place before a special occasion. Things can go wrong and you may not recover as quickly as you thought you would. Many women find that their shape changes after a hysterectomy so you may want to get back into shape before a celebration.

If you have a choice, go into surgery as fit as possible. This is a great time to stop smoking once and for all. If you've always exercised, you'll have an easier time. Always tell your doctor which medications and supplements you are taking and ask if you can take preparations like Traumeel or Arnica; they don't want any surprises in the operating theatre. See that you have comfy, loose-fitting garments to wear after surgery. Accept that you can't have sex for at least eight weeks after the procedure. Allow yourself time to get used to the idea of being without a womb and if you feel weepy, weep.

If you are perimenopausal be prepared for the usual symptoms and accept that you might have to tinker with various hormones before you find some that suit you. Start with very mild exercise when your doctor says you can and build up to your old regimen gradually. Remember that most women have time to get used to menopause gradually, but if you are only in early perimenopause or not yet menopausal and your ovaries have been removed, you will be plunged into menopause. If you have realistic expectations about your surgical menopause, you will deal with it much more easily.

Surgical terms
Hysterectomy – surgical removal of the womb

Hysteroscopy – a procedure whereby an instrument is passed through the mouth of the womb to allow the inside of the womb to be viewed

Myomectomy – a procedure whereby a fibroid is surgically removed. It is frequently the chosen treatment for premenopausal women because it usually helps to preserve fertility

Laparoscopy – a procedure whereby a surgeon using small incisions inserts a small instrument (laparoscope), often through the navel, into the abdomen, looks at the problem and then treats the patient. This is sometimes called 'keyhole' surgery

Laparotomy – a technique whereby the surgeon makes a cut in the abdomen and removes the fibroid

Colposcopy – a procedure whereby the cervix is examined with a high-powered magnifying lens and a light inserted into the vagina

Bilateral oophorectomy – removal of the ovaries

Endometrial ablation – the lining of the womb is burnt away

Embolisation of fibroids – an advanced X-ray technique where the blood supply to the fibroid is cut off, so that it shrinks

EMPOWER YOURSELF

- Lifestyle changes can help reduce hot flushes and night sweats.
- Ask your doctor for non-hormonal options for your hot flushes if HT is contraindicated.
- Some stress reduction programmes may alleviate distress caused by hot flushes and night sweats.
- Sometimes a combination of an antidepressant and a sleeping pill may work well for women who are battling with hot flushes and night sweats and they can't take HT.
- Check the following site for a full list of drugs that may affect the action of tamoxifen: http://www.pharmacytimes.com/publications/issue/2009/2009-03/2009-03-10041/
- Always get a second, or even third, opinion before you decide to have major surgery like a hysterectomy.
- Be sure that you are making properly informed choices.
- If you become prematurely menopausal or if you have your ovaries removed, you will almost certainly need some ET, **if it is not contraindicated**.
- Have an in-depth discussion with your doctor before surgery about your different ET options. Reread the HT guidelines in Chapter 4; they also apply here.

7
The heart of the matter

Andrea was very agitated. Wringing her hands, she said to me: 'I feel so afraid. I had a bout with breast cancer and though I'm now in remission, I have an absolute terror of a relapse. I live in a very health-conscious way. I eat all the right foods; I exercise and try to live sensibly.

'I am really battling with menopausal symptoms like mood swings, depression, hot flushes, night sweats, bad headaches and a pounding heart. I can't sleep and I have constant anxiety. I have no desire for sex and when I have it it's painful.

'My estradiol levels are very low but I really don't want to take hormone therapy. I would like to try something alternative to see if that will help my hot flushes. On a recent visit to my physician I found that my bad cholesterol level is high and my gynaecologist tells me that I'm more likely to die of a heart attack than of breast cancer and he wants to put me back on conjugated equine estrogens, but my oncologist is absolutely opposed to my taking HT! I am confused and scared.'

I was not surprised that Andrea was feeling anxious. She was trying to take responsibility for her health but was receiving hugely conflicting advice. Her story is pertinent both to the question of heart health and to that of cancer.

Research has shown that estradiol, as explained in Chapter 2, is a steroid or growth hormone, which means in some women it may cause breast cells that have the predisposition to become cancerous to increase. Research has also shown that women who take estrogen for longer than the recommended time and at an older age may be at greater risk for breast cancer, so it seems sensible not to increase the risk by taking HT. The fact that estrogen is a steroid hormone also impacts on the issue of heart health because just as estrogen causes good cholesterol (HDL) levels to rise, it may also cause bad cholesterol (LDL) levels to rise. The Women's Health Initiative (WHI) study showed that taking estrogen does not necessarily improve heart health; on the contrary, it might aggravate potential heart problems, especially in older women. So it didn't make sense that Andrea should take something that might both increase her risk of breast cancer and actually raise her already high cholesterol levels and increase her risk for heart attack or stroke.

'Cardio' means the heart and 'vascular' means the blood vessels (veins and arteries). In this chapter, I use the phrase 'heart disease' because heart and vascular diseases are interrelated.

The popular theory for most of the last century was that before menopause women were much less vulnerable to cardiovascular disease than men. This idea led the medical profession to believe that this was because women's hearts were protected by estrogen, and when their estrogen levels fell after menopause, they were at risk. Therefore, doctors felt, it was logical to assume that if women replaced their falling levels of estrogen they would protect their heart health.

Of course, the manufacturers of hormones were delighted with this development and several large, well-designed research studies confirmed these assumptions. The best known of these was the Postmenopausal Estrogen/Progestin Interventions Trial (PEPI). When it was reported in the *Journal of the American Medical Association (JAMA)* in 1995, the results of the study clearly showed that postmenopausal women may benefit from a regimen of HT because, among other things, it seemed to improve certain risk factors for heart disease; levels of HDL (good cholesterol) were raised and *fibrinogen* levels were lowered. Fibrinogen is a protein present in the blood which can cause a heart attack when its levels are raised as increased levels cause blood clots. You may have heard your healthcare practitioner referring to a *myocardial infarction*. This is simply a heart attack, which happens when parts of the heart muscle die because the blood supply to the heart has become obstructed.

In light of this type of research, women felt that much of their anxiety about HT could be allayed and that they were taking responsibility for their health by taking either estrogen or a combination of estrogen and progestogen, and they were encouraged in this belief by their doctors. However, in 2002, as you know by now, there was trouble in paradise. The results of the Heart and Estrogen/progestin Replacement Study (HERS) caused some consternation. HERS was a well-designed, double-blind, randomised placebo-controlled trial of 2 800 women who already had heart disease. It also included only women who still had their wombs and the aim was to examine whether HT would protect them from further heart disease. The results showed that after four years of taking estrogen and progestogen daily, the overall risk of heart disease was not reduced in this group of women.

More problems were to come. The WHI study, which is discussed at length in Chapter 3, showed that there was an increased risk of stroke in women taking estrogen and progestogen, and that these hormones offered no benefits in relation to heart disease. The figures per 10 000 were seven more heart attacks, eight more strokes and 18 more blood clots. In 2004 the estrogen-only arm was stopped because the study showed that there was an increased risk for stroke and, as in the combined trial, there was no perceived benefit for heart disease, so it was decided that the risk of a stroke outweighed the benefits. As I wrote earlier, these results turned the medical establishment upside down. Why had they been so mistaken?

Firstly, many of the earlier trials on heart disease did not represent women fully and the information gathered was assumed instead of being based on clinical evidence. One problem was that many old-school doctors relied on observation and anecdotes to guide their treatments. Another interesting fact is that a large number of the women who die of heart attacks have not shown any previous symptoms, so doctors assumed, without clinical evidence, that heart attacks in menopausal women were caused by a drop in their estrogen levels. The PEPI trial served to confirm these assumptions.

Furthermore, because doctors assumed that women didn't suffer from heart disease before their menopause, they were not carefully tested and examined for it. Finally, with more effective diagnostic techniques, such as *magnetic resonance imaging* (MRI) scans, it became clear that the arteries of some young women (in their late twenties and early thirties) who were nowhere near menopause were showing signs of the damage that precedes heart disease, indicating that estrogen was not actually protecting them to the extent that their doctors believed.

But the doctors who had spent so many years prescribing estrogen to women to prevent heart disease were not convinced. After the WHI was published, many gynaecologists criticised the trials. Their objections were that the women studied were too old and only a small proportion had significant menopausal symptoms. They failed to accept, however, that the trials enrolled more than 8 800 women aged 50 to 59, of whom more than 20 per cent reported moderate to severe vasomotor symptoms (hot flushes and night sweats). They believed that the WHI and HERS trials failed to show that estrogen protected against heart disease because the subjects already had some kind of heart disease. So while they agreed that estrogen might be bad for those older women, they thought that if ET was started immediately after menopause it would prevent arteriosclerosis. They were determined to prove that younger women would benefit. This was called the timing hypothesis.

In 2007 their thesis seemed to have been vindicated by a new sub-study from the WHI. This study, called the WHI-Coronary-Artery Calcium Study (WHI-CACS), done about 1.3 years after the WHI study was completed, found that younger women who use ET at the onset of menopause are less likely to have calcification of their arteries (see pages 154–156) than their contemporaries who are not taking ET. It is important to note here that the calcification of these women's arteries was only measured after they completed the WHI study, not before. This suggests that younger, postmenopausal women on ET have a reduced risk for heart disease. Those who recommend ET as a preventative for heart disease greeted this research with delight. The International Menopause Society (IMS) issued a press release saying that the results of this study were encouraging and stated that 'women can be reassured that estrogen therapy is cardioprotective until at least 65'.

However, not everyone agreed. Some doctors cautioned restraint and advised gynaecologists not to extrapolate too much from this data. While it is clear that short-term HT to alleviate menopausal symptoms at the onset of menopause is probably not risky, and may even help to reduce the risk of heart disease, there is no evidence that this initial advantage would extend to older women were they to continue to use ET.

In fact, although the coronary artery calcium scores were reduced in these younger women, there is no evidence to show the effect of estrogen on blood clots, since these events are more likely to happen in older women. Coronary artery calcium scoring is a special X-ray test, *computed tomography* (CT), which helps to check whether there is a build-up of plaque on the walls of the arteries of the heart (coronary arteries). This test is used to see whether or not you are at risk for heart disease, and if you are how severe it is. Many experts believe the data in this sub-study is insufficient to prove this categorically because at the end of the estrogen-only trial, *only* the women in the younger 50 to 59-year age group and not the older women were measured. In spite of these reservations, many doctors support the timing hypothesis and once again members of the media are picking up on these enthusiastic statements and writing things like: 'Hormone therapy actually prevents heart attacks in women who start close to menopause'.

It is dangerous to make a blanket statement like this. Heart disease may already be present in a younger menopausal woman, but may not be evident without appropriate screening. A newly menopausal woman who is overweight and has high blood pressure may already be at risk for heart disease, and giving her ET may aggravate her risk. On the other hand, her healthy contemporary who has none of these problems may benefit, especially if she has had an early surgical menopause and HT is not contraindicated. Once again we come back to the indisputable fact that every woman should be evaluated as an individual and her medical history and potential risk factors should be taken into consideration. There is compelling evidence that the timing hypothesis has a big role to play in reducing or increasing the risk for heart disease. Ongoing research suggests that estrogen may be protective against heart disease in women in the very early stages of atherosclerosis, because it may have an action known as 'positive remodelling', which seems to help the blood vessels widen, **but** is harmful as they age and the plaque has already built up. Estrogen may also slow down the development of atherosclerosis in younger women, but older women are not so well protected and estrogen seems to be related to instability of coronary plaque in the arteries, which may then cause a rupture, resulting in a heart attack or a blood clot.

More research is needed to determine whether timing different types of estrogen can play a protective role in heart disease.

In the meantime, two ongoing studies, the Kronos Early Estrogen Prevention Study (KEEPS) and the Early versus Late Intervention Trial with Estradiol (ELITE) will provide more information. The KEEPS trial is a large five-year, double-blind, randomised placebo-controlled study to determine the response of women receiving transdermal estrogen, oral estrogen (CEE) or placebos. The ELITE study will study the effect of oral estradiol with intravaginal progesterone given to women who are less than six years into menopause, as opposed to those who have been menopausal for 10 years or more. These studies are due to be completed in 2012 and 2013 respectively, and the results should be very helpful in aiding doctors and their patients' decisions about the benefits and risks of HT and the most beneficial time to start it.

More research is needed to determine whether timing, different types of estrogen, and perhaps even micronised progesterone, can play a protective role in relation to heart disease. In the meantime, as we wait for definitive results, it is vital to look at how ageing affects the cardiovascular system and to try to understand how changes in hormone levels affect many middle-aged women who put on weight and may develop insulin resistance as a result. These women probably exercise less as well, so all those factors may increase their risk of heart disease.

The new evidence from the WHI and the HERS trials clarified why so many women who were on HT were also taking cholesterol-lowering drugs. Instead of protecting their hearts, the 'magical' estrogen was causing an increase in both good and bad cholesterols. In addition, it seemed that oral estrogens were causing an increase in C-reactive protein (CRP), which as I explained in Chapter 4 is a sign of inflammation and may cause heart disease when the level is raised.

Delia is very health conscious and was extremely worried after a recent visit to her gynaecologist, who had told her to take a hormone containing 2 mg of estradiol and 1 mg of norethisterone acetate (a progestogen) daily, because he felt it would shrink a cyst that she had in her ovary.

'The problem is that my GP had put me on a cholesterol-lowering drug because my cholesterol was over eight, which I told my gynae, but he didn't seem concerned. I felt very confused because I had read that recent research showed that estradiol raised the levels of both bad and good cholesterol. I was also worried because I had heard that the new dosage recommendations for HT were much, much lower than they had been previously.'

In fact, as you read in Chapter 4, a starting dose of no more than 0.25 mg to 0.50 mg of oral estradiol is recommended. I couldn't understand why a healthcare practitioner would recommend such a high dose of estrogen, given all the recent research. In perimenopausal women it might be a good idea to try an oral contraceptive, which stops ovulation and calms the activities of the ovaries, which in turn may cause the cysts to shrink, but there is no evidence that HT makes the ovaries less active. But in this case even that would have been irrelevant – Delia was clearly postmenopausal; her estrogen levels were less than 37 pmol/l (< 10pg/ml) and her FSH levels were high. As I explained in Chapter 1, in perimenopause your FSH levels rise in reaction to your falling levels of estrogen. After menopause your estrogen levels usually drop and stay low.

In Chapter 8, I will discuss the most conservative way to approach the problem of ovarian cysts. Delia was also concerned about her high levels of cholesterol and we know that although estrogen raises the level of the good cholesterol, it also raises the levels of the bad cholesterol and triglycerides, high levels of which are markers or warning signs of future heart disease. Finally, it may have been safer to give Delia her HT in the form of a patch or gel, since there may be lower levels of C-reactive protein and less of a risk of clots if HT is taken through the skin.

PREVENTING AND TREATING HEART DISEASE

Lifestyle is a vital factor in preventing heart disease. Around 90 per cent of coronary heart disease can be prevented if you live a healthy life. The American Heart Association (AHA) has very strong recommendations about lifestyle and thoroughly reviews the latest available scientific evidence on preventing and treating heart disease in women. It makes practical suggestions about ways to prevent heart disease or to lower the risks, discussing and describing the most effective treatments, all based on sound clinical evidence. The AHA realised that because so much medical research had concentrated on heart disease risk in men, many women were not aware that heart disease, not breast cancer, was their number one killer and did not know enough about risk factors for heart disease, so they began a campaign to promote awareness of these risks and reduce the number of deaths in women. This campaign is called *Go Red for Women*, which aims to empower women to take responsibility for their heart health. I have read and summarised their 2011 *Heart Disease Prevention Guide*.

Before we look at the various treatments, let's look at ways in which you can alter your lifestyle to keep your heart healthy. It should be no surprise that the number one risk is cigarette smoking. If you still smoke, it's really time to stop! The incontrovertible fact is that toxins in cigarettes, like lead, nicotine and cadmium, poison your system, cause cancers, prevent the absorption of calcium, interfere with your hormones and lead to the hardening of the arteries. Hardening of the arteries (*arteriosclerosis*) is caused by fatty materials known as plaque being deposited or collecting on the artery walls (*atherosclerosis*), or by the artery wall becoming scarred or thickened. As this happens the blood flow may be interrupted, and this can get worse if blood clots (*thromboses*) form round the larger deposits of these fatty materials. When your arteries become hardened or less elastic and the blood flow to the heart is affected, you can have a stroke or suffer a heart attack.

A stroke happens when the flow of blood to the brain is interrupted, killing off or damaging brain cells in varying numbers, depending on the kind of stroke. This happens when an artery is blocked or when the wall of the artery has become weakened and bursts. In one type of stroke (*ischaemic*), blood clots or plaque form in these hardened arteries, causing a blockage by breaking away from the artery wall, travelling throughout the body and ending up in an artery in the brain, where they interfere with or stop the blood flow, causing the death of the brain cells. This is called an *embolus*. The other kind of stroke is caused by a weakened artery in the brain bursting and causing bleeding (*haemorraghic*).

An excellent way to prevent heart disease is to exercise for a minimum of 30 minutes a day 5 days a week.

It is important to remember that certain hormones may increase the risk of stroke. The WHI study showed that there was an increased risk of stroke with estrogen and progestin, as well as with estrogen alone. In 2007, results from the Estrogen and Thromboembolism Risk (ESTHER) study suggested that oral estrogen, but not transdermal estrogen, may increase the risk of a *thrombosis* (blood clot) and that some less androgenic progestogens (see Chapter 4) and micronised progesterone may be safer than the more androgenic progestogens as far as risk of blood clots is concerned. Other studies show that women on tamoxifen are at greater risk for stroke, clots in the lungs and a clot in the deep veins (*deep-vein thrombosis*). Discuss these concerns with your healthcare practitioner if you are taking any of these medications.

An excellent way to prevent heart disease is to exercise for a minimum of 30 minutes a day at least five days a week, and work up a sweat. Calculate 150 minutes of moderate exercise or 75 minutes of vigorous exercise weekly. You've already read that exercise is helpful in reducing hot flushes and making menopausal women feel less symptomatic, and it's clear that it really does help to maintain good general health, keep your weight at a healthy level, and help to reduce fat levels, because you build up muscle and burn fat when you exercise. It is also known that fat women are at a higher risk for heart disease and high blood pressure.

So it follows that as well as exercising, you should have a healthy, varied diet of fruits and vegetables, good proteins, wholegrains, nuts and legumes, fish (especially oily fish at least twice a week), low- and non-fat dairy products, healthy fats (such as olive oil and avocados), and alcohol only in moderation. Your diet should severely limit sodium (salt), trans fatty acids, sugar, saturated fats (such as butter and margarine), which can cause a build-up of bad cholesterol and high triglycerides, which in turn can result in hardening of the arteries. Being overweight can also trigger insulin resistance, which can be a precursor of diabetes, which research has shown increases the risk of heart disease. I will discuss this in detail in Chapter 10 when I look at the issues of food and weight.

Other lifestyle factors that may help to prevent heart disease are a reduction in stress levels as far as possible and the ability to deal with the kind of problems that may cause unhappiness and depression. If you are seriously depressed you should seek help and find the appropriate treatment. There are also supplements like omega-3 fatty acids, antioxidants and folic acid, which I wrote about in Chapter 5, that may help heart health. Niacin and nicotinamide have also been shown to be helpful, but the jury is still out on the efficacy of all these supplements and a lot more research needs to be done before they can be recommended without reservation as being effective. Finally, you may lead an exemplary life and still be at risk because of hereditary factors. Those genes you inherited from your parents and grandparents play a very important role. I have seen women who live like athletes but have cholesterol levels of over 10, while others can spread on the butter and munch on hamburgers and still have textbook levels!

Your doctor will keep several factors in mind when he or she assesses your risk for heart disease. Based on your answers your risk for heart disease can be established going forward over a period of 10 years. There are many tools, which have been derived from very well-known research called the Framingham Heart Study. This study created a risk assessment tool based on your age, gender, whether you have diabetes, your total cholesterol levels, your HDL cholesterol, blood pressure and whether you smoke. Your healthcare practitioner will explain to you which tool is best to use and how to calculate your individual risk.

ALL ABOUT CHOLESTEROL

Everybody talks about cholesterol but do you really know what role it plays in your health? Cholesterol levels are a very important marker of heart disease risk. Cholesterol is a fatty substance that is found throughout your body: in your cells, blood, tissues, brain, muscles and liver. It is present in most of the protein we eat – meat, chicken, fish, eggs and dairy products. Your liver produces cholesterol and also synthesises it. When we think of cholesterol we often think of it in negative terms; in fact it is essential for healthy living. It plays a vital role in cell repair, in the storage and production of energy, and as I explained in Chapter 2, all sex steroid hormones come from cholesterol. So from this point of view we need cholesterol to live. The problems occur when the levels of certain cholesterols in your bloodstream become too high.

There are a few terms that you will hear when you visit your healthcare practitioner. The first of these is *lipoproteins* (a lipoprotein consists of a molecule of fat and a molecule of protein). These are substances found in the blood that transport cholesterol. The two that we are concerned with are LDL (*low-density lipoproteins*) and HDL (*high-density lipoproteins*). The next term is *triglycerides*. All of these perform important functions in the working of your body. LDL is usually called 'bad' cholesterol because although when its levels are normal it does an essential job of carrying cholesterol away from areas where it isn't needed to areas where it can best be used, if the levels of LDL become too high, it starts to stick to the walls of the blood vessels or arteries and forms deposits of the fatty material or plaque (*atherosclerosis*) that I described earlier. This can lead to hardening of the arteries – *arteriosclerosis*. The job of HDL, the 'good' cholesterol, is to carry cholesterol and triglycerides to the liver, which converts them so that they can be used again in different parts of the body. If they are not needed, the liver uses the bile to get rid of unwanted cholesterol, so obviously higher levels of HDL are good because they help to protect your body from excess cholesterol.

Many cardiologists will recommend a scan of your carotid arteries, which are the major arteries running on either side of your neck to your brain, supplying it with blood. If the walls of these arteries are clear and free from plaque (the fatty material that builds up), then even if your cholesterol levels are raised, you are probably not at such high risk for heart disease. cIMT means carotid intima media thickness. This is tested in order to measure the thickness of the plaque in your carotid arteries. The test is non-invasive and is not harmful. Using an ultrasound probe, the width of this plaque lying between the two layers of tissue that make up the carotid artery, the intima and media, is determined and the results are shown on a computer. The reason to measure this is that depending on its thickness, blood flowing through your carotid arteries will have more or less space to flow through and if the flow is obstructed you will be at greater risk for heart disease and stroke, as I explained earlier. New research suggests that women who transition rapidly into menopause, as with a surgical menopause for example, seem to be at greater risk for cIMT thickness.

In order to make sure that you are not at risk for heart disease your doctor will suggest that you have a group of blood tests called a *lipid profile*, where your blood will be tested to measure your total cholesterol, HDL, LDL and triglyceride levels. This test should be done after you have fasted for 12 hours so that any foods you have eaten won't interfere with the results. The results should be within the accepted healthy levels, and if they aren't, you and your doctor will work out the necessary lifestyle changes and/or treatment. For middle-aged women, depending on your age and risk factors, the best results would read as follows:

- Total cholesterol less than five (<5 mmol/L (<195 mg/dL))
- LDL less than three (<2.6 mmol/L (<100 mg/dL))
- Triglycerides less than two (<1.7 mmol/L (<150 mg/dL))
- HDL greater than one (>1.5 mmol/L(>60 mg/dL)).

Donna was looking great; slim, healthy and fit. I complimented her on her appearance and she told me that when she reached her mid-forties she became concerned as her weight had gradually crept up over the past few years. She had read that exercise was the answer, so she began walking three times a week for 40 minutes at a time and then upped the ante and started running, but was very disappointed to find after six months that her weight stubbornly remained the same. 'I saw my GP,' she said, 'secretly hoping that he'd say I had a thyroid problem,' but to her surprise, because she was a healthy eater, he said that although her thyroid was fine, her cholesterol was higher than it should be at 6.7 mmol/L and she needed to lower it. He said he would give her eight weeks to try a combination of diet and exercise to see whether she could bring it down and if it still tested high when she returned, they would discuss medication.

Donna saw a dietician who told her that her body mass index (BMI), which is a red flag for type 2 diabetes, was too high and she would need to lose at least 7 kg. The dietician also said that losing weight might help to bring her cholesterol down as long as she increased and maintained her exercise routine. She explained that although Donna was eating healthy foods, she was having too much of them. Donna felt that she needed to be monitored and visited the dietician weekly so her progress could be checked. She upped her exercise time and started running five times a week. After two months she had lost 8 kg and over the next two months another 2 kg. Her cholesterol dropped to 4.6. She then decided she was happy with her weight loss and could maintain this on her own by eating small portions and being aware of what she ate and drank. She said she eats when she's hungry and never when she distracted or down, she chooses the low- fat, sugar- free options and doesn't snack like she used to. Her GP said he was happy for the moment with her cholesterol levels but that she should continue to monitor them.

Statins

Today doctors believe that it is important that your LDL (bad) cholesterol levels are as low as possible. Although I have used the suggested targets for those women who have not previously had any type of heart disease, cardiologists prefer even lower levels of 1.8 mmol/L (70 mg/dL) if a woman has already had a heart attack. Very recent research even suggests a level of 1.3 mmol/L (approximately 50 mg/dL) for people at very high risk for heart disease.

If you have only slightly elevated levels of the first three and lowered levels of the last, your doctor may decide that if you can reach the correct levels with lifestyle changes such as losing weight, stopping smoking and increasing your exercise regimen, she or he will monitor you again and see if your test results have improved. If you have very elevated levels, or levels that are only slightly elevated but you have risk factors for heart disease such as a family history, or if you are a smoker, overweight or drink more than two glasses of alcohol a day, your doctor will probably suggest a cholesterol-lowering drug, the most effective of which are called *statins*. These are drugs that act on a certain enzyme in the liver, causing a lowering of cholesterol in the blood. They can be taken for many years and have very few bad side effects apart from some muscle and joint pain in some cases. Research has shown that different statins have different effectiveness and side effects, so it is important to discuss this with your doctor. I know that as a result of reports in the media, some women are afraid to take statins, but be reassured, long-term research has shown that statins are still the safest and most proven way to reduce bad cholesterol in women. Remember that if you are prescribed a statin, it is not a blank cheque to go crazy with high fatty foods and unhealthy habits. You need to take your statin and follow a healthy lifestyle programme.

Red yeast rice

A word of warning about red yeast rice; many women tell me that they prefer to use a 'natural' statin. As I wrote in Chapter 5, you should take care when using a medicine that has not been regulated. Analyses of red yeast products have shown that certain of these may not be reliable in lowering cholesterol and may be harmful. This is because they contain statin-like components, including lovastatin, called monacolins. Monacolins are 'naturally occurring' statins and should not be harmful if taken in standard doses. For example lovastatin (Mevacor, Altoprev, Lovachol) is available as a regulated prescribed statin medication. The problem arises because these products have not been properly controlled by medicine control councils and may contain very inconsistent amounts of monacolins, so sometimes you will get almost no statin-like compounds and at other times you will get large amounts, which can cause harmful side effects. Another concern is that some products using red yeast rice were found to contain a contaminating substance called *citranin*, which is *nephrotoxic* (poisonous to kidney cells) and could cause kidney damage. Citranin occurs when the rice has not been correctly fermented; a recent study found this toxin in seven out of nine products. Speak to your doctor and choose a product that has been medically approved and suits you.

HIGH BLOOD PRESSURE

Other problems that might put you at risk for heart disease are high blood pressure and diabetes. I will deal with the latter in detail in Chapter 10 on weight and weight loss, so here I will just focus on *hypertension*, which is the medical term for high blood pressure. When you have a check-up your doctor will always check your blood pressure. As your heart beats, it pumps the blood through your body and as it flows, it exerts pressure on the walls of your arteries. Your blood pressure is highest when your heart pumps out the blood and drops when the heart rests between beats. The former is called *systolic* pressure and the latter, *diastolic*. This is why you are told your blood pressure is for example 120 over 80; it means the systolic pressure over the diastolic pressure. It is written 120/80 mmHg. Your blood pressure usually stays more or less the same when you are awake. Certain factors – like your teenage children, fear or illness – may cause it to rise, and it is usually lower when you sleep, which is why if you get up very quickly you may feel giddy or experience a rush of blood as the pressure normalises itself. Normal blood pressure ranges from 120–129/75–84.

High blood pressure (*hypertension*) means that the top number and the bottom number are higher than normal, and doctors would classify a top number over 140 and a bottom one of over 90 as high. This means that your heart is pumping out your blood at a higher level and working harder, which can cause heart disease or, more commonly, stroke. As you get older your blood pressure tends to rise, which is why so many older women are on medication for high blood pressure. Several things, including your diet (too much salt and too many fatty foods), water retention, being overweight, certain hormones and illnesses can affect your blood pressure.

Lifestyle plays a big part in reducing blood pressure. Your blood pressure can be lowered if you eat lots of fruit and vegetables, lean meat, low-fat or non-fat dairy products, wholegrains and reduce your sodium (salt). This diet is rich in potassium, calcium and magnesium. This was shown in an eating plan called the DASH diet (http://dashdiet.org/). Stress and tension can also cause high blood pressure because agitation causes your heart to beat faster. New research, which examined over 9 000 men and women in 11 different countries with an average age of 53, found a huge benefit in simply lowering women's blood pressure to prevent future heart disease and urged doctors to be aware of this and to monitor blood pressure regularly. There are several different types of medication that can help to lower your blood pressure and your doctor may prescribe some or all of the following: *diuretics*, which help to prevent water retention; *ACE inhibitors*, which help to bring your blood pressure down; and *beta-blockers*, which help to regulate your heartbeat by calming your body's responses.

To prevent blood clots from forming, which may cause a stroke, your doctor may also prescribe anticoagulant medications. These are used to decrease the clotting ability of your blood. If you are at risk for heart disease, your doctor and cardiologist may recommend that you take an aspirin or half an aspirin daily, but you should not embark on this course without the knowledge, recommendation and agreement of your healthcare practitioner. Just because you can buy aspirin over the counter doesn't mean it's harmless; there may be many side effects, including internal bleeding and stomach upsets, as well as kidney failure. If pure aspirin upsets your stomach, coated aspirins are also available.

OTHER RISKS FOR HEART DISEASE

Your cholesterol levels and your lifestyle are not the only markers that may indicate to your healthcare practitioner that you are at risk for heart disease. Advances in research are revealing new risks. You've already read in Chapter 4 that taking oral estrogen raises the levels of *high sensitivity C-reactive protein (hsCRP)*. Sometimes it is abbreviated to just CRP. This protein is produced by the liver only when you are experiencing severe inflammation, injury or disease. It is part of the normal immune response to problems in your body. Research has shown that although hsCRP levels may be raised when you have a heart attack, it is not clear what role it plays in heart disease – whether it is just a marker of the disease or whether raised levels may be a risk factor for heart disease. However, there is a growing body of evidence that it provides additional information about inflammation in the arteries and that it may be a warning signal, especially if your levels are greater than 2.6 mmol/L(100 mg/dL). In a very big study, the JUPITER study (Justification for the Use of

Statins in Primary prevention: An Investigation Trial evaluating Rosuvastatin), which investigated 17 000 subjects using either a statin or a placebo, results suggested that statins might also reduce hsCRP. But the investigators also noted the importance of a healthy lifestyle in reducing hsCRP; namely losing weight, not smoking and exercising.

Another marker seems to be high levels of *homocysteine*, which is an amino acid that helps to make protein and build and maintain tissues. The reason we want to lower these levels is that recent research seems to show a strong link between high levels of homocysteine and the risk of stroke and heart disease. It seems that high levels result in a build-up of bad cholesterol in the arteries, causing hardening. High levels combined with smoking and high blood pressure make your risk of heart disease even greater. However, it is still uncertain whether high levels of homocysteine are the cause or the result of inflammation in the arteries (atherosclerosis) as studies have not shown that reducing the levels of homocysteine reduces the risk of stroke or heart attack. Some alternative healthcare practitioners recommend certain supplements like folic acid and beta-carotene to reduce homocysteine levels, though neither have been shown to be effective in this regard and a recent, very large meta-analysis of eight large randomised-placebo controlled studies involving over 37 000 people examining the benefits of folic acid supplementation versus placebo showed that taking folic acid routinely had no significant effect either positively or negatively on heart disease, overall cancer, or mortality (the age at which a person dies). Nevertheless it seems that it is safe to supplement with folic acid in the recommended amounts.

A further problem may be high levels of something called *fibrinogen*. Fibrinogen helps the blood to clot, which is absolutely vital for survival, but when the levels of fibrinogen in the blood become too high, the clotting mechanism can become a danger and cause clots to form in your arteries. As is the case with C-reactive protein, the presence of fibrinogen may indicate inflammation in the walls of your damaged arteries, which is why high levels in your blood may act as a warning flag for heart disease. Lifestyle and certain hormones can cause your fibrinogen levels to rise, but guess what the number one cause is – smoking! I know I am repeating myself but the evidence is too compelling not to keep mentioning the huge risk that smoking poses to your health.

Earlier I wrote about lipoproteins. A new lipoprotein called *lipoprotein(a)* or Lp(a) has been identified. It seems to be formed when a particular protein in the body attaches itself to a molecule of LDL. The bad news is that when LDL carries this specific protein, it appears to interfere with your body's ability to dissolve blood clots, and when this happens you are at increased risk for stroke because of the interrupted blood flow.

Recently a big meta-analysis caused great alarm when it suggested that calcium supplements might increase the risk of heart disease because they raised levels of calcium in your blood and increased calcium deposits in your arteries, though this did not seem apply to healthy postmenopausal women. Recent recommendation from the Institute of Medicine (IOM) for calcium supplementation in women is 500 mg daily for women under 50 and 1 000 mg daily for those older than 50. Many experts believe that your calcium supplement must be taken in conjunction with the appropriate amount of vitamin D (400–660 IU daily). It is also important to remember that many women can achieve the recommended doses of elemental calcium through their diets (Chapter 9) and it's unlikely that if you eat healthily and get enough calcium from food sources (making sure your dairy products are fat-free or low-fat) that you will need to supplement with more than 500 mg daily, if at all. A moderate daily supplement of 500 mg of elemental calcium to make up for any calcium deficit in your diet should be safe. However, in a sub-study of the WHI that examined coronary artery calcification in women aged between 50 and 59 who took the suggested doses (1 000 mg calcium and 400 IU vitamin D daily), it was found that they did not have higher levels of coronary artery calcified plaque than those women who were taking placebo. This is reassuring but, since the research is conflicting, more studies are needed so discuss your calcium and vitamin D supplementation with your doctor.

The menopause transition and increased risk for heart disease

Research has shown that certain factors related to menopause may increase a midlife woman's risk for heart disease, such as premature and early menopause, increased weight, the way fat is distributed, estrogen levels and HT – the type, the way it is taken and when it is given. Studies now show that hot flushes and night sweats may play their part as far as variations in heart rate and cortisol levels are concerned. Other research shows that during the menopausal transition women have a changed lipid profile, with rises in total cholesterol and LDL (bad cholesterol), while other studies show that the protective effects of HDL (good cholesterol) may be reduced as women move into menopause, so it is very important that your doctor monitors your cholesterol levels.

These results are conflicting, which is why dealing with midlife women's health is so complicated. A new analysis from the WHI suggests that women who have hot flushes early on in their menopausal transition are at lower risk for heart disease, lower risk of stroke and all causes of mortality than those women who only experience these symptoms later in their menopause. The reason may be that when younger women experience hot flushes, these signify healthy blood vessels but later in life the blood vessels may not be as healthy. The study also showed that persistent hot flushes throughout the menopausal transition did not affect heart disease risk. These results don't seem to apply to night sweats, so there is a lot of speculation as to whether these different symptoms are caused by different factors but once again the issue of individuality is most important. This was also corroborated in other research that suggested that women who had any type of vasomotor symptoms (hot flushes and night sweats) seemed to have less calcification in their arteries, though these results depended on the amount and length of time they had these flushes and night sweats, and when they started HT.

But menopause is complex, and the wide range of information can be bewildering; a different study shows that women with severe hot flushes are at risk for calcification of the arteries, while another study indicated that women battling with night sweats may be at some risk for heart disease, though this risk doesn't appear to be related to hot flushes. In yet another study, it seemed that severe hot flushes didn't affect the actual thickening of the lining of the arteries, but only the way in which the inner lining of the blood vessels (the endothelium) functions. Hot flushes and night sweats, depending on when and at what stage of your menopause transition you get them, may be useful in predicting your risk of heart disease. I believe that future research will show that hot flushes, while normal and to be expected in most women, may possibly be a red flag for heart disease in some postmenopausal women and not in others, depending on their individual health profile. It may become important for doctors to add the information of whether you have severe or moderate hot flushes to the list of factors that could put you at risk for heart disease. In the light of these confusing findings, it is very important for you to be monitored in order to identify risk factors for heart disease and live sensibly, regardless of whether you suffer from hot flushes or not.

All of these studies I describe above, are part of a large body of research examining the mechanisms and effects of hot flushes on heart disease. The problem is that hot flushes usually occur at an age when women start to be at greater risk for heart disease, so it is important to understand whether hot flushes and night sweats signal ageing blood vessels and underlying problems relating to early heart disease and other health issues. Because the above results don't apply to all women, as always, the individual approach seems the way to go. Regardless of your menopausal symptoms you should work in partnership with your doctor to understand and be aware of heart disease risk factors, having appropriate tests and treatment when necessary. Because there is so much new research it is not yet clear what future strategies will be most effective in dealing with these issues, but it seems certain that a healthy lifestyle and giving up smoking, drinking moderately and exercising, as well as taking cholesterol-lowering drugs when indicated, should help keep these risk factors at bay.

Know your risk factor levels

Remember that these numbers are only guidelines as to optimal levels you should have. They may depend on your age, ethnicity, gender and your individual risk factors at present.

- Blood pressure not greater than 120–129/75–84 mmHg
- Total cholesterol less than 5.0 mmol/L (<200 mg/dL)
- LDL 'bad' cholesterol lower than 2.6 mmol/L (<100 mg/dL)
- HDL 'good' cholesterol higher than 1.5 mmol/L (>60 mg/dL)
- Triglycerides lower than 1.7 mmol/L (<150 mg/dL)
- Fasting blood glucose of less than 5.6 mmol/L (<100 mg/dL)
- Body Mass Index 18.5–24.9 kg/m^2
- Waist circumference less than 80 cm (<31.5 inches)

EMPOWER YOURSELF

- You should always be treated as an individual. All the personal risk factors, such as your lifestyle and family history, whether you smoke or are overweight, have diabetes, plus any others, should be taken into consideration and carefully discussed.
- If you're a smoker, stop smoking immediately.
- Be aware of the risks involved in heart disease and take control of your life.
- Women who are having heart attacks don't often complain of chest pain; they are more likely to report discomfort or pain in their necks, one or both arms, the middle of their backs or their jaws. They often describe palpitations, a feeling of indigestion, cold sweats, light-headedness, shortness of breath, stomach pain and often nausea, which may be combined with vomiting.

- Symptoms of a stroke may include a very severe unexplained headache, a sudden numb feeling or weakness in your face, arm or leg, down one side of your body. There may be confusion; problems speaking or comprehending a conversation; problems walking; feeling dizzy and losing coordination or balance. Migraine sufferers may experience some of these symptoms, but always be alert if they are different or more severe than those you usually experience.
- If you're anxious about taking a particular medication don't be afraid to question your practitioner or get a second opinion. You might not want to take a risk that your practitioner deems acceptable.
- Until there is more evidence, HT should not be used to prevent cardiovascular disease as there are unambiguous studies that show that there are other drugs, like statins, that really work.

8

The C word: cancers in menopausal women

As a very active mother of three, Bonnie's life was hectic but she enjoyed every minute. At 45 she was healthy and took care of herself. Early one morning during her shower she was very disturbed to find an unusual lumpy area in her breast. She immediately called her gynaecologist and was given a cancellation appointment the following morning. He examined her breast and diagnosed fibroadenosis – a term doctors use to describe a benign condition of the breast that can cause lumpiness, enlargement, tenderness and sometimes pain. It describes a group of benign lumps or growths called fibroadenomas. A fibroadenoma is a smooth, rounded, solid lump, sometimes called a tumour, which can develop outside the milk ducts. It is made up of the fibrous and glandular tissue in the breast. It usually has a rubbery feel and moves easily in the breast when touched. They are often found in younger women but can occur at any age as they may be caused by hormonal changes in the body. Since most women have lumpy breasts – some more than others – fibroadenosis is not usually a cause for alarm, but doctors can confirm their diagnosis by sending the patient for an ultrasound or even a fine-needle aspiration to confirm that the cells are benign.

Bonnie listened carefully and told her gynaecologist she still felt very anxious. He then asked whether she had a family history of breast cancer. When she replied she did not, he assured her there was no cause for further worry and that his examination of her breast was quite adequate. Since she trusted him – she had been his patient for many years and he had delivered her three children – she was reassured. But that afternoon one of her children had a sore throat so she visited her GP and mentioned the story of her breast. The GP saw she was uneasy and offered to examine her breast. Alarmed by what he felt, he suggested a mammogram. Bonnie wasn't keen, as her gynae had told her not to worry and she didn't want to pursue the matter. The

GP refused to accept her decision and insisted she make an appointment for a mammogram.

The radiologist was alarmed by what she saw in the mammogram and advised Bonnie to immediately have a fine-needle aspiration. The results showed that she had Invasive Ductal Carcinoma (IDC). Though many of these cancers are low grade and not aggressive, hers was particularly aggressive. Bonnie had a mastectomy and chemotherapy. After 12 years there has been no recurrence and she has just celebrated the birth of her first grandchild.

Bonnie was lucky; she had a GP who had known her for many years and whom she trusted. This doctor was aware that the risk for breast cancer increases in midlife women and insisted that she have it checked, even though Bonnie wasn't keen to have a mammogram – perhaps she was subconsciously frightened of what she might find. Most of us are terribly afraid of cancer, even more so than of heart disease, which is strange since research has shown that cardiovascular disease kills far more women than breast cancer does, but fear is irrational.

Andrea's story told in Chapter 7 graphically illustrates the fact that the issues of heart disease and cancer are vital to middle-aged women, especially as far as HT is concerned, but it is cancer that really frightens us. Even as I write these words, I feel anxious and hesitant about writing about cancer. I am almost superstitious. Why go into this? Why mess with it? The spectre of cancer is so terrifying. We have friends who have died of it and know others who are battling with it. We may also know some who are in remission. However, if we can try to conquer these fears and give ourselves the chance to understand the dynamics of cancer and heart disease, how to lower our risks, especially if we are vulnerable, and to be aware of the risks, so we can increase our chances of living to a healthy and happy old age. As we age the risk factor for cancer increases, and it's very important to understand how it may occur so we can live in a way that may help to prevent it, or at least, decrease the risk. Since middle-aged women are more vulnerable to certain types of cancer, I think it is important to give a laywoman's perspective on these illnesses.

There are, of course, hundreds of different types of cancers, but the ones that I write about are those that seem to be associated with women in menopause: breast cancer, endometrial cancer and ovarian cancer. I have also included a section on colorectal cancer, which becomes more prevalent in midlife. In fact, these are all very complicated diseases; for example the subject of breast cancer deserves a book all on its own. My object here is to give a general overview to help you understand a little more about these cancers, to be aware of the risks and to see that there are treatment options available. There are many really good cancer associations and access to the Internet and media in the twenty-first century allows women to be much more enlightened, to understand the nature of their cancer and how they can participate in their treatment and recovery. The bulk of the information in this chapter is about breast cancer because it is the most widely researched and the most common cancer in middle-aged women. There are excellent websites and information centres with toll-free lines available (some of these are listed with the references at the end of the book).

As is evident in this book, I am not keen on too many diagrams but I think that in order to help you conquer the fear of breast cancer and to arm yourself with knowledge, I will use a couple of diagrams to show where breast cancer usually begins and where it travels. Breasts are of major psychological and physical significance for most women. They are the symbols of beauty and femininity, the sign that we have changed from girl to woman and then to mother, as we nourish our children from our breasts. The image of a woman cradling her baby at her breast is as old as humanity. This is why when our breasts are cancerous or removed we feel so bereft and why breast cancer has so many psychological implications.

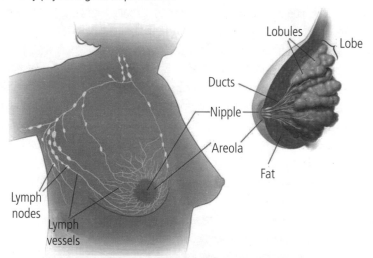

**The parts of the breast and the lymph nodes
and lymph vessels near the breast**

Source: 'General Information about Breast Cancer'. National Cancer
Institute. US National Institutes of Health (www.cancer.gov)

Our breasts are specifically designed to make milk. They are made up of different tissues – fatty and connective – and groups of tiny milk-producing glands. They are divided into sections called *lobes*, which contain even smaller lobes, known as *lobules*. It is in these lobules that milk glands are found. When we breastfeed, the breast milk flows out of the breast through tubes (*ducts*) to our nipples.

As you can see in the diagram on page 162, the breast also has tiny vessels, which are very similar to veins. These vessels are called *lymph* vessels because they belong to the *lymphatic system* and carry a clear fluid that cleans the tissues throughout the body. The role of the lymphatic system is to guard our body from infection, and to help in this function there are little areas called lymph nodes throughout the body, including in the armpits, neck area, near the collarbone and in the groin and chest, where lymph fluid collects. These *lymph nodes* collect materials like bacteria and cancerous cells that are harmful to the body and prevent them from entering the bloodstream. So when a lot of harmful material is gathered in the nodes they can become swollen and painful, a sign of infection or that something is wrong, which is why your doctor feels for swollen lymph glands when you complain of feeling ill. But be aware that a malignant node is generally painless.

The cells that make up the tissues in our bodies are constantly growing and dividing as new cells are needed, but sometimes the way in which the cells form new cells goes awry and there is a spate of new cell growth when new cells are not needed because the old cells haven't died. This mass of cells in the tissue becomes a lump or growth (*tumour*) and this is what can be felt or detected by means of a screening. At different times during your cycle your breasts may feel lumpy because of the rise and fall in your hormone levels. Some women only have lumpy breasts at certain times of the month and others always seem to have lumpy breasts, which shows you that not all lumps are dangerous or malignant.

These non-threatening lumps are called *benign* and generally only one out of 10 breast lumps is *malignant*. The most common cause for a breast lump in most menopausal women is a cyst. The lumps you should worry about are the ones that are diagnosed as malignant. These little masses of cells may start out very small indeed, so small that they cannot be felt in a breast examination, which is why healthcare practitioners, especially those involved in dealing with cancers, believe in a screening process called *mammography*, which helps them to identify and deal with the cancer in its earliest stages.

MAMMOGRAMS AND ULTRASOUNDS: SCREENING FOR BREAST CANCER

'That's it!' said Leigh triumphantly. 'I never need another mammogram, thank goodness. It was a horrible experience.'

'Why not?' I asked in amazement.

'I've just been for my annual check-up and my gynaecologist says she can pick up any changes in my breasts with her yearly examination. She also gave me information which showed that radiologists couldn't claim scientifically that there was a better survival rate for women who had regular mammograms than those who didn't!'

I was dumbfounded. I knew immediately what she was talking about. In medical research there is an independent non-profit organisation called the Cochrane Collaboration, which reviews the available research on different healthcare interventions and then reports its findings so that healthcare practitioners can see whether the research is valid or not. In 2001 a Cochrane review stated that the research that was currently available did not show that there was a survival benefit if there was mass screening of women and that furthermore the available evidence did not show that women with breast cancer lived longer if they had been screened. It suggested that those who recommended screening and those who wanted to be screened should consider these findings carefully.

All hell broke loose among those who felt that the review was incorrect, because many of the studies and the statistics they had reviewed were faulty, so it created a misleading impression about the efficacy of screening for breast cancer. As I explained in Chapter 3, it is all too easy for doctors to take what they want from a report and present it to their patients as the truth to reinforce their own opinions. It is true that mammograms may be done by inadequately trained radiographers and that there can be misdiagnoses, which cause either tremendous anxiety when a woman is told there is a problem when there isn't (*a false positive diagnosis*), or possibly even death when a woman is told she is fine when she is not (*a false negative diagnosis*). We should understand that screening as a tool, however effective, can be misused.

Believers in mammography responded to this review in depth, stating that they understood that no study is perfect but that many of the criticisms cited in the review were incorrect and that in fact there had been careful control of the statistics, which they believed to be valid in spite of their drawbacks. They said that in general the research showed that mammograms are effective in reducing deaths from breast cancer.

In 2004 researchers from the American Cancer Society, reviewing the randomised trials of over 40 years, concluded that the trials generally showed that mammograms substantially reduce death from breast cancer and that while there are still problems like false positives, which means that a lump is diagnosed as cancerous when it is benign, or false negatives, which is when a patient is told she is in the clear when she is not, the 20 per cent reduction shown overall is statistically very significant in both absolute and relative terms. In January 2005 another Cochrane review examined randomised controlled trials conducted with a follow-up time of nearly 20 years and came to the conclusion that regular physical examinations and yearly mammograms are very effective in detecting recurrences of cancer and in reducing the mortality rate of breast cancer survivors.

When I wrote about mammograms in 2008, I thought the debate had been laid to rest. I was wrong. The controversy around mammograms still rages. In 2009 the US Preventative Services Task Force (USPSTF) suggested that annual mammograms may not be necessary in women younger than 50 and that these women should generally only have a mammogram once every two years. There is a strong body of opinion that welcomed this report; the clinicians in this camp believe when younger women have mammograms, they are 10 times as likely to be overdiagnosed and overtreated. They raise the issue of harm caused by false positive diagnoses, anxiety on the part of the patient and unnecessary radiation, ultrasound and biopsies. Issues of affordability and access for poorer women to mammograms also play a part in the debate.

These opinions have elicited some of the most heated commentary in medical journals that I have seen for a long time, since those who advocate annual mammograms from the age of 40 are equally adamant. They cite several studies showing that early detection may reduce the risk of death by invasive breast cancer; the American Cancer Society recommends annual mammograms from the age of 40 because it seems not only do they reduce death from breast cancer but if detected early, the cancers may also be less aggressive. Those who are in the pro-annual mammogram camp believe that early detection may also reduce the need for mastectomy and chemotherapy and describe studies suggesting that in women aged 40 to 49 with a family history of breast cancer, annual mammograms could be lifesaving. Finally, in February 2011, further analysis of the USPSTF recommendation came up with very different results from the studies analysed, suggesting that annual screening in younger women (40 onwards) does save more lives.

These different arguments may be pretty convincing in statistical and medical terms, but how can we make sense of it? Let's imagine that you have a small cancerous lump in your breast that is less than 1 cm in size. It is called a *ductal carcinoma in situ* (DCIS), meaning a cancer in a specific part of the breast duct that has not invaded the surrounding duct. These cancerous cells are confined to the inside of the ducts and because they have not become invasive, which means they have not broken through the wall of the breast ducts to affect other breast tissue, there is no risk of the cancer cells spreading.

DCIS cannot usually be felt as a breast lump or other breast change, and so most cases are found by routine screening with mammograms. If this DCIS is detected by screening and appropriately treated, the recovery rate is excellent because it has not spread. In fact, research has shown that recovery may be over 95 per cent, because steps can be taken to prevent it developing into invasive breast cancer and treatment for DCIS is usually very successful. However, if the DCIS is not detected and therefore not treated, approximately between a quarter and half of all these areas of DCIS will develop into invasive breast cancer. And the chances of survival can be 40 per cent less!

As cancers grow they become more aggressive and start to invade the surrounding areas, which in the case of the breast, would probably be the lymph nodes and then the bloodstream. This movement, when a group of cancer cells starts to travel and damages other organs or tissues or forms other secondary growths, is called *metastasis*.

From my personal perspective, I believe a woman's personal preferences play a part in her decision to have a mammogram or not and they should be taken into consideration, based on her individual risk profile. I tend strongly towards the view that annual mammograms from the age of 40 may lower the risk of death from breast cancer; there has been a steady decline in the rate of breast cancer death in the last 20 years. This may be attributed in part to women taking less HT and better cancer treatments, but it is also strongly related to early detection of cancers. Though there is a theory that even low-dose radiation may be risky, there is not gold standard evidence that the amounts of radiation in screening outweigh the benefits of early detection.

I believe that all women over 50 should, if they can, have an annual mammogram. Women of any age should have an annual mammogram if they are taking HT or if they are at high risk, have the BRCA gene mutation (see page 173) or a family history of cancer. Breasts of postmenopausal women are less dense, which means that their mammograms are more effective. But obviously if you already have become menopausal in your forties, you may be a better candidate for a mammogram than a 50-year-old woman who is still having regular periods. If you have not yet reached menopause but have decided to have an annual mammogram, a study has shown that it is best to have your mammogram in the first week of your menstrual cycle.

If you have very dense breasts, you should expect to have an ultrasound as well. If you are very anxious because you are at high risk it is a good idea to have an annual mammogram and then an ultrasound every six months. Research has shown that for women who are at very high risk for breast cancer, *magnetic resonance imaging* (MRI), when performed in venues specialising in breast cancer screening, is much more sensitive than mammography, though, like all techniques, it has its drawbacks and is, of course, very expensive.

However, an annual MRI may be recommended for women who have a BRCA altered gene, those women who have not been tested but who have a first-line relative with a BRCA positive cancer, and who have had three or more false negative biopsies. Use of this diagnostic tool has expanded and MRI is now also used in certain specific cases after a woman has been diagnosed for breast cancer to determine the extent of the disease and as guidance for both biopsies and the localisation of the cancer. It can also be used to evaluate whether the treatment recommended is being effective.

THE DREADED MAMMOGRAM

Mammograms strike fear into the hearts of many women. Some women have had one and found it so uncomfortable that they swear they will never have another; others have been put off by gruesome descriptions of mammograms being like having your breast slammed in the freezer door or lying on a cold concrete floor while your breast is squished between two weights. Still others are worried about the amount of radiation they might be exposed to when they have their annual mammogram.

The truth is, a well-performed mammogram is no more than slightly uncomfortable. You will be taken into a private room and told to undress from your waist up. Here your breasts will be positioned on a plastic shelf. You will need to stand in two different positions, your breasts will be sandwiched, but not in any way that should hurt – if it is unbearably painful ask the radiographer to stop. If you know your breasts are very tender, take a painkiller before you embark on the process.

Try not to have a mammogram just before your period when your breasts may be very full and tender. Some women find it comforting to take a close female friend or relative with them and others may want to be with their partners or husbands. My view is that whatever makes you feel most at home should be the rule. Here's a tip: I have found that if you stand on tip-toe so that you let your breasts lift on to the little plastic ledge of the mammography machine it feels much more comfortable. It is a bit undignified but most of us have felt far worse during gynaecological examinations and if you are really uncomfortable you should find a centre that specialises in breast screening, firstly because experts will probably interpret the results better and secondly because the woman who does your examination will probably make you feel more at ease.

If you are worried about exposure to radiation it will probably help you to remember that mammograms require very small doses of radiation. Discuss these concerns, if you have them, with your radiographer.

Since I first wrote about mammograms, digital mammography has become more common. This kind of mammography uses the same technique as film screen mammography, but the image is recorded directly into a computer. The image can then be enlarged or highlighted. If there is a suspicious area, your radiologist will then use the computer to take a closer look. If digital mammography is used your radiologist may read your mammogram with the help of computer-aided detection (CAD) programmes, and can then transmit your mammogram to your doctor via email. This procedure may be more effective on younger women with dense breasts.

Once your mammogram is over you will be asked to wait while the radiologist looks at the pictures of your breasts. If all looks clear, she or he will probably tell you to get dressed and will then spend a little time with you, telling you that all is well and suggesting when your next visit should be. Usually your breast tissue changes after you have had children – this is called an *involuted* breast, which means that it has sort of collapsed inward, so the fatty tissue is not too dense. You may have very dense tissue because you are hormonal or on HT (research shows that HT regardless of type seems to increase density), or because you have had a breast implant or reconstruction. If so, and the image doesn't look clear, or the radiologist sees something that looks out of place, she or he will suggest you come along to another room where an ultrasound machine is set up. Your breasts will be scanned to see the area of concern more clearly. There may be a tiny lump or there may be small areas of calcium that are clumped together, which might also be a sign of cancer.

The scan doesn't hurt at all, I promise you. You lie on a bed next to a screen and the radiologist spreads a gel over your breasts and moves an ultrasound probe, a flat object, with light pressure over your breasts while watching the screen to see more clearly what's going on. To you it will look like a map of the moon, but to the expert it will give a clear indication of whether there's something to worry about. The only problem is that if the radiologist hasn't explained why you are there, you may feel a bit panicked. Stay calm. Often the scan is just routine, to make absolutely sure that any shadowy areas that are shown in the mammogram are no more than denser bits of tissue.

The problems begin when the doctor sees that there is indeed an abnormal mass. But remember that many suspicious findings may not be cancerous; perhaps only one in five or even fewer will be problematic. A needle biopsy will usually be performed. This should be done by a specialist radiologist in a specialist radiological suite, using either a mammogram or ultrasound for guidance. An oncologist friend says that doing a 'blind' biopsy is like sticking your hand into a haystack and trying to find a needle.

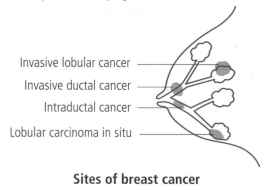

Invasive lobular cancer

Invasive ductal cancer

Intraductal cancer

Lobular carcinoma in situ

Sites of breast cancer

By kind permission of Dr Carol-Ann Benn

There are several ways to determine if the lump is malignant. The specialist will use the ultrasound and a needle to take a sample of tissue and the cells, which will be sent to a pathology laboratory to see if they are harmful. There are two types of needle biopsies. The *fine-needle biopsy* is most effective in collecting cells from cysts and lymph nodes and can also be used for solid masses. A *core-needle biopsy* is generally performed on a breast lump to collect both tissue and cells. The needle used for this procedure is slightly thicker but neither procedure, in the hands of an expert, should be too painful. If it is unbearably painful, there is something wrong – and not with you!

The specialist may also suggest another form of biopsy where either a bit of the lump or the entire lump is removed so that the pathologists can examine the tissue carefully. A surgeon at a hospital does this procedure. This surgery is performed only if the material collected from the core-needle biopsy or fine-needle biopsy comes back as inconclusive, doesn't have typical characteristics, or doesn't fit with the clinical findings of the specialist. A biopsy can also be performed if the suspicious area is in a place that is hard for a needle to reach. From the pathology point of view, if you have cancer, your samples should be checked to identify the type of cancer cells, their build-up and how aggressive they are, as well as seeing if the cells carry a number of receptors, namely estrogen, progesterone and Human Epidermal growth factor Receptor 2 (HER2), because this might affect your treatment options.

I am not saying that once you have an annual mammogram you can abdicate your responsibility to yourself and your health. Living well is one of the first lines of defence, as is an understanding of the possible risk factors in your particular situation. It would also be sensible to know how to examine your own breasts once a month.

HOW TO EXAMINE YOUR OWN BREASTS

Decide when you want to examine your breasts and make it the same time each month. Remember that breast tissue reacts to hormone changes in your body so your breasts could feel a little lumpy or tender just before or during your period, or if you are on HT, or are perimenopausal and experiencing the wide fluctuations of estrogen levels that I discussed in Chapter 1.

Some women like to examine their breasts in the shower, others in the bath, or while lying in bed. It's up to you. Probably the best way is to get your doctor to give you a thorough clinical breast examination. Then feel over your breasts yourself so you know how they feel after they have been given the all clear. This will help you to be more confident when doing a self-breast exam and something feels different: a harder lump, or one that wasn't there before.

Be alert for *any* changes in your breasts. A change can be an important warning sign. Look at your breasts in a mirror, hold each one in your hand and look down at it to see if you can detect any changes in shape (I'm not talking here about weight gain or loss). Are there any strange rashes or dimpling? Has your nipple changed and moved inwards or is the skin around the nipple tender or inflamed, itchy or painful? Is the skin crusty or an angry red? Is there any fluid or discharge coming out of your nipple? Raise your arms and check again that everything still looks the same.

Now get into the bath or shower, or lie down, and gently move the first three fingers, held flat and together, in a circular motion over your entire breast from the top to the bottom and from over your cleavage to under your armpits, exerting a gentle pressure and feeling deep into the breast tissue.

Use the right hand to examine the left breast and vice versa. Ideally you should do this examination both standing and lying down.

Having said all that, I must admit that I am useless at breast exams. I immediately think that a rib is a sinister lump and I can never remember what my breast felt like from one month to the next. If this is the case with you as well, get your GP to examine your breasts thoroughly. But even if you are uncomfortable examining yourself, you must be alert to any of the changes in your breasts that I have mentioned above.

RISK FACTORS FOR BREAST CANCER

The first thing to be aware of here is that 50 per cent of women who get breast cancer have no obvious risk factors at all, which is my opportunity to say that no woman should ever, ever blame herself for getting breast cancer. Plenty of healthy women, living as well as possible, get breast cancer. If you are at a high risk because of your family history, you can take responsibility for your health and see that you are monitored and screened regularly. There are steps you can take to lower your risk profile and live as healthily as possible. However, blaming yourself and immersing yourself in guilt can only impede your recovery. Everyone is going to have risk factors for some illness or another. The National Cancer Association has created a breast cancer risk assessment tool that is based on research called the GAIL model. It is somewhat like the FRAX tool, which calculates your risk for osteoporosis, and I have cited the website in Empowerment Points at the end of this chapter.

One of the strongest risks for breast cancer, which I will explain later, is your age. Your genetic make-up will determine whether you suffer from certain illnesses like diabetes, cardiovascular disease or cancer. In your make-up there is a predisposition that will determine what will happen to you and it may happen no matter how healthily or unhealthily you live. In any case, as we get older and live longer, we are at greater risk for some kind of cancer or another as the cells in our bodies age. I am appalled at those alternative medicine writers and practitioners who put this kind of burden on women with cancer. You are who you are, and ultimately your genetic make-up may be the culprit, not you. Of course relaxation techniques and appropriate living can improve your immune system and your chances of recovery, but the burden of recovery should not be placed on you alone. Work in partnership with your surgeon, oncologist and counsellor. Allow yourself to work through the grief, rage and fear, and don't hide those feelings. You have not wished cancer upon yourself!

This is also probably the place to mention alternative and complementary cures. If you have read Chapter 5 you already know my bias, but 'natural' cures may be devastating for cancer patients in terms of the false hope, the cost and the often harmful effects, and because they promise to work and don't, which could deprive the cancer patient of valuable time and exposure to conventional medicines that have generally been proven to work.

The same rules should apply when assessing alternative cures as with conventional treatment. What is the evidence that they work? What are the interests of those involved and what are their medical qualifications? I accept that many people have had horrific experiences with conventional doctors but I have heard equally horrific stories about alternative healers. Be aware and don't allow despair to make you gullible. Also, don't forget the power of the placebo effect that I discussed on pages 104–105. Those who offer these 'cures' should allow the most thorough scrutiny possible. Anecdotal evidence can never replace sound scientific evidence. If supplements make you feel better, take them. Just remember to discuss what you're taking with your oncologist – any potent natural medicine can cause serious side effects or interfere with some of the conventional treatments you are taking. I recommend that you look at the articles on complementary and alternative cancer cures on www.quackwatch. com, one of my favourite sites for logical, balanced comment on this subject.

Here are the factors that may increase your risk of getting breast cancer (remember even if you have one or more of these risks you may never get it at all).

Age

Age is the strongest risk factor for breast cancer. Like most cancers, the risk of developing breast cancer increases as women get older. Nearly 80 per cent of breast cancer occurs in women older than 50. This happens because there are changes in your breast cells which can cause cancer, and obviously the longer we live, the more time there is for this to happen. This is why I recommended earlier that women over 50 have annual mammograms. You can't stop ageing but you can have regular screenings.

Family history of breast cancer

This is high on the list. Approximately less than 10 per cent of breast and ovarian cancers are inherited, which means that they are caused by an altered gene that has been passed on from parent to child. Remember, you **do not actually** inherit cancer but you **may inherit a higher risk of getting it**.

Family history of breast cancer refers to any first-line relative – your mother, sister, daughter or father – who may have had it. Information about this is especially important if these relatives had breast cancer before they were 40; this is called early breast cancer. You should also mention if any of your second-line family members on either your father's or mother's side – such as a paternal or maternal grandmother, aunt, or even first cousins – had breast cancer.

Information about your family history of breast cancer and ovarian cancer becomes even more important if there are three relatives on the *same* side who have had or have breast cancer. If you have had a bout with cancer, such as endometrial cancer, you may also be at high risk for breast cancer. *Genetic make-up* is therefore a risk factor. The reason for members of one family being susceptible to breast cancer may be in their genes.

BRCA1 and BRCA2

There is a lot of talk and confusion surrounding two genes called *BRCA1* and *BRCA2*. Every person has these genes and normally they play an important role in preventing breast and ovarian cancers. But sometimes a change may occur in these genes and they do not work as they should in controlling the growth of the cells. Instead, they allow the cells to grow at an abnormal rate, which may lead to cancer. We inherit two copies of each and every gene – one from our mother and one from our father. So, if either one of your parents carry an altered BRCA1 or BRCA2 gene, you have a 50 per cent chance of also having this altered gene. This does not mean that you are definitely going to get breast cancer or ovarian cancer but it does mean that it increases your possibility of developing either of these. Certain groups of people have been found to be more likely to carry these altered genes, for example people of Ashkenazi Jewish descent, some groups in Holland, Sweden, Iceland and members of Afrikaner families. Other population groups have also been found to be more likely to carry these altered genes.

Thanks to ongoing medical research there is a simple blood test available that can determine whether you are a carrier of one of these altered genes. But it is very important to understand that unlike a mammogram or other screening tests, this test is specifically for people who are thought to be at high risk for breast or ovarian cancer.

Anyone considering this test should first meet with a qualified specialist (a genetic counsellor or oncologist) and do a thorough evaluation of their family history to be sure that this genetic testing is the right path to take. People can determine whether they carry an altered BRCA gene that may be responsible for the cancers in their family, and if they do carry an altered gene they can develop a strategy with their doctors and discuss the options that are available to decrease their cancer risk, as well as ensuring that they have ongoing monitoring that will help detect the cancer early, when the prognosis may be better.

A downside is that no screening or testing is infallible and some people become terribly anxious when they realise that they carry an altered gene that increases their risk of cancer, and they may act impulsively without considering all the available options, or they may not feel ready or able to take the steps that may protect them. Remember that scientists are continuing to discover new genetic markers for breast cancer, so if you know that you have these factors your doctor will help you decide what you want to do.

Risk-reducing surgery for women with a mutation of the BRCA gene: Is it an option?

Lori was 38 when both her ovaries and womb were removed after she was diagnosed with early-stage ovarian cancer and tested positive for the BRCA1 gene mutation. Luckily she had completed childbearing and had two lovely little girls. Because she was plunged into menopause she found she experienced many menopausal symptoms: weight gain, dry skin, hair loss and dry eyes. Her hot flushes were quite mild but since her doctor had prescribed an antidepressant containing venlafaxine, she believed this was helping these as well as her mood swings. She had been reading widely on the subject of early menopause and was worried that because she had lost her ovaries she was at risk for heart disease, but was very frightened that she might get breast cancer if she started taking ET. Her local health shop recommended bioidentical hormone creams, estradiol and progesterone, saying they were the 'safest' way to go, but her GP was horrified when she discussed this option. Lori was perplexed: 'I honestly don't know what do. I want to protect my health; I have two small children and I am so anxious about what is best for me, but I find the information out there confusing and contradictory.'

Lori is a modern woman. She coped bravely and sensibly with the blow life dealt her and took responsibility for her health. As I wrote in Chapter 4, unless a medicines control board has approved bioidentical hormones, it is not wise to use them. Lori's womb has been removed so she would be able to take estrogen-only therapy, if it were not contraindicated, without a progestogen. There are studies showing that it may be safe for some at-risk women who have had premature menopause to take ET, but this should **only** be done after extensive discussions with an oncologist where **all** risks and benefits are considered. If Lori's specialist believes she is not a candidate for ET, she should help Lori focus on a strategy to lower her risk for heart disease and Lori may also want to discuss whether she could use a local vaginal estrogen, under careful supervision.

The decision to have surgery to reduce the risk of breast and ovarian cancer is a very complex and emotional one. A recent study analysed women at 22 research genetics centres in the USA and Europe to understand the relationships of bilateral mastectomy and/or bilateral oopherectomy with ovarian and breast cancer risks. The research showed there was a lower risk of breast cancer in the group who had a mastectomy, and lower risk of ovarian cancer, breast cancer and death from these cancers in those who had their ovaries removed.

The problem is that either of these surgeries profoundly affect women. Removing the ovaries in women, especially younger ones, is associated with death at an earlier age and risk for heart disease. However, there are medications that can deal with heart disease risk. Women with early surgical menopause often have much more severe symptoms than those who have had a natural one. Because of their high genetic risk they are not great candidates for ET, especially in the long term. Some research has shown that short-term ET in these young women may not increase the risk of breast cancer, but the anxiety remains and these studies are not long term. Constant monitoring would be necessary, especially if the woman had elected to keep her breasts (as it would be even if she had had the mastectomy but kept her ovaries). The issue would also be what type of gene mutation it was; it seems that women with the BRCA2 mutation are at greater risk for estrogen receptor-positive breast cancer than those who have the BRCA1 mutation – their breast cancer is usually estrogen receptor-negative. The different options should always be thoroughly discussed with the appropriate medical specialist; all relevant issues, such as your individual risk profile, should be factored in and assessed before the decision is made as to whether both ovaries and breasts should be removed, or just the breasts or just the ovaries.

HUMAN EPIDERMAL GROWTH FACTOR RECEPTOR 2 (HER2)

Connie was having a romantic, island holiday with her husband. They had blocked these days off so that they could have some quality time in their busy lives, because she said they never seemed to have any time to be close together. During a romantic interlude, she was slightly surprised to notice that the nipple on her left breast had become slightly indented and during foreplay, when her husband touched her nipple, she felt no reaction. She was not worried and had a fleeting thought that her menopausal nipples were not as perky as they used to be and perhaps this was something that happened as you got older. At 54, she was very health conscious and had regular annual mammograms.

She returned from Europe glowing with health and thought no more about it till a few days later when she realised that her nipple was sore. Connie began to be a bit anxious; two of her friends were already dealing with breast cancer and she realised her nipples had never hurt before. Because she was hyper-aware of breast cancer and had just been discussing it, this seemed to be a red flag and by the Friday, she was sure she felt a lump next to her nipple. She was due for her mammogram in a month's time but her anxiety had grown during the weekend and on the Monday she phoned the receptionist at her breast care centre, who said she could come in immediately as they had a cancellation.

The radiologist examined her breast and said that he was concerned and advised a biopsy. Connie takes responsibility for her health; she had had benign breast cysts for many years and been told not to do unnecessary biopsies, so she called her specialist and asked what he thought. He told her to go ahead. When the results came back, she was told that she had a HER2 cancer that tested positive for estrogen and progesterone. Connie's tumour grew rapidly: on the Tuesday it was 2.5 cm (1 inch) and by the Thursday when she had her mastectomy, it was 3.5 cm (1 ½ inches).

After her operation, Connie underwent three months of chemotherapy and was chosen by her oncologist to participate in a major trial called ALTTO (see page 193) to see how effective a new drug called lapatinib (Tyverb) was when compared with the results of trastuzumab (Herceptin) in treating HER2 cancer. Eighteen months after she discovered the lump, her cancer appears to be in remission and she has just gone on another romantic holiday.

Although HER2 is **not** a risk factor for cancer because the genetic abnormality is in the tumour and **not** in the person, I have placed the information here because many women ask me about it and I want to use this opportunity to discuss receptors, particularly estrogen receptors, which are relevant for women with breast cancer. In order to understand HER2 cancer, you need to know something about receptors and growth hormones.

Firstly, it is important to understand that the life cycle of each one of the millions of cells in our body is programmed to behave in a specific way but sometimes this process can be changed by various factors, one of which I will explain below. In the development of cancer a key factor is a change in the growth rate of the cell. Now let's go back to receptors. In Chapter 1, I explained that receptors are special groups of cells that are present in the organs and tissues, and respond to messages from the different hormones in your body. Your doctor will tell you about these receptors when they explain your breast cancer pathology report. There are receptors for the female hormones estrogen and progesterone present in your breast cells. These cells respond to messages from these hormones. Estrogen or progesterone will 'tell' the receptors to increase normal breast cell growth, where for example, it can make the cell repair or reproduce itself, or they can cause abnormal breast cell growth. Remember that each of these receptors only responds to their own specific protein or chemical, like the right key opening the right lock. Some of these chemicals I mentioned above are called *growth factors* and they attach to these receptors and stimulate cells to grow.

The HER2 gene is responsible for making HER2 protein. HER2 is one of the proteins found on the surface of certain cells. So we could say that HER2 is a receptor for a **particular** growth factor called *human epidermal growth factor*, which occurs naturally in the body.

Usually the HER2 protein plays an important role in normal cell growth and development. It transmits signals directing cell growth from the outside of the cell to the nucleus inside the cell. Sometimes, however, there is a genetic alteration in the HER2 gene that causes human epidermal growth factor to attach itself to HER2 receptors on breast cancer cells and stimulates the breast cancer cells to divide and grow. The problem starts because some breast cancer cells have a lot more HER2 receptors than others. When this happens, the tumour is described as being HER2 positive. It is thought that about one in five women with breast cancer will have HER2-positive tumours. This excess of HER2 is due to an altered gene, which can occur in many types of cancers, not only breast cancer. It is very important to understand that this altered HER2 gene is only present in the breast cancer cells, not in the rest of the cells in the body, and cannot be passed on to other family members.

The problem with HER2-positive breast cancer is that it tends to grow more quickly than other cancers, so you may have heard the specialist talking about your cancer being more 'aggressive'. When this happens, tests can be done to find out whether you have HER2-positive breast cancer. Usually the specialist oncologist will have a sample of cancer tissue from previous biopsies or your surgery. Testing may also have been done for HER2 in your initial surgery.

If you test positive for HER2, a drug called *trastuzumab* (trade name Herceptin) has been developed and can be effective against this type of cancer. Recent research also suggests that Herceptin may help reduce the risk of the cancer coming back or recurring in women with early breast cancer. It is currently known that chemotherapy and/or hormonal therapy can also reduce this risk. A number of research trials looked at giving Herceptin as a treatment at the same time a woman received chemotherapy, to see if this further reduced the risk of cancer recurring. The results of these trials were very promising; the cancer came back in fewer women who had Herceptin combined with chemotherapy, compared with women who only had chemotherapy.

There are some minor side effects of Herceptin which may be related to a small allergic reaction to the drug. It is generally well tolerated. These side effects usually lessen after the first dose. As I will discuss later in the section on treatment, chemotherapy and/or hormonal therapy can reduce the risk of breast cancer returning and as you can see, research has shown that Herceptin in combination with chemotherapy may help reduce the risk of the cancer recurring.

You may remember reading about several cases in different countries where women took their medical aids to court to ensure that this particular treatment, which is very expensive, would be paid for by their medical aids and they won. Unfortunately this battle continues, so you should have a frank discussion with your oncologist about this. Your own specialist will advise you about the best available treatment.

THE HORMONE CONNECTION

It seems clear that there is a strong causal relationship between estrogen and breast cancer, so a long exposure (more than five years) to estrogen and high doses of estrogen are listed as potential risk factors. In addition, research shows that an estrogen plus progestin combination may increase your risk. Therefore, the following are risk factors:

- **Early menarche**, which means that you got your first period at an unusually young age, so your body has been exposed to estrogen for longer than normal.
- The longer exposure to estrogen also applies to **late menopause**.
- **Long-term hormone therapy** speaks for itself. If you're putting estrogen into your body you are increasing your exposure to it. This also applies to high doses of estrogen therapy (ET). The jury is still out concerning the length of time a woman may safely use ET but it seems as though a period of less than five years does not increase the risk. But ET may increase the growth of breast cells, breast density and breast pain, and it is thought that estrogen-progestogen therapy may make the interpretations of mammograms more difficult.
- Recently investigators following up on over 12 000 women who had been part of the original WHI study confirmed that **estrogen plus progestin therapy (EPT)** is related to increased breast cancer risk and while the cancers found in women not using HT were similar to women using it, those using EPT had more cancers in their lymph nodes and seemed to be at greater risk of dying of breast cancer. However, the risk of breast cancer increases with the length of time it is used, with both EPT and ET.
- It is also shown that when you stop using HT your risk of breast cancer decreases over time.
- **A late first pregnancy** is also a risk factor because in the first place you've had long-term exposure to estrogen, then during your pregnancy you have large amounts of estrogen coursing through your system at an age when you are starting to be at higher risk anyway.
- **If you've never had a baby** you could be at higher risk. This almost seems contradictory, but it relates to the hormone prolactin that is involved

in pregnancy and the production of milk, which inhibits the production of estrogen. The interruption of estrogen production in a woman's life for a significant amount of time is thought to be protective.

- **Dense breast tissue** is also related to hormones and studies of women with dense breast tissue show they are at more risk for breast cancer and should be particularly aware of this when opting to take HT. This is a risk factor because if your breast tissue is dense, it is more difficult to spot any abnormalities either during a clinical examination or a mammogram and many women who are on HT have much denser breast tissue. Interestingly, women who have had cosmetic plastic surgery of the breast, such as breast enlargement with implants or breast reduction, do not have increased risk of breast cancer, though mammograms need to be done more carefully on these women.

LIFESTYLE

Kim called me because she was really battling with terrible hot flushes and very bad night sweats. She had had a mastectomy a year previously at the age of 47, when estrogen receptor-positive breast cancer was discovered. To her horror, a few months later, she was diagnosed with cervical cancer, and had to have a total hysterectomy, where both her ovaries were removed. She was plunged into menopause. She was prescribed tamoxifen for at least five years. She certainly couldn't take HT and was worried about taking an antidepressant in case it interfered with the tamoxifen. As we talked, I listened to her husky throaty voice and the slight cough that followed her every laugh and asked her whether she was a smoker. 'I am,' she said, slightly abashed. I started on my usual spiel about why smoking just isn't okay but she quickly interrupted me: 'I know, I know ... it's no good telling me that. I'm just not ready to stop.'

I told Kim not to despair since there are antidepressant options that don't interfere with the action of tamoxifen and suggested she talk to her doctor about these.

The glaring red flag that came up when I chatted to Kim was that she was a heavy smoker. Though previously there did not seem to be a relationship between smoking and breast cancer, new research has shown that smokers are at greater risk for dying of breast cancer. In addition, smoking is an established risk for cervical cancer. Before she did anything else, Kim needed to quit. Unfortunately she couldn't take a well-known medication that might have helped her stop smoking because it contains bupropion, which may affect tamoxifen's actions. I understand that smoking is so addictive that it is very hard to stop, especially when you are dealing with all the emotional baggage that comes with cancer, but your health and survival may depend on quitting.

In this section, I have named some lifestyle risk factors that are associated with breast cancer. I believe that it is vital for women to understand their role in helping to reduce their risks for breast cancer. These risks include:

- **Being extremely overweight after menopause.** This is a risk because the enzyme aromatase, which is in the fatty tissues, can produce excess estrogen. Obviously your diet plays a part here since an unhealthy diet can lead to excess weight and part of an unhealthy diet is eating too many hydrogenated fats, which have been shown to put you at risk. (Hydrogenated fats are oils that have become solid during cooking, releasing trans fatty acids that are associated with raised cholesterol levels.)

  It is important to eat well. Choose a diet that is low in saturated fats (fried food and red meat) and high in vegetables including broccoli, cabbage, Brussels sprouts, kale and cauliflower and fruits. A good rule of thumb is to make sure that your daily diet includes something red, something yellow, something orange and something green from the fruit and vegetable families. (See Chapter 10 for more information on diet and weight.)

  Recent research into a type of breast cancer known as *triple negative breast cancer*, which is when the cancer is not estrogen receptor or progesterone receptor-positive and is not HER2, shows that obese women are more likely to suffer from this type of cancer than women who are thin. Triple negative breast cancer appears in between 10 and 20 per cent of women with breast cancer and has a poor prognosis because there are no specific medications that can target it.

- **Lack of exercise** contributes to excess weight and general unhealthiness, so this is a logical risk factor. Research has shown that **drinking more than two glasses of alcohol a day** is also very risky. The reason for this is that alcohol may increase the levels of estrogen in your blood or interfere with the way it is broken down and used effectively. This explains why a new study suggests that alcohol is strongly associated with estrogen receptor-positive breast cancer, while another showed that moderate to heavy drinking after breast cancer might increase the risk of a recurrence or even death. This seems to apply more strongly to overweight or postmenopausal women who are more susceptible to the effects of alcohol. If your liver doesn't do its job properly because of excess alcohol, it may not be able to get rid of harmful substances that may cause cancer.

- **Smoking** – as I explained earlier, has reared its ugly head as a lifestyle risk factor, since new research suggests that women who smoke are at much greater risk of dying from breast cancer than those who don't smoke. It has also been found that if you smoke your reconstructive breast surgery may not work; the flap may break down.

Recent research shows that a healthy lifestyle lowers your risk for invasive breast cancer after menopause, even if you have a family history of breast cancer. However, the problem is that even though you can take responsibility for your daily breast health, most cancers are so tiny when they start out that even an expert can't detect them with a physical examination. We know from research that it is better for us to treat cancers as early as possible, before they become aggressive or invasive. In fact, it's just common sense that a smaller tumour would probably be easier to treat, which is why I believe in regular screening.

STRATEGIES FOR DEALING WITH BREAST CANCER

Julie, who was in her forties, found out over the phone that she had cancer. She was told that she would be having surgery the following morning and would meet her surgeon for the first time in the pre-op ward of the hospital. When she ventured a protest she was told brusquely that it was her breast or her life! Within 24 hours she suffered both the trauma of learning she had cancer and a radical mastectomy (where the whole breast is removed, as well as some pectoral muscles, the chest muscles that move the arm).

For a year following the surgery she was in a deep depression, her balance had been altered, she felt ugly and she had had no counselling to help her deal with her trauma. Whenever she told the oncologist how down she felt, her feelings were brushed aside. 'You're alive,' she was told. 'What more do you want?' She was left with an underlying unresolved anger and felt depressed, guilty and ashamed that she wasn't more grateful to her 'saviour'.

Julie had every right to feel ill-treated. A year after the surgery she visited another oncologist and a surgeon who took the time and trouble to explain the process of breast reconstruction and performed the surgery that reconstructed Julie's breast. The surgeon dealt with her angst and despair, listened to her without judging her and helped her to find professional counselling.

It is now five years since her bout with breast cancer and though Julie is aware of the risks, she is living well and happily. I have included this story because I passionately believe that all women with cancer should be treated with dignity and respect; their partners and families should be involved; they should be entitled to clear and unambiguous explanations of their disease; they should have the right to question their doctors as much as they want to; and they should never be made to feel ignorant or helpless. They should also always be given the opportunity to get a second opinion on treatment decisions. A sympathetic atmosphere and appropriate counselling should be an integral part of the treatment and no woman should be bullied or rushed into a hasty decision about a mastectomy or other surgery. By the time the cancer is diagnosed it has been around for a while and it is far better to be allowed to make a careful and informed decision than to feel helpless, angry and patronised. Being treated with respect will help you to take control and be a partner with your specialist in fighting your cancer.

When you get the bad news, make an appointment to see your oncologist or cancer specialist. Make a list of questions. This applies to all medical consultations. I always tell my clients to keep a piece of paper and pen handy before an appointment and to write down anything that comes into their minds about their problem, no matter how trivial they might think it is. When you are shocked and emotional you won't be able to think clearly and if you write down whatever comes to mind during the time before the appointment with your specialist, you will be able to address issues that you might otherwise forget or suppress during the consultation. Ask about anything and everything. It is your body and your life, and you have the right to question your doctor. Never feel embarrassed or anxious about wasting his or her time. If you aren't satisfied with an answer or don't understand something, that's fine, ask for clarification. The doctor's job is not to be judgemental about your perceived level of intelligence; it is to help you heal as quickly as possible.

Take your partner or husband with you to the consultation. I think that the support of your family and friends is vital at this time. You set the boundaries and don't be afraid to ask for exactly what you want. I think children handle trauma such as a mother's illness better when the information they are given is straightforward and there are no hushed whispers and mystery surrounding the problem. Uncertainty is terribly frightening for a child.

Treatment options

Depending on the type of cancer you have and how advanced it is, there are different treatment options. Usually you will have some kind of surgery to remove the lump and the infected area. You should discuss the type of surgery with your specialist surgeon and the choice will probably depend on the size and position of the lump, the size of your breast, and what you hope for from the surgery. This is a good time for your surgeon to refer you to a plastic surgeon to discuss your options for reconstructive surgery. Many surgeons now work in conjunction with a plastic surgeon since research has shown that for many women immediate reconstruction seems to lessen the trauma of a mastectomy or lumpectomy. However, not all patients are good candidates for this upfront procedure and therefore it is very important for you to discuss it with your surgeon and ask about the risks involved.

During surgery for breast cancer it is common to leave a clear margin of 1 cm around the lump. At the same time the surgeon may surgically remove some of the sentinel lymph node under the armpit on the side of the breast that has the cancer to ascertain whether the cancer has spread. The sentinel node is the first node into which the duct in which the cancer is found drains. If the sentinel node is affected, your surgeon may remove more glands from the armpit to identify further involvement. Further treatment should be tailored to the needs of each individual. Cancer treatment should not be of the 'cookie cutter' variety. In the first place, treatment may differ depending on whether you are peri- or postmenopausal. So if a friend has had breast cancer and her treatment was different from yours, don't panic; your treatment will be the most effective for your particular cancer or your own circumstances.

Radiation therapy, which is when the cancerous area is blasted with high doses of X-ray, may be suggested after the surgery, usually after breast-conserving surgery such as a lumpectomy or segmentectomy, or after the chemotherapy to make sure that all the cancer cells are killed. Sometimes a woman may have radiation therapy or chemotherapy before the surgery if she has a large and aggressive tumour, to help shrink it and keep the cancer localised. In other cases she may first be given one of the two medications I write about below before her operation.

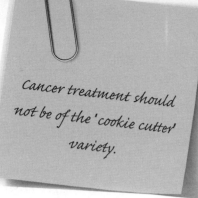

Cancer treatment should not be of the 'cookie cutter' variety.

After surgery some women will be given chemotherapy, which is a chemical treatment usually given as an intravenous treatment and sometimes as a pill, travelling through the bloodstream and killing the cancer cells in the body. The course usually takes several months (three to six months) and some women may have bad side effects, but once again, your individual coping mechanisms will dictate this. You may have heard the word *adjuvant* therapy – it simply means medical treatments given after surgery. If your doctor talks about *neoadjuvant*, it means medical treatments given before surgery.

If you have an estrogen receptor-positive (ER+) or a progesterone receptor-positive (PR+) tumour, or both, which means that exposure to one or both of these hormones the cells in the tumour to grow, a logical step would be either to suppress your estrogen or block the estrogen receptors throughout your body. This can be done surgically with a total hysterectomy and oophorectomy, where your womb and your ovaries are removed (see Chapter 6), or by giving you hormone treatment. This is not the HT that I have talked about throughout this book but a sort of 'anti'-hormone treatment or hormone blockade that is called *adjuvant endocrine therapy (adjuvant hormone therapy)*. It stops your own internal estrogen from reaching the estrogen receptors or stops your body from making estradiol. So women on this treatment may take tamoxifen as well as chemotherapy, or may not have chemotherapy at all and just take tamoxifen or an aromatase inhibitor, which blocks the enzyme aromatase from converting the androgens in your body to estrogens. It is thought that cancers develop in places where the activity of this enzyme is highest, like the breast.

As I explained in Chapter 4, tamoxifen is a selective estrogen receptor-modulator or SERM, which is now often called an estrogen agonist/antagonist (Eaa). This means it has an estrogen effect in certain areas of your body that will benefit you, and block unwanted estrogen effects in other parts of your body, so that the amount of active estrogen is not increased. Another SERM is called raloxifene (Evista); many studies have examined the risks and benefits of this medication, and have shown that it can lower the risk of invasive estrogen receptor-positive breast cancer. Unlike tamoxifen, it doesn't increase the lining of the your womb or the risk for endometrial cancer, but one of its bad side effects is that it increases the risk for thrombosis or clots, including deep-vein thrombosis and pulmonary embolism, so women who are at risk for blood clots or have a history of them should not use this medicine.

Another hormonal treatment involves *aromatase inhibitors* (AIs). *Letrozole* (trade name Femara), *anastrozole* (Arimidex) and *exemestane* (Aromasin) work by blocking an enzyme, aromatase (see Chapter 2), which is responsible for making small amounts of estrogen in postmenopausal women. The AI hampers the production of estrogen and actually reduces the total amount of estrogen in a woman's body so that less estrogen can reach the breast cancer cells. Aromatase inhibitors are used in postmenopausal women because they prevent the action of the enzyme aromatase, but they cannot prevent premenopausal women's ovaries from making estrogen. The problem with an AI is it makes you estrogen deficient, so it can give you a wide array of debilitating menopausal symptoms, including severe hot flushes and night sweats, weight gain, sleep problems, forgetfulness and breast sensitivity. One medical scientist referred to it as 'menopause plus' and suggests that your doctor try different AIs, if you are prescribed them, to see which one has the fewest side effects for you. AIs seem to have fewer risks than tamoxifen and raloxifene as far as blood clots are concerned and of course no risk for endometrial cancer.

An additional treatment option is *fulvestrant* (trade name Faslodex), which is an estrogen receptor antagonist. Unlike the estrogen agonist/antagonists discussed above, it doesn't just block the action of estrogen on the estrogen receptors, it eliminates this action and may be a good treatment option for those women whose breast cancer has progressed or recurred after treatment with tamoxifen and/or an AI. Fulvestrant is given as a monthly intramuscular injection (the medicine is injected directly into your muscle) and side effects include hot flushes, mild nausea and fatigue.

Another hormone-blocking treatment is *luteinising hormone-releasing hormone analogue* (LHRHa), such as *goserelin* (trade name Zoladex), which suppresses the LH (see Chapter 2 to remind yourself about LH) from your pituitary, which means that the production of estrogen from your ovaries is greatly reduced. LHRHas are now being tested as adjuvant therapies in addition to tamoxifen and only for premenopausal women.

The bad news is that while these treatments are dealing with your cancer, they may also be causing some very nasty side effects. You can understand why: tamoxifen blocks certain estrogenic effects; chemotherapy can induce menopause-type symptoms; and the removal of your ovaries will plunge you into menopause, causing all the symptoms of dropping estrogen levels that I discussed in Chapter 1. This is why tamoxifen is usually prescribed for no longer than five years, since long-term treatment with it may put you at risk for blood clots, endometrial cancer and sometimes the formation of cataracts. On the upside it may prevent bone loss and may have a beneficial effect on your cholesterol levels.

Unlike tamoxifen, AIs don't cause cancer of the womb and seldom, if ever, cause blood clots. But they can increase a woman's fracture risk because they remove almost all estrogen from a postmenopausal woman's body. Women using an aromatase inhibitor should discuss this risk with their doctors and have a bone density test to see whether they should also be taking a medication to strengthen their bones. There may also be certain side effects with aromatase inhibitors, such as joint pain and muscle aches. Research is still under way to determine the length of time women should be taking this treatment, but the usual period of time is also five years.

Women who use an aromatase inhibitor often battle with a dry vagina (vaginal atrophy), which can cause urinary problems and affect your sex life. The problem is that estradiol is the treatment that works best to alleviate this but you're taking these medications to suppress the actions of estrogen. Women who battle with cancer may also suffer debilitating hot flushes and night sweats, due to surgery, chemotherapy, depletion of estrogen or the suppression of estrogen receptors. The treatment of these symptoms is often very problematic. Using an antidepressant medication (SSRI or SNRI) off-label may help, both from the perspective of mood and the lessening of symptoms, but you should be careful not to take one that may interfere with your cancer treatments (pages 129–130). If you have disturbed sleep due to night sweats, ask your doctor about using the SSRI in conjunction with a sleeping medication containing *zolpidem*. Many women find even the smallest dose (5 mg) helps them sleep better.

Vaginal dryness cannot be solved with SSRIs and even though many oncologists believe that they shouldn't be giving these women ET, they are aware of and deeply sympathetic about the terrible symptoms affecting their patients' quality of life, especially when they're dealing with cancer and all it entails. Have a frank discussion with your specialist to see whether they are prepared to let you use a small dose of vaginal estradiol, either in the form of a pessary or an estrogen-containing ring, for a short time. Some doctors prefer you to use an estriol cream. However, there is no gold standard evidence-based research definitively saying there is no risk for breast cancer sufferers who use them. The most important caveat here is that you must be regularly monitored if you decide to use local vaginal estrogen; you may even be tested to see whether the tiny amount that may reach your system is affecting your blood estradiol levels.

There have been conflicting results in some randomised controlled trials about the use of HT in breast cancer survivors, and it is generally recommended by most menopause societies that HT and clinicians should be **extremely** careful before recommending any HT options, including tibolone (Livifem).

Researchers are constantly searching for new treatment options and at the moment one of these third-generation SERMs, *bazedoxifene*, is in Phase 3 trials (see Chapter 9) and is being explored as a potential agent to reduce the risk of, or delay, the development or recurrence of cancer. This is because it binds to both the two different estrogen receptors (alpha and beta) that I wrote about in Chapter 2, so it acts on the estrogen receptors in the skeletal tissue, helping to lower bone turnover (Chapter 9) but inhibits the activity of the estrogen receptors in the tissues of the breast and womb. This means that it does not lead to thickening of the lining of the womb as can happen with tamoxifen. Some studies are now under way to see whether a combination of bazedoxifene and conjugated estrogen may help menopausal symptoms in women who have breast cancer and also eliminate the need for a progestogen in women who still have their womb. In a recent study, *lasofoxifene*, another new SERM, shows promising results in lowering the risk of breast cancer and the risk of fractures; more long-term information is needed on both these SERMs.

Medical scientists are still looking for the perfect estrogen agonist/antagonist (Eaa). Some believe that this will be available within the next 10 years. Doctors hope this will have all the benefits of estrogen – especially as far as hot flushes are concerned – without the risks, and that in some cases they will be able to be combined with different types of estrogens. They will not be able to be used by women who are at high risk for clots, either deep-vein thrombosis or pulmonary embolisms.

Other adjuvant therapy treatments for advanced HER2 breast cancer include lapatinib and trastuzumab, which I mentioned earlier in Connie's story. Lapatinib is usually used in women with this kind of cancer who have already had chemotherapy. It is an *antineoplastic* drug and so you understand the meaning of this word, let's unpack it. A *neoplasm* is a new and abnormal growth in the tissue in some part of the body. The growths of the cells in the neoplasm are usually very fast and uncontrolled. Neoplastic is a way of describing a neoplasm, so antineoplastic is something that acts against the neoplasm.

The trial Connie described is called ALTTO (Adjuvant Lapatinib and/or Trastuzumab Treatment Optimisation), which has a huge sample number; well over 8 000 women in 50 countries worldwide. It will last for a year and the women in the trial will then be followed for 10 years after the date they started the medication. The study will examine whether lapatinib is effective in helping women with HER2-type breast cancer survive longer and whether it will prevent recurrence in early breast cancer. These women would first have had 12 to 18 weeks of chemotherapy. Lapatinib will be compared with four other treatments; trastuzumab by itself for a year or lapatinib only for a year or trastuzumab followed by a break for six weeks and then lapatinib for either 28 weeks or 34 weeks, or lapatinib and trastuzumab together for a year. Some results have already been published showing that in the lapatinib and trastuzumab arm of the trial, women had a better survival rate and their quality of life was improved, but in the Neo ALTTO study, which looked at the same treatments, though not in women who had had surgery first, preliminary results showed that lapatinib alone may not have such a promising effect. Some women may have some side effects with lapatinib, which include dry skin, diarrhoea, nausea, heartburn, fatigue, loss of appetite, mouth sores and some hair loss.

Trastuzumab is a *monoclonal antibody*. This is a small molecule that is made in a laboratory and has been specifically engineered to attach itself to certain areas in a woman's cancer cells. Antibodies are produced by your body's immune system in response to a threat like germs or other things that may threaten your health. Because your body doesn't always see cancer cells as a threat, monoclonal antibodies have been specially made to attach themselves to the cancer cells so that your immune system can be alerted to this threat. Trastuzumab has been made to target a particular type of cancer, HER2. The side effects of trastuzumab become less severe as treatment continues, but feel like flu with chills, fever, aching muscles and nausea. The most severe side effect could be heart disease issues, which might affect up to 4 per cent of the group of women receiving it in conjunction with some chemotherapy. Before you begin this drug your oncologist will refer you to a cardiologist to check your heart function.

BREAST RECONSTRUCTION

One of the biggest issues for most women who are told that they must have surgery is the removal or surgical excision of a breast or both breasts. Luckily plastic surgery has made such huge advances that many women who have had surgery for breast cancer can have their breasts reconstructed.

Reconstructive surgery means plastic surgery to restore or preserve the shape of the breast. In the past, surgeons and oncologists would recommend that women wait until after the completion of all their treatments before having their breast reconstruction, but today plastic surgery techniques are so advanced that immediate reconstruction – carried out at the same time as the breast surgery to remove the cancer – may be a good option for some women. This is called onco-reconstructive breast surgery.

There are several reasons for this. From a surgical perspective most plastic surgeons agree that the *aesthetic* result, the way the breast will look, is generally better when the surgery is done at the time of the mastectomy or lumpectomy. At one time reconstruction was only offered to women who had mastectomies; now, even if you've only had a small part of your breast removed, plastic surgery is available to restore balance and symmetry between the two breasts.

Sybil was in her late eighties when she was diagnosed with breast cancer, but she did not want the life-saving mastectomy procedure. When her surgeon asked her why not, she replied that she had been told she was too old to expect breast reconstruction. She had had a long and happy marriage and, as a deeply religious woman, she believed that when she died she would be reunited with her beloved husband. She explained to the surgeon that her husband had loved and admired her body, especially her breasts, which had been part of the very good sexual relationship they had enjoyed. She did not want to meet him again without one of her breasts.

The surgeon reassured her and said that she always worked with a plastic surgeon and they would make sure that she had a breast reconstruction at the time of her mastectomy without increasing the length of the operation. Sybil came through the treatment well and was very pleased with her 'new' breast. She lived a happy and cancer-free life for the next five years, and died peacefully in her sleep at the age of 94.

Research has shown that there may be a real psychological benefit in beginning the reconstructive process at the same time as the initial surgery. For some patients it may be life affirming at a very frightening time. Some women have found that after a consultation with their plastic surgeon they choose to have the kind of breasts they've always wanted and decide to have a breast reduction or breast enhancement after their lumpectomy or mastectomy.

So here is rule number one: When you have your first consultation with your surgeon you should ensure that you are referred to a plastic surgeon for an evaluation and a thorough discussion of your options in breast reconstruction. Many surgeons work in conjunction with a plastic surgeon and are very comfortable with this type of working relationship. There are those surgeons who believe, as Julie's surgeon did, that their job is to chop out the cancer and save your life, but since it is likely that you will still be alive 10, 15 or many more years after your initial surgery, others believe that in addition to treating your cancer you should also be offered a good quality of life. It seems that women who have breast reconstruction have a better self-image than those who don't. Breast removal without reconstructive surgery may adversely affect your self-esteem, your femininity, your sensuality and your sexuality. Not all women choose to have reconstruction, but all women should be equipped with enough information to make an informed decision.

You and your surgeon will decide when to do the reconstruction. Some surgeons will opt for immediate reconstruction if it is safe and feasible, because there is less scar tissue, which makes the plastic surgery easier, and there are good psychological benefits for some women. Other women prefer to deal with their cancer and have the appropriate treatments first. Once they have been cleared by their oncologists, they may then decide to have further surgery for a reconstruction. Once again, it depends on your personal decision and your oncologist's recommendations. Be aware of what suits you best. It is very important that before surgery your surgeon should discuss all your options with you and describe all the risks and benefits involved rather than 'push' you to have immediate reconstruction. Take your time to consider all the pros and cons.

There are upsides and downsides to reconstructive surgery, and it's important to remember that no matter how good the reconstructed breast is, it won't look as good as the original, though it can be pretty close. The upside of reconstructive surgery is that if you decide to have it sooner or later, it is an option that may help you to look and feel better and to wear the clothes you want to wear. Some women who have opted for this feel more at ease sexually and better psychologically. Women who decide not to have immediate breast reconstruction can use an external prosthesis, which is a specially designed unit that resembles a breast, which you put into your empty bra cup. There are many specialist shops that can help fit you with this and with a bra that suits you. There may be some trial and error until you find the one that suits you best.

There are two main methods of reconstruction. In implant reconstruction implants are placed under the chest muscle. In *flap reconstruction* the plastic surgeon uses your own body skin, muscle and fat from your tummy or elsewhere to reconstruct your breast. The two donor areas that are most commonly used are the back (*latissimus flap*), which is a relatively small operation, and the abdomen (*TRAM* or *DIEP flap*). The abdominal tissue flaps are the more popular option in eligible patients, though it requires more intensive surgery. The ideal patient is in good health, has some extra abdominal skin and fat without being significantly overweight and can tolerate a longer time in surgery and an extended recovery period. The use of implants may mean an easier recovery and is also a popular choice. Many surgeons think that when your own tissue is used, the reconstructed breast looks better and feels more realistic than a breast with an implant, but the complications of the flap reconstruction outlined above persuade some women, particularly very athletic or thin women, or those with careers on the line, to opt for the implant. Some surgeons think that if possible women who are going to be treated with radiation should have flap reconstructions, because the materials that make up the breast prosthesis do not radiate well. Often patients who require radiation therapy will start with the less invasive implant surgery and have a flap procedure once they have completed the cancer treatments.

There are no simple rules and the best reconstruction option for each patient should be carefully considered. The reality is that if you feel good about yourself, then whatever you've chosen is the right choice for you.

For implant reconstructions, the surgeon often starts with a temporary implant, known as a *tissue expander*, which will be put into your breast and gradually inflated in the surgeon's office until the size of the reconstructed breast matches that of the other breast. At a later date this tissue expander will be replaced, in a brief outpatient procedure, with a permanent implant. The advantage of this method is that each surgery is relatively quick, with a limited recovery time. In very thin patients, implant reconstructions are often excellent.

Finally, if your nipple and areola have been removed, they can be reconstructed under local anaesthetic about three months after the reconstruction. Some women say they can't be bothered about replacing the nipple, but many find they are much happier when their breast looks complete.

There are other types of cancers that affect women and I will cover these briefly, just to keep you informed and to enable you to recognise some of the warning signs and to know what questions you should ask your doctor and what questions they should be asking you.

Cervical cancer

Your cervix is the lower part of your womb that connects to your vagina. The best way to detect cervical cancer is by having a Pap smear once a year. In this procedure some of the cells of your cervix are scraped off painlessly and sent to a laboratory to be checked. Some cervical cells can look abnormal but are not cancerous or pre-cancerous. If there are abnormal cells, your cervix can be checked by a procedure known as a *colposcopy*, during which the cervix is examined with a powerful microscope that enables the specialist to look down your vagina. Colposcopy is only necessary to diagnose a premalignant condition (something that may or is likely to become cancerous.) Generally colposcopies in this area are done to see and treat CIN (*cervical intraepithelial neoplasia*) lesions, changes in the cervix that are not malignant.

Please note that even if you no longer have a cervix because your womb and cervix were removed after a Pap smear revealed abnormalities, you *must* still have an annual Pap smear to check for something doctors call *skip lesions*. These are unusual but it is wise to be cautious, so if you have had a hysterectomy for reasons other than an abnormal Pap smear, and are in a long-term, monogamous relationship, most experts suggest that you have a vault smear every 10 years, just to make sure all is well.

There is a lot of discussion about how often women should have a Pap smear, but even older monogamous women can have *human papilloma virus* (HPV), especially when they are becoming menopausal. I recently read of a case where a monogamous woman in her early fifties had tested positive for HPV after years of negative tests. This woman was obviously very upset and thought that her husband had been unfaithful to her, though he swore he hadn't. The medical experts explained that he was probably telling the truth. Some research suggests that there are perimenopausal women who can suddenly present with HPV even after years of having negative Pap smears. This is described as the second peak and is quite common in women of this age. They may have had an HPV infection in the past which lay dormant for many years and then reappeared. This may be because hormone fluctuations can affect a woman's immune system. Many midlife women find that their immune systems, which were previously strong, become less so. The healthy immune system has kept a prior HPV infection down but when it becomes compromised in some way, perhaps due to illness, the HPV virus may raise its ugly head again.

Of course there is always the possibility that this woman's husband had been messing around and this should obviously be taken into consideration. Some women also have affairs and should be tested. There are many different factors to be considered; for example, it is rare for older women who have had Pap smears year after year for a long period of time to get cervical cancer, but it has been shown that because of the state of the vagina, which becomes dryer after menopause, false positive tests may result, which can be distressing and lead to unnecessary treatment. Based on your individual risk profile, your healthcare practitioner should always take a sexual history, noting any new risk factors for HPV, and update it at your annual check-up. If you have had a lifestyle change, don't be afraid to admit it. Different countries and medical organisations have different recommendations, so based on these your doctor should help you decide how often you need to have a Pap smear. It is probably safe for older women following two-three consecutive negative Pap smears to have one every three years.

Women are at risk for cervical cancers if they *smoke*, have had *many sexual partners*, or have a *partner who has had many sexual relationships*. This is because they are at greater risk of catching the HPV, which is acquired through sexual intercourse and which research has shown to be strongly associated with cervical cancer and cancer of the vulva (the external genital parts that lead into your vagina). HPV is one of the strongest factors implicated in the risk of getting cervical cancer. Many women have HPV and while doctors believe that this virus must have infected women with cervical cancer, it is very important to understand that **not** all HPVs cause cancers. HPVs are a group of more than 100 types of viruses called papilloma viruses because some of them can also cause warts, or papillomas, which are benign tumours.

However certain 'high-risk' types of HPV can cause cancer of the cervix. These types include HPV16 and 18. About two-thirds of all cervical cancers are caused by HPV16 and 18. Currently there is no cure or treatment for the HPV infection, but the infection can disappear without treatment because a woman's immune system will successfully fight the virus. The good news is that there are now two vaccines available: *Gardasil*, which protects against HPV6, 11, 16 and 18, and *Cervarix*, which protects against HPV16 and 18.

Although these vaccines are recommended for women younger than 26, some research suggests that women who are at risk, such those who are very sexually active and have multiple partners, should be vaccinated. There are several trials under way at the moment to develop vaccines to broaden cancer protection by including protection against HPV31, 33, 45, 52 and 58.

Apart from ensuring that you have a Pap smear once a year, you should be aware of the following signs that might indicate cervical cancer: painful intercourse, bleeding after sex and pain while urinating (though these could be attributed to a dry vagina from an estrogen deficiency), lower back pain, abnormal bleeding, or an unusual discharge from your vagina. If you change your partner or are at a high risk for carrying HPV, some doctors will test for HPV together with the Pap smear. If you have daughters, they should be vaccinated against HPV, probably when they reach puberty, to decrease their risk of cervical cancer.

Once you have been diagnosed with cervical cancer, spend some time with your oncologist discussing your treatment options. The colposcopy that I described above will have alerted your doctor to anything abnormal; the biopsy that follows it will have taken a section of the tissues and cells so that they can be examined by a pathologist to confirm your doctor's diagnosis. If the lesions are malignant, your doctor will recommend a hysterectomy, which may have to be an extended hysterectomy, in which the womb, the top of the vagina and the surrounding lymph glands are removed. Your doctor may call this *Wertheim's hysterectomy*. If a woman's reproductive years are over, an oophorectomy (removal of the ovaries) will also be performed (see Chapter 6). The surgery may be followed by the appropriate cancer treatment – radiation or chemotherapy. Research has found that radiation therapy may be very effective.

Endometrial cancer

The endometrium is the lining of your womb (see Chapter 1). It is a well-documented fact that endometrial cancer, cancer of the lining of the womb, is usually associated with *unopposed estrogen* or *excessive levels of estrogen*, where the lining of the womb builds up because you are on an HT regimen of estrogen only and do not have the monthly bleed associated with progesterone (see Chapter 1).

Even if you are on continuous, combined HT, don't be lulled into thinking that you are not at risk. An imbalance in the estrogen and progestin you are taking can still cause the lining of your womb to become too thick. If you still have your womb, you should have an annual vaginal ultrasound examination to evaluate the lining of your womb.

It is interesting that the risk of endometrial cancer increases with the number of years you have been on estrogen-only therapy. You remain at risk for several years after you have discontinued the hormone therapy. So today it is standard practice, if you still have a womb, to take a progestogen along with estrogen. Research has shown that taking the two together, which is called *continuous combined therapy*, may be safer than taking them sequentially, which means taking the estrogen first for a couple of weeks followed by the progesterone. A progesterone-releasing intrauterine device inserted into your uterus is another option because this can be very effective in preventing a build-up of the lining of your womb. In Chapter 4, I wrote that if you are taking HT and you have a womb, you must be monitored regularly. The same applies to women who have kept their wombs and are taking tamoxifen – studies show that these women are at greater risk for endometrial cancer and should be checked when this is prescribed, and then annually by means of a transvaginal ultrasound.

All women who have kept their wombs, especially those on HT, should have an annual gynaecological examination. You should also have yourself checked if you are experiencing unusual bleeding, if you have problems when you urinate, if sex is very painful, or if you have pain in your pelvis. If you are not on HT you may have *vaginal atrophy*, which is the drying up of your vagina and which may account for some of your symptoms. The pelvic examination will reveal this. Your gynaecologist should examine your pelvis to see if your uterus has become abnormally enlarged. She or he should then, as a matter of course, do a transvaginal ultrasound, which will show if there are any abnormal features in your uterus.

During the ultrasound examination your doctor will measure the lining of your womb to see if it is thicker than the normally accepted range. He or she will then decide whether further investigation is needed and will take a sample of the lining by inserting a *pipette*, which is a thin, flexible tube, into your womb and removing a small amount of the lining. This sample will be sent to the lab, where a pathologist will examine it to see if there are pre-cancerous or cancerous cells.

Some doctors may prefer to do a D&C (*dilation and curettage*; a surgical procedure performed under general anaesthetic, where the neck of the womb is stretched – dilation – and a surgical instrument is used to remove the lining and contents of the womb – curettage), but this is more invasive and hence the need for an anaesthetic.

But there are some doctors who are now qualified to do an outpatient hysteroscopy (Chapter 6) that will allow you to recover more quickly since you don't need a general anaesthetic. This is probably a more controlled and accurate way of obtaining tissue for evaluation from suspicious areas. Note that if you are taking tamoxifen you should have the lining of your womb screened every six months. If you have bleeding, your doctor should take a sample of the lining and may do this using a *hysteroscopic-directed biopsy*, either as an outpatient procedure or under general anaesthetic.

If your cells are shown to be pre-cancerous or cancerous your doctor or specialist will discuss the different treatment options with you. If the cells are pre-cancerous but you don't show any risk factors – you are not on unopposed estrogen, you are not overweight, you don't smoke or drink to excess, or have high blood pressure or diabetes – your doctor may monitor you within three months, or may prescribe a high-dose progestogen.

If the cells are cancerous the treatment follows much the same route as treatment for cervical cancer. Surgery is performed after careful clinical evaluation of the stage that the cancer has reached. This will determine the extent of the operation. Samples of tissue from the organs that have been removed will be checked for cancerous cells. After surgery, depending on what you and your oncologist have decided, you will have the appropriate cancer treatment, which might involve radiotherapy or chemotherapy, or both.

Colorectal cancer (colon cancer and rectal cancer)

Many midlife women who take their health seriously and are meticulous about having their annual mammograms are strangely careless when it comes to screening for colon cancer. Yet colon cancer is third highest on the list of deaths from cancer. The good news is that regular screening and detecting the early stage cancers that start in the tissue lining of the bowel could drastically reduce this death rate. These often manifest as *polyps*, which are small, benign growths on the lining of your colon and *rectum*. The colon is the part of your digestive system where water, minerals and nutrients are absorbed from undigested food, before it is eliminated; it is approximately 1.85 m (6 ft) in size. The rectum is the last part of the large intestine, which leads to your *anus*, where stools are kept until you are ready to evacuate them; it is about 15.24 cm (6 in.) in size.

Many midlife women battle with irritable bowel problems and as you will see below, some of these symptoms are similar to the symptoms of colon cancer, so it is really important to check out any changes in your bowel habits. Some of the symptoms of colon cancer are diarrhoea, constipation or a feeling that you have not emptied your bowels completely, or blood in your stools (sometimes this blood can be due to piles or haemorrhoids but don't assume this; in any case you should deal with that problem too). You may also feel bloated, fuller than usual and have frequent pains from gas or cramps. In addition, your weight may suddenly drop, you may vomit frequently and may feel constantly exhausted. If you are battling with these symptoms, your doctor will send you to a specialist who will take a family history and do a rectal examination, which isn't pleasant.

Some doctors will then decide to make an appointment for you to return to have a *sigmoidoscopy* in their rooms. This involves inserting a sigmoidscope – a tube with a light and small video camera at the end that is connected to a display monitor – into your anus so they can examine your rectum and colon. Before this procedure you will have to clear out your digestive system and your doctor will give you a series of instructions to follow the day before, including drinking only clear liquids and taking a laxative. This test, which takes up to 20 minutes, will allow the doctor to see your whole rectum but only part of your colon. It is uncomfortable, but you should not need to be sedated for it.

Your doctor may prefer you to have a *colonoscopy*. Before this procedure you will have to clear out your digestive system and your doctor will give you a series of other instructions to follow and a laxative to help you. You will be sedated during the procedure, which should take about half an hour. During the colonoscopy your doctor will examine your colon by inserting an instrument called a colonoscope, which is like a longer type of sigmoidscope, into your anus so that they can see what's going on in your rectum and colon on the display monitor that is attached to it. They are able to pass instruments down the colonoscope to enable them to take some tissue samples, or to remove smaller polyps so they don't have a chance to grow and possibly become cancerous. You will need someone with you to take you home after the procedure, and since air is inserted into your colon you may feel a bit bloated and have some discomfort. Your doctor may prefer you to have an X-ray test first called a *barium enema*, where a white chalky liquid coats your colon and rectum and highlights any abnormal areas. Like both of the above tests, you will need to clean out your bowel the day before and not eat after 10 pm that night. If any problems show up on the imaging, your doctor can then recommend a colonoscopy.

These tests may reveal several different types of cancers. The most common is *adenocarcinomas* (growths that form in the glandular tissue cells of the colon and rectum that make mucus, and may become cancerous); most colorectal cancers are of this type. However, there are other types, including gastrointestinal stromal tumours, carcinoid tumours, lymphomas and sarcomas, which your doctor will describe in detail. The treatment will depend on the type and stage of the cancer you have (how advanced it is, and where it has spread). The treatment options include surgery of different kinds that may remove the cancer. If your specialist is concerned that some cancer remains, you may have chemotherapy or radiation treatment.

The problem with colon cancer is that because it usually takes so long to develop, the symptoms only occur in the advanced stage.

The problem with colon cancer is that because it usually takes so long to develop, the symptoms only occur in the advanced stage, so it is vital to have regular screening, since this may prevent colon cancer, and the recovery rate is very good if it is detected early. Risk factors that you can't avoid for colon cancer include age (most cases of it are detected after 50), a personal history of polyps or adenomas, or a bout of colon cancer when you were younger. If you have Crohn's disease or ulcerative colitis, which are called inflammatory bowel disease (IBD), you are at risk. IBD is different from irritable bowel syndrome, which doesn't carry the risk of colorectal cancer. Other risks include a family history of colorectal cancer and your ethnic or racial background. Ashkenazi Jews are very prone to this type of cancer, due to some genetic mutations, as are African Americans. Another risk factor is type 2 diabetes. However, there are lifestyle risks that are strongly linked to colorectal cancer and you can make a difference here. Eat sensibly; your diet should not be high in red meat and processed foods. A regular exercise routine is a must; follow the recommendations in Chapter 7. Maintain a healthy weight, drink in moderation and don't smoke.

I understand that most of us feel reluctant to be screened for colorectal cancer since many of the tests are unpleasant, but I would strongly recommend that as you transition into menopause these tests become as important as your annual mammograms. From 50 onwards, experts suggest the following: sigmoidoscopy, every three to five years. Earlier screening will probably be recommended if you have a strong family history of colon cancer. Have a *Faecal Occult Blood Test* (FOBT) every year. This test shows, under a microscope, whether you have blood in your stools but is not the gold standard for detecting colorectal cancer; it just acts as a red flag. Your doctor may ask you to give two or three samples on consecutive days. It may be wise to have a colonoscopy every 10 years too. If you have a strong family history of colorectal cancer you should start all screening earlier and your healthcare practitioner should help you plan for these check-ups.

Ovarian cancer

Sandy has a pretty, pixie-like face; she would have been blonde except that she lost all her hair while undergoing chemotherapy. She was a good example of the difficulty of diagnosing ovarian cancer.

*For many months Sandy had been experiencing stomach problems. None of the medications prescribed by her GP seemed to bring her relief. She found that although she was not putting on weight, her stomach had become so bloated that she was unable to fasten her jeans or the waistband of her skirts. By the time she ended up at a gynaecologist specialising in ovarian cancer she had seen several doctors, including her GP, her regular gynaecologist and a gastrointestinal specialist who did a series of tests, including those for heart failure, liver failure and lung problems. All came up negative. Feeling absolutely desperate and terribly unwell, she begged her sister to get her an appointment with her own gynaecologist. He did an ultrasound and saw that her abdomen was full of fluid. He drew off some of this fluid and when it was tested, found it to have certain ovarian cancer biomarkers. This doctor referred her to the specialist in ovarian cancer, who for the **first** time since she had seen all these doctors gave her an internal examination, and actually felt the lumps that were present; a primary indication that all was not well.*

Sandy's story may not have a happy ending since she now has Stage 4 ovarian cancer, but what all women can learn from it is that when you see a gynaecologist, he or she must do an internal examination especially if you are complaining of any of the following symptoms, which are described below but are so important that I'm repeating them: continuous stomach pain or pain in your pelvis, persistent ongoing bloating (not bloating that comes and goes just after you've eaten) and an increased abdominal circumference, even though you haven't gained weight, difficulty eating and feeling full too quickly. In addition to these you may have changes in bowel habits or urinary symptoms and at the same time feel extremely tired and have back pain. Don't be embarrassed to have these checked and, if they persist, get a second opinion.

The words ovarian cancer strike dread into the hearts of most women and their doctors. The reason is that the survival rate of women with ovarian cancer is poor. It is a deadly and silent cancer, and is often only detected when it is quite far advanced. Because your ovaries contain reproductive tissue the cells are programmed to grow, but when this programming alters, abnormally fast growth of cells and tissues takes place. These little growths may be benign, which means that they stay in one place in the ovary and don't move into the surrounding areas, but in some cases the growths are cancerous and start to invade the neighbouring tissue.

You may have been told by your gynaecologist during an examination that you have an *ovarian cyst* (a sac filled with fluid). You may want to look back at Delia's story in Chapter 7. The rule is that all ovarian cysts in postmenopausal women should be investigated. If they are benign, there is no problem. It is only when the cysts are malignant that doctors worry.

The most common reason for ovarian cysts is that a little egg-containing follicle in the ovary, which I described in Chapter 1, grows bigger and doesn't burst – sometimes it releases the egg, sometimes it doesn't. In the normal course of events this little follicular cyst will shrivel up, but sometimes it just remains. If the cysts are benign, the best treatment is conservative. In other words, your doctor will keep an eye on them with regularly scheduled vaginal ultrasound examinations. There are other little cysts in the ovary called *endometriotic cysts*, which are filled with blood and can become very painful, but they are not necessarily dangerous. When these are noticed on an ultrasound scan your doctor will make an informed decision about how to deal with them. Some specialists will do a blood test called a CA-125, which screens for cancer. This test shows a certain substance, present in cancerous cells, that has been released into the blood. However, some doctors are wary of a result that shows raised levels of CA-125 because other conditions, such as gastrointestinal cancer, can also cause this elevation. In any case, an ultrasound scan of the ovaries is much more sensitive. Your specialist will carefully examine the ultrasound features of the ovary together with the CA-125, which will guide them as to whether it is malignant or not.

Ovarian cysts are not usually cause for alarm unless they are increasing rapidly or have certain abnormal features that show up on an ultrasound. If you tend to get them you may find that once your ovaries stop their reproductive function after menopause, you may no longer be troubled with them. If you are perimenopausal and battle with painful ovarian cysts, many doctors prescribe an oral contraceptive, which stops you ovulating, so that your ovaries 'quieten down'. If you are still having your periods, you may find that ovarian cysts often disappear within a couple of menstrual cycles and if your doctor is concerned, he or she can repeat the transvaginal ultrasound within a couple of months to see whether the cyst has disappeared or if there is a change in appearance.

The strongest risk factor for ovarian cancer is those women with a family history (mother, sister or daughter) of the disease. Second-tier relatives, like aunts and grandmothers, also constitute a risk but it is not as high. Some women who have a genetic mutation in their BRCA1 and BRCA2 genes and are susceptible to breast cancer may also be at risk for ovarian cancer. It is thought that women who have never had children may be at greater risk for ovarian cancer than those who have. Your risk for ovarian cancer increases with age. However, it is now thought that long-term users of the low-dose oral contraceptive (more than 10 years) may be protected from ovarian cancer because this pill stops ovulation. Don't forget though that there may be an increased risk of breast cancer among long-term oral contraceptive users, so we need more research to clarify this.

Research about the role of HT in increasing the risk of ovarian cancer is contentious, and the association, if there is one, between HT use (more than five years) and ovarian cancer is very rare. Some observational research has shown that HT, regardless of length of use, dose, route of administration or whether it is EPT and ET, is associated with an increased risk of ovarian cancer in women who use it as opposed to those who do not, though this risk decreases once therapy is stopped, but until further definitive data is provided it seems that the absolute risk is very small.

Sometimes ovarian cancers may be misdiagnosed, so be aware of certain symptoms such as swelling and bloating, which may occur as the tumour grows in the ovary. A woman may feel nauseous or suffer other symptoms that are usually associated with indigestion, like gas and bloating, and a general feeling of being too full, which often results in a loss of appetite. She may also suffer from diarrhoea or constipation.

Be alert for ongoing symptoms of indigestion that aren't cured with the appropriate medicine. A gynaecologist friend remarked that he remembered an old professor at medical school telling the class of the many times he had seen 'ovarian cancers drowning in a sea of antacids'!

A biopsy should **never** be done on the ovaries. The most effective way for your doctor to determine if the growth is cancerous is to do a laparotomy, a procedure I wrote about in Chapter 5. The incision in this surgery should not be a bikini cut but a proper up-and-down cut. At the time of this procedure the surgeon will determine whether there is a malignancy. Once this is identified, specific surgery is performed, usually a total hysterectomy, which includes the womb, fallopian tubes and ovaries.

The apron of fat which hangs from the large bowel is also removed (*omentectomy*) and any other tumours greater than 1 cm or those that can be felt during the surgery, which may mean removing some of the bowel. The surgeon will send all the removed tissue plus the fluid that was in the cavity (*washings*) for diagnosis and staging. Staging is a process to see how far the cancer has spread, especially if it is not obvious to the surgeon during the surgery. Staging is very important because it helps the surgeon and the oncologist to decide on the correct form of follow-up treatment, depending on the extent and type of cancer. If an expert does not do this type of surgery then any cancer that has spread outside the ovary may be missed and not properly treated.

Some gynaecologists who don't have the ability to perform this meticulous routine or the knowledge to diagnose this type of cancer want to be conservative and try not to do this extensive surgery, but it is very dangerous and the patient may then require repeat surgery and/or additional therapy.

I mentioned that if you are diagnosed with breast cancer you should consider your options carefully. If you have been diagnosed with ovarian cancer, my sense is that speed is of the essence; usually because by the time it is diagnosed it will be quite far advanced. Ovarian cancer patients usually have chemotherapy after surgery, but because there are different types of ovarian cancer your oncologist will decide on the most effective course of treatment and will inform you whether radiation therapy would be beneficial in your particular case.

Paget's disease

Many women don't know that Paget's disease is also a type of breast cancer. It usually shows up as an irritation of the nipple, which looks like some kind of skin problem because the area is inflamed, red, crusty and may sometimes ooze, so dermatologists and other doctors may mistake it for some kind of common skin dermatitis and prescribe a cream to soothe it. Be alert. Paget's disease means that there is cancer in the milk ducts of the breast that has spread to the nipple.

Vaginal cancer

Many peri- and postmenopausal women suffer from itchy and dry vaginas caused by low levels of estrogen. If you have this problem and the condition is not helped by the application of topical estrogen or an estrogen ring, you need to make sure that there is nothing untoward going on by making an appointment for a thorough vaginal examination and the accompanying screens, because vaginal cancer may occur in middle age.

EMPOWER YOURSELF

- Know about the symptoms for the different cancers and have regular health check-ups and screening.
- The Breast Cancer Risk Assessment Tool was updated in 2011 and may be a useful guideline if you are worried about breast cancer. Discuss it with your doctor. (http://www.cancer.gov/bcrisktool/about-tool.aspx#gail)
- Don't be embarrassed to challenge your doctor if you have unusual symptoms; no one knows your body better than you do. Better to feel stupid than sorry.
- Don't rush into surgery without considering all the options and getting a second opinion.
- Make a comprehensive list of questions before your consultation. Some people get flustered or anxious when facing their doctors. Take someone with you to make notes, or use a tape recorder. It is impossible to assimilate all the information you will be given when you are in a highly emotional state.
- Live as healthily as possible but don't ever blame yourself if you get cancer.
- Be sure to have an annual gynaecological examination. An annual mammogram is a must if you have specific, individual reasons, are older than 50, or are on HT. For peace of mind, if you are at high risk for breast cancer, arrange to have an ultrasound every six months in addition to your annual examination.
- Work in partnership with your oncologist to get the best out of your treatment. If something worries you or you don't understand some point of information, don't be afraid to ask over and over again until you are satisfied that you understand what's going on.
- Once you are diagnosed, get good counselling. Having a safe place to let off steam, scream, weep and shout will help you deal with those overwhelming feelings.
- A brilliant cancer glossary can be found at http://www.cancer.org/Cancer/CancerGlossary/index.aspx

9
The bare bones: menopause and osteoporosis

Nina is a pretty, vivacious woman in her late fifties; small boned and petite, she glows with health. She started having very irregular periods when she was 40. When she told her gynaecologist, at the time, he didn't seem worried.

'He told me that it was normal and when I went back to him at 42 because my periods had stopped altogether, he told me once again that it was normal. I trusted him so I did nothing about it.'

The next time she saw him he did some hormone tests. 'He told me that I had no estrogen in my body whatsoever but that since I was so young he felt it was only the onset of menopause.'

Once again he did nothing, and she stayed with his practice for the next five years. Then she started hearing her friends discussing their menopausal symptoms. Many of them were going to the same gynaecologist, a different one from the one she consulted. 'They raved about him and, because they seemed to know so much about menopause, I felt I should be seeing the doctor from whom they had learnt everything.

'I changed doctors but I didn't really like his practice; the waiting room was overcrowded, he never spent quality time with me and when I saw him, he kept interrupting my appointment to talk to other patients on his constantly ringing phone. It was like being part of a factory assembly line. To be fair, he did tell me to have a bone density test, which had never been suggested to me before. I had the scan and then thought nothing more about it.

'Five months later I ran into some friends who were talking about their bone density scans and I realised I hadn't heard anything about my results, but thought this was probably because my bones were normal. I never imagined there could be a problem because I felt so well, but I thought I'd better phone my doctor and ask.'

> Nina called the doctor's receptionist, who took the file through to the doctor. 'He obviously had someone with him. I heard the receptionist give him my file. When he was talking to me he used my name all the time, which made me very uncomfortable because I knew he had a patient with him. I asked for my bone scan results. I heard him riffling through papers, then he suddenly said: "Oh my God! You've got very bad osteoporosis in both your hip and spine. You must go onto to a bisphosphonate immediately!"
>
> '"What's osteoporosis?" I asked him – I'd never heard of the condition. He explained briefly and irritably. I was really upset and asked him why no one had come back to me with my results, which were obviously serious, in the five months that had passed since I had my test.
>
> He said impatiently: "This is a huge practice; my nurses can't waste their time phoning everyone with their results." I thought he had a point as far as cases where the results were normal were concerned, but if results came back which showed that something was seriously wrong, I felt it was his responsibility to inform his patients. I ended up at a specialist bone clinic. Today I take Fosamax once a week and my bones aren't bad at all.'

It is clear that Nina was treated very badly. Her first doctor didn't explain to her that a woman's periods become erratic in perimenopause or test her hormone levels. Even when she told him that her periods had stopped completely he still didn't test any levels and, in addition, gave her wrong information based on his assumption that because she was young she was not yet in full menopause.

When her next doctor eventually had her hormone levels tested and saw that the estrogen levels were very low, he never explained about the different levels of estrogen. To say that she had 'no estrogen whatsoever in her body', is as you know from Chapter 1, absolute nonsense. He never suggested that she have a mammogram or a bone density scan. He didn't check her levels of vitamin D or see whether she was getting enough elemental calcium.

Although he advised her to have a bone density scan, her doctor didn't even bother to look at the test results or inform her that she had bad osteoporosis. He also took no responsibility for his negligence, which could have had serious consequences if Nina's condition had been left untreated.

He violated patient/doctor confidentiality by naming her and discussing her condition in front of another person who may have known her.

The worst part of Nina's story is that so many years elapsed while she was losing bone density, so she never treated the problem with calcium, vitamin D, hormones or bisphosphonates (drugs that slow bone loss). I think the doctors *assumed* that because she was young, did not drink or smoke, and exercised regularly, that she was not at risk. Remember, osteoporosis is a silent disease and often the first sign that there is a problem is when a woman finds she has a fracture, especially a vertebral fracture (fracture of the vertebrae in your spine), which can happen without pain and without falling. Another way that your doctor may diagnose osteoporosis is height loss over the years. A wrist fracture can occur at quite an early age and may be a warning sign of early osteoporosis. In any case there are several ways to diagnose osteoporosis and merely looking at a patient isn't one of these. Ways to determine whether there is a problem are to do a thorough medical history, a physical examination and a bone density scan, in conjunction with a fracture risk calculation and, in some cases, to take blood tests.

Osteoporosis is a hot topic in menopause. Some practitioners now refer to it as *bone fragility*. It has become very controversial because until recently the gold standard treatment for peri- and postmenopausal women with osteoporosis was estrogen replacement therapy, but the WHI study challenged this thinking and ideas changed. The study showed that women who were taking HT had an overall 24 per cent reduced risk for total fractures but that the other problems – increased risk of stroke, heart disease and breast cancer – did not seem worth the gain in bone density. Furthermore, other research shows that a couple of years after a woman stops taking estrogen the improvement in bone density is lost.

Books about osteoporosis seem to follow the same trend as many books about menopause. They are very dense and there are pages and pages of scientific information about osteoclasts and osteoblasts. As I researched this chapter I realised that osteoporosis is a rather dry subject, but you do need some technical information in order to understand it properly. Once again, knowledge is power. Once you have grasped the facts you will be empowered and able to take charge of your health in this area, so persevere, even if you have to read some of what follows a couple of times.

UNDERSTANDING BONES

The human skeleton is made up of bone, which develops in babyhood and carries on growing until we reach our peak bone mass in our mid-twenties.

The phrase 'bone mass' refers to bone density, which is the quantity of bone in a certain area. Imagine two pieces of Emmenthal cheese exactly the same size. The one has large holes and only a little cheese, the other has small holes and a lot of cheese. The latter is denser than the former.

When bones are at peak density, they are at their optimal strength. Bones are made up of a protein called *collagen*, which provides the framework of the bone, and a mineral substance called *calcium phosphate*, which adds strength to the bone and makes the framework harder. We have two types of bone: *trabecular*, which is spongy and softer, and *cortical*, which is very hard. Trabecular bone is found at the ends of long bones and in the spine, while the cortical bone on the outside makes up the shaft of the bones. This combination of hard and soft materials makes bones more flexible and stress resistant.

Because bone is made up of these tissues, it doesn't remain static when we reach peak bone density in our twenties. Throughout our lives, the bone tissue is breaking down and then being built up again. Interestingly, the body ensures that the bone material is distributed in areas that are under the greatest stress. As we get older, in areas where there has been a lot of wear and tear, and that need to be repaired or strengthened, the older bone material is replaced with new bone material. Obviously the old bone can't just stay there so the body breaks down the old bone tissue and ensures that it is removed by cells in the bone known as *osteoclasts*.

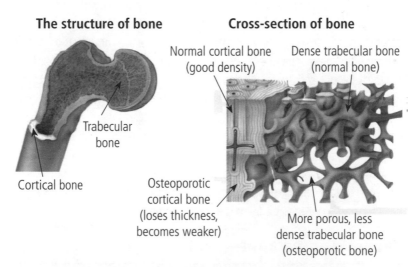

The structure of bone

Cross-section of bone

Normal cortical bone (good density)

Dense trabecular bone (normal bone)

Trabecular bone

Cortical bone

Osteoporotic cortical bone (loses thickness, becomes weaker)

More porous, less dense trabecular bone (osteoporotic bone)

Diagram showing normal bone and osteoporotic bone

Based on drawings from a poster produced by Hologic, SA Scientific.

During this process, which is known as *resorption*, calcium and phosphorus are released into the blood. Once this has occurred the new bone material replaces the old material, using other bone cells known as *osteoblasts*. This process is called *formation*, and the two actions together are called *bone remodelling*. The greatest amount of bone turnover takes place in the trabecular bone, which as I wrote above, is mainly in the vertebrae of the spine and in the ends of the long bones like the femur, which fits into your hip joint.

The osteoclasts break down the old bone tissue, then the osteoblasts take over, building the new bone tissue before it is absorbed into this new layer of collagen and bone minerals, where it becomes an *osteocyte*. It is actually the osteocytes, embedded in the bone, that send out the messages to the body that a specific area needs to be remodelled for one reason or another, such as stress, damage or wear and tear. Osteoclasts and osteoblasts have another very important job: they regulate the supply of calcium in the body.

As I wrote in Chapter 5, calcium maintains the cell structure and is a mineral that is essential for bone formation and cardiovascular, nerve and muscle functioning. It is also very important in metabolising food, so too little calcium may mean that you put on weight. Because it is such an integral part of a healthy body's functioning, calcium needs to be maintained, not only in the bones but also in the blood. Calcium imbalance, too much (*hypercalcemia*) or too little (*hypocalcemia*), can lead to a wide variety of symptoms. Too much induces a feeling of exhaustion, weight gain, high blood pressure, dehydration, depression, an irregular heartbeat and, in extreme cases, coma. Too little results in muscle cramps, irregular heartbeat, low blood pressure and sometimes seizures.

Resorption and the process of remodelling, which continues throughout the life of the body, is controlled (once again) by the hormones, in particular *parathyroid hormone* (PTH), which regulates calcium and phosphorus in the blood, and estrogen, testosterone and *calcitonin*, which influence the activity of the osteoclasts, the cells that break down bone material.

THE IMPORTANCE OF ESTROGEN

This is probably the best point at which to write a bit about the vital role that estrogen plays in maintaining women's bone density and the reason why, in the peri- and postmenopausal years, we lose bone so quickly. While we are young, healthy, reproductive adults with normal circulating levels of estrogen, the places in our body where bone is remodelled (the remodelling sites) are controlled by estradiol.

As I wrote above, estrogen influences the activity of the osteoclasts, whose job it is to break down bone material. Because the estrogen limits their activities, we don't lose bone in the normal course of events, but as we become peri- and postmenopausal and our estrogen levels fluctuate and drop, this carefully regulated activity of bone resorption speeds up. The osteoclasts at sites all over the body begin to get overactive, breaking down more bone material and releasing more calcium and phosphate into the blood. The body can't deal with too much calcium phosphate because there isn't enough calcium and vitamin D naturally in our bodies to replace the minerals we are losing. Because we are losing more bone material than we are replacing, our bones become fragile and our risk of fracture is greatly increased. This is why doctors may recommend that women who have an early surgical menopause, causing a sudden drop in their levels of estrogen, should consider taking estrogen therapy if it is medically allowed. Research has shown that premature menopause often leads to rapid bone loss and a higher risk of osteoporosis and fractures.

Osteoporosis is a condition in which bones may fracture with very little force and sometimes no force at all. It is one of the major contributory causes of death in elderly women and a powerful reason for the diminished quality of life of women who suffer hip or vertebral fractures and/or multiple fractures as a result of this silent disease. Women who have osteoporosis die at an earlier age than those without it and suffer enormous pain and distress as a result of their crumbling bones. If you are going to live a long and healthy life you need to be extremely aware of the risks for this disease and try to prevent it if you can.

As I mentioned, if you are fortunate enough to have peak bone density, you have a much lower risk of fracture, but as we age, both bone density and bone strength decline. When bone loss occurs, it affects the bone density, which in turn affects the strength of the bones. Because we lose bone density and strength as we get older, we need to be able to predict whether we are at risk for fracture and take steps to reduce this risk.

BONE MINERAL DENSITY AND BONE STRENGTH

Apart from the actual density of the bone (the amount of bone material packed into a certain volume of bone), there are three other aspects relating to bone mineral density (BMD) and bone strength. These are: the micro-architecture (the three-dimensional structure of the bone, which can be determined under a microscope and indicates whether the structure is sound or not); the mineralisation of the bone (when bone tissue or material is broken down, releasing calcium and phosphate); and the bone-remodelling rate (the rate of resorption and formation of the bone material).

Bone density contributes to bone strength, so we need to determine it by means of a bone scan called *dual energy X-ray absorptiometry* (DEXA), which measures the bone density of two different types of bones: those in the lumbar spine, which is made up of the five vertebrae in the lower back, and those in the total hip and the femoral neck of the hip, which is where most hip fractures take place. The femur is the long bone in the upper part of the leg. The bone has a head and shaft, which fit into each other at the femoral neck like a ball into a socket.

THE DEXA SCAN

Known also as the DXA scan, the DEXA scan takes measurements of your bones by means of a special X-ray machine while you lie on a flat bed. Be reassured, the radiation level of this machine is extremely low. The test produces a *T-score*, which shows how the measurement of your bone density differs from the normal peak bone density of a young, healthy adult. Your bone density is normal if your T-score is -1 to +1. You have *osteopenia* (now called low bone density) if your score is less than -1 (< -1) and more than -2.5 (> -2.5). If you have low bone density you are more likely to be at risk for fractures than if your bone density was normal. If you have osteoporosis your score will read -2.5 or less than -2.5 (< -2.5).

Some doctors believe a good rule of thumb is to have a bone scan when you become perimenopausal or as near to that time as possible, but today the DEXA is usually used as part of the whole fracture risk assessment (see below). A sensible healthcare practitioner would be likely to recommend a DEXA if a woman has suffered a low trauma fracture; the kind where you slip and break your wrist or trip and fracture an ankle. It is also advised if you are a premenopausal woman who hasn't had a period for more than six months, if you're on long-term cortisone or have breast cancer and are taking a treatment like anastrozole (Arimidex) that blocks your estrogen receptors (Chapter 7). Before starting you on a treatment, your doctor should probably do a basic screening – blood and urine tests – to make sure the correct medication is prescribed.

But remember, if you have a surgical or chemical menopause, if you stop your hormone therapy or if you develop a thyroid problem you should have a bone scan within the year to check that all is well. It is important to ensure that the healthcare practitioner who reads your DEXA results has been properly trained to interpret these readings. Osteoporosis can be diagnosed without a DEXA scan if you have a fragility fracture and are considered to be at risk according to certain criteria discussed below. Your age when you have a DEXA is relevant, for example if you are 65 or older a low bone density measurement on the DEXA means you are at greater fracture risk.

Beware those who tell you that they can determine your bone density by performing a heel scan, which is called *peripheral site measurement* in medical terminology. This scan is usually done with smaller, much less accurate machines on your heel bone and is often administered by people who are not trained in this area, such as pharmacists. This is not a validated tool to measure fracture risk. Bone density tends to vary from one part of the body to another, so this measurement is not as accurate as a measurement taken at the hip or spine, since changes in your heel may happen long after they have occurred in your spine.

Because the DEXA is only two-dimensional it can't show the actual structure of the bone, but it is theoretically possible to examine the structure of bone with an ultrasound scan to determine its quality as well as its density. This can only be done for diagnostic purposes since the ultrasound can't be reproduced. Your doctor may measure the breakdown of bone in your body by doing a blood test and a urine analysis. This is a *bone turnover test*. Bone turnover reflects what is happening in bone at a moment in time – if bone turnover markers are elevated, this suggests that bone loss is occurring. These elevated bone markers can be useful in certain cases to assess fracture risk when the BMD measurement alone does not give a clear diagnosis. Combining the BMD measurement and bone marker levels may help the assessment of future fracture risk.

A pathologist should also be able to measure the calcium, phosphate, parathyroid hormone (PTH) and vitamin D in your blood and the levels of creatinine and calcium in your urine. These tests are done to exclude other causes of bone loss that may require correction. These levels are markers, much like cholesterol levels in monitoring for heart disease, which tell the specialist about the activity of your bones and whether you are at increased risk for fractures.

International bodies recommend that you should have your bone density measured in the following instances: when you are over 65; if you are postmenopausal and have medical conditions that can cause bone loss (see below); when you are postmenopausal and over 50 and have had a fracture; if you are abnormally thin; if you smoke; if you drink more than two glasses of alcohol daily; if you have a parent with a hip fracture; or if you have rheumatoid arthritis.

In an ideal world it would be good if you could have a premenopausal bone scan, so that when you have a DEXA after menopause, your doctor can monitor the amount of bone you are losing over time.

RISK FACTORS FOR OSTEOPOROSIS

Although the assessment of bone mass plays an extremely important part in diagnosing osteoporosis, it is very important to understand that like most other conditions, there are multiple risk factors that can cause osteoporosis. Knowledge of all these risks plays an important role in the diagnosis and treatment of osteoporosis. The World Health Organisation (WHO), together with the International Osteoporosis Foundation (IOF) and several other interested bodies developed an easy-to-use fracture risk assessment tool (FRAX) for doctors to use with patients where the DEXA scan may not be readily available or affordable. They studied patients in Europe, Asia, North America and Australia to develop it. If you are one of the lucky ones who can have a DEXA scan, the accuracy of the diagnosis made by your doctor can be even further improved if they also take your other risk factors into consideration.

The *FRAX risk calculator* uses both a woman's clinical risks and her bone mineral density at the femoral neck of her hip to work out her possible fracture risk over 10 years. This means that if you have more risk factors in conjunction with low bone density you may be at greater risk for a fracture. The FRAX asks 12 questions that are related to your risk. As with all these risk tools, there are some limitations to FRAX: it doesn't include all risk factors and is only meant for patients who are not on medication for osteoporosis, so your healthcare practitioner should be aware of these. However, this tool will continue to be updated. If you are interested to read more about FRAX there is plenty of information available on the Internet. Just remember to check that it is a reliable site.

A DEXA scan alone may not be enough to make a clinical judgement about fracture risk. Indeed, without assessing other risk factors, up to 75 per cent of patients who need treatment for osteoporosis may be missed! I have listed these risk factors and explained why they may put you at risk. Doctors should be aware of all these risks when they take your medical history.

- **Age**. As you age you are at greater risk for fracture, especially hip fracture; in fact, your risk doubles about every eight years after you turn 50.

- **Family history**. As with heart disease and cancer, family history and genetic make-up play a huge part in determining your future bone density. It is thought that more than 50 per cent of women are at risk for osteoporosis because they have first-line relatives like a mother or sister with the disease. So if you know your mother has battled with osteoporosis you need to be more alert and live the kind of life that will lessen this risk. If your parent had a hip fracture you are at also increased risk.
- **Small-boned women** may be at greater risk, like Nina in the case study, and Caucasian women.
- **Previous fractures** (apart from skull, finger, toe, facial bones and ankles) are a serious risk, either hip or vertebral, and if you have a fracture after perimenopause you are twice as likely to get another one.
- **Transition into menopause** also increases your risk because of the rapid bone resorption that happens when your ovaries start to produce less estrogen. This is why women who experience early menopause are at greater risk for low bone density than their contemporaries who went through natural menopause.
- **Lifestyle**. As with most of the conditions I have written about in this book, lifestyle plays an important role in your level of risk for osteoporosis. Heading the list is, of course, **smoking**. Not only do the toxins in cigarettes block the absorption of calcium, but smokers have lower estrogen levels, which contributes to overactive osteoclasts. Smokers often have an earlier menopause than non-smokers, they lose bone more quickly and research has shown that they have an 80 per cent increased risk of fractures. Women who are **heavy drinkers** are also at risk for osteoporosis, which is logical because they often eat poorly and have low body mass, while excessive alcohol interferes with their body's absorption of calcium and vitamin D. Because estrogen plays such an important role in controlling bone metabolism, anything that interferes with your estrogen levels, like excessive drinking, will affect your fracture risk.
- **Falling estrogen levels**. Anything that lowers your estrogen level can put you at risk. So *surgical menopause* and/or early menopause, which was Nina's problem; not having your period (*amenorrhoea*) for a number of reasons such as chronic stress; not ovulating; and *high prolactin levels*, which as you recall inhibit estrogen production, are all risk factors.
- **Low body weight**. If you are extremely thin, you are also at risk. Anything that contributes to low body weight, like excessive dieting, eating disorders or fanatical exercising, will also put you at risk for this

disease, since the absence of fatty tissue will affect your estrogen levels (see Chapter 1).

- **Lack of exercise**. You are also at risk if you never exercise because, as you will read, appropriate exercise is actually bone strengthening.
- **Certain medication**. Certain medicines like anti-epileptic medication, long-term cortisone treatment, drugs that thin your blood, thyroid medication, aromatase inhibitors and GnRH agonists (discussed in Chapter 7) and chemotherapy may also put you at increased risk for fractures.
- **Vitamin D deficiency** is a risk factor.
- It is important to know that there are **several illnesses** that put women at risk for osteoporosis. These include kidney and liver disease, thyroid disease, bone cancer and rheumatoid arthritis. In fact, anything that because of inflammation and infection causes a high level of C-reactive protein or homocysteine in the blood can put you at risk for osteoporosis. In medical language, these two markers of the immune system, which you read about in Chapters 4 and 5, are called *cytokines* and affect the process of bone material breakdown.

If you go back and look at all these risk factors, it is encouraging to see how many of them are under your control, which means that even if you are at risk for osteoporosis you can change your lifestyle to reduce your risk of fracture.

REDUCING YOUR RISK FOR OSTEOPOROSIS

There are some easily achievable ways of lowering your risk for osteoporosis. Apart from living and eating sensibly, there are other things you can do to look after yourself. Firstly, if you smoke – stop. If your alcohol intake is excessive, stop drinking or if you are disciplined, reduce it to no more than one glass daily. As I have written, too much alcohol can increase your hot flushes and put you at risk for cancer. Complete abstinence may not be necessary but, as you will read in Chapter 10, it's just sensible for peri- and postmenopausal women to be temperate if they drink.

Exercise

Exercise is essential if you want to lower your fracture risk and here the kind of exercise you choose is very important. Your bones are living organisms composed of cells and tissue. The cells in the bone 'talk' to each other about how much stress is being put on the bone, so that they can respond to this stress by building new bone. If the appropriate amount of stress is exerted, new bone will be built, so any exercise that puts stress on the bone is beneficial to bone strength. However, there is a downside. If too much stress is put on the bone and the body responds by breaking down and trying to build the new bone, the bone builders may not be able to cope, so you will find yourself with a stress fracture, which occurs as a result of too much exercise or too much pressure on a certain area, like the pounding action on the ankle bone when marathon runners run too long and too hard.

It is interesting to note that astronauts who spend significant time in space lose bone density because of the weightlessness of space. Because of the zero gravity, there is no stress on the bones to encourage the formation of new bone, but the body continues its work of breaking down the bone materials. Astronauts who have been tested have lost some bone in their spines and quite a bit more in their hip areas.

Before you embark on an exercise programme, especially if you haven't exercised before, you should check with your doctor that it's okay to go ahead. Be moderate. Take it gradually and work up to your desired regimen. Probably the most effective type of exercise for peri- and postmenopausal women is walking. A large body of research has shown that it is beneficial not only for the weight-bearing bones but for the skeleton as well. Women who walk regularly for a minimum of 30 minutes at least four times a week will generally have better and stronger bones than those who don't and, as an added bonus, walking is also an excellent way of increasing your metabolism. I have always recommended that peri- and postmenopausal women do some weight-bearing exercise. In this case your body is the weight, so it's not too complicated to include brisk walking, jogging or running in your exercise programme.

I believe that exercise should be varied, like your diet, because apart from the boredom factor, I think that it is important that you exercise all parts of your body for optimum results. Resistance or strength training twice a week is another kind of exercise that ensures that all the muscles in your body are strengthened, which in turn is beneficial for your bones, because apart from anything else you may fall less often as your muscles become stronger. Join a reputable gym with good trainers or find yourself a well-recommended personal trainer and check their qualifications carefully. Get an expert to design your weight-training programme and be suspicious if there are too many repetitions; more than 10 to 15 is too many. The initial weights should be set low so that you don't strain yourself. Don't be overambitious. You can add more weight gradually but never so much that you hurt yourself or have to lift the weights in an inappropriate manner. There are right and wrong ways to lift weights and your trainer or instructor should be able to show you the correct way. Go slowly; it takes time to build your muscle and nothing worth doing well comes quickly or easily. Don't forget to cool down and stretch once you have finished.

Another important type of exercise is something that increases your flexibility and balance. Fracture risks are increased when women become older and fall more often because they lose their balance. Either Pilates or yoga would be an excellent addition to your exercise regimen, and both of them, if correctly taught, are ideal for middle-aged women as they help posture and balance. Pilates uses a technique called core stabilisation, where the muscles that support your spine and upper body are strengthened with the use of special machines and carefully designed exercises. It is a gentle but thorough form of exercise and helps improve your posture, coordination, balance and flexibility.

Yoga also increases your suppleness and flexibility through a series of floor exercises that don't jar your joints. Both types of exercise stress the importance of breathing correctly, balancing, focusing your mind and using carefully controlled movements. If you have been diagnosed with osteoporosis it is very important that you take care not to fall. As I mentioned above, certain exercises will help you improve your balance, but pay attention to your environment to ensure that there are not objects you could trip over, such as floor rugs. Don't wear heels that are too high and compromise your balance. Keep a small light burning and the way cleared to the bathroom when you get up to go to the loo at night. See that the tiles in your bathroom aren't slippery when wet; place some bath mats with rubber bottoms strategically when you get out of the bath or shower.

SUPPLEMENTS AND OSTEOPOROSIS

In both Chapters 5 and 7 I wrote about vitamin D and calcium supplementation. The recommended levels have changed quite radically over the past few years. In earlier editions of this book, my recommendations were quite a bit higher. However, because there was so much confusing information about these two supplements, the Institute of Medicine (IOM) recently presented a comprehensive report, which analysed and reviewed the data and published some new reference values. There will always be disagreement when this happens but the medical experts and organisations I trust are on board with these, so at the time of writing I am happy to pass their suggestions on. In a perfect world healthy eating is the best way to obtain calcium because of all the essential vitamins and minerals that are found in high-calcium foods. Research has shown that dairy products are the best sources of calcium. Four cups of dairy products, such as milk, yoghurt and cottage cheese, would give you about 1 000 mg of elemental calcium and the good news is that it makes no difference whether they are whole, low-fat or fat-free dairy products.

Four cups of dairy products, such as milk, yoghurt and cottage cheese, would give you about 1 000 mg of elemental calcium.

However, you will recall that in Chapter 5, I wrote that most peri- and postmenopausal women don't get enough calcium in their diets and must supplement this. So if you're not eating enough calcium-rich foods – milk and milk products, especially cheese; sardines with bones; dark leafy greens like kale and broccoli; sesame seeds; oranges and soybean products – you should take a calcium supplement. If you have a reasonably healthy diet, you can probably assume that you are getting about 500 mg of calcium daily, so you could supplement with about 500 mg of elemental calcium. If you really are unhealthy, or your specialist recommends it for a variety of reasons, supplement with about 1 000 mg of *elemental* calcium daily, but no more. Calcium carbonate seems to contain the most elemental calcium and is better absorbed with food, but you can take calcium citrate if you prefer it, either with meals or on an empty stomach. Just see that it contains enough elemental calcium – the actual basic calcium that is available in the tablets.

There are all sorts of calcium products in the marketplace but research indicates that calcium carbonate and calcium citrate are the most effective types. If the calcium is a good brand it will tell you whether to take it with or without food. This is important, but I know how stressed women can get, so it is probably okay to take it when it suits you rather than not take it at all. Try to take your dose with food if that is recommended.

Make **absolutely** sure that any calcium you take is combined with an adequate amount of vitamin D, which is essential for calcium absorption because it helps your body to use this vital mineral most effectively. Though in the past few years experts suddenly started recommending supplementing with high levels of vitamin D, there has been a shift. The IOM report shows that in healthy women, levels of vitamin D (25 OH vitamin D) should not be lower than 20 ng/ml. Other medical experts disagree and would like to see them higher, as suggested by the task force in the Endocrine Society 2011 clinical practice guideline, who prefer levels consistently above 30 ng/ml. Discuss this with your healthcare practitioner. It is probably fine if your levels are between 20 and 30 ng/ml. Many postmenopausal women's levels of vitamin D may be lower than this and you can check by asking your healthcare practitioner to do a test to determine whether your levels of this essential nutrient have dropped below 20 ng/ml. The recommended dose of vitamin D with calcium is now between 400 and 600 IU daily. Because, in addition to your diet, you also get vitamin D from exposure to sunlight, many factors need to be considered when determining how much vitamin D supplementation you need. For example, you get different amounts during summer and winter. Women older than 70 may need more vitamin D (800 IU), as do women who are very covered up. Those who have darker skin probably have lower levels of vitamin D. You need hours of sun exposure to make enough vitamin D, and overexposure to the sun is ageing and dangerous. It is much simpler to make sure that whatever supplements you are taking contain enough of this vitamin.

In Chapter 5, I mentioned that soy isoflavones might have a protective effect on bone. Some small studies suggest that when you use these, there may be some small increases at the spine and hip when compared with placebo, and others have shown that soy isoflavones are effective in maintaining the bone mineral content in women who are in late menopause, but many trials show that they do not protect women in early menopause against bone loss or prevent it. It's clear that more research is needed to determine whether isoflavones help maintain or build bone density. It's your call. Talk it over with your doctor. If you have decided to take soy for menopausal symptoms, as well as a preventive treatment for osteoporosis, you must be monitored either by having a DEXA scan with an appropriate follow-up time, or a urine analysis, which will allow your healthcare provider to see whether you are losing calcium and creatinine.

Many peri- and post-menopausal women complain about joint pain and resort to glucosamine and chondroitin supplements to help relieve the problem. Glucosamine and chondroitin are natural substances found in and around the cells of cartilage. Together they help protect the cartilage. It seems that glucosamine may play an anti-inflammatory role, while chondroitin is thought to keep the cartilage strong and resilient (see Chapter 5). The results of a recent long-term study, Glucosamine/Chondroitin Arthritis Intervention Trial (GAIT), under the aegis of the National Institute of Health (NIH), showed that these supplements did not provide relief from osteoarthritis pain to all the participants in the trial, nor did they bring relief to those who had mild pain, but a much smaller subgroup study showed that those who had moderate to severe pain experienced significant relief, which means that further research is needed to confirm these findings.

TREATMENTS FOR OSTEOPOROSIS

The next section is quite technical, but I truly believe that all women should understand how the medication they are taking works, and what their choices are. There are very effective and powerful agents available to prevent the breakdown of bone material. These can be *anti-resorptive*, which stops bone resorption activity; *anabolic*, which means a medication that stimulates the formation of bone; or *dual acting*, which does a bit of both.

The question that you and your doctor will need to decide is when it is best to start treatment. Your specialist will probably tell you that you need it if you are postmenopausal and have any of the following: a vertebral fracture or a hip fracture; a T-score that is -2.5 or less; or if you have low bone density based on a T-score of between -1.0 and -2.5 in conjunction with some of the major risk factors.

The first category includes bisphosphonates, SERMs (see Chapter 4), estrogen and calcitonin. Before I write about these different treatments, it is important to understand something about bone biology that recently came to light. Research found that there was a connection between the osteoblasts and the osteoclasts; whatever you do to the one happens to the other. This connection is known as 'coupling'. This is relevant because of the way medication prescribed for osteoporosis works and will make sense later in this chapter when I describe newly available medications.

Hormone Therapy

I have already discussed estrogen and it is clear that even a very small amount (0.014 mg) of additional estrogen protects the bones. Bone loss will accelerate when you stop HT. At a conference at the end of last year, I heard some interesting research showing that when women stopped their HT they were at much greater risk for hip fractures, and that the protection the estrogen gives bone disappears within two years after stopping it. The NORA (Nordic Research on Ageing) study showed that women who used HT had high T-scores, but women who stopped HT after five years had similar bone scores to women who had never used HT (see the section on DEXA scans above to refresh your memory on T-scores). The thought is that when you stop HT, it is very important for you and your doctor to reassess your individual risk of osteoporosis and decide how you intend to go forward and what bone protection regimen may be best for you. The risks of HT may outweigh its benefits, so if you don't have menopause symptoms, don't take HT to prevent osteoporosis. However, if you really can't take other treatments for osteoporosis and you are quite early on in your menopause, the use of HT may be the way to go, depending again on your individual health profile and whether in your case the benefits outweigh the risks.

This is probably a good place to mention tibolone (trade name Livifem). As you saw in Chapter 4, this product has a combination of weak estrogenic, androgenic and progestogenic effects on your body and is often recommended for women with osteoporosis because it has been shown to increase bone mineral density. There are worries about tibolone and its associated risks with stroke in older women, so there will need to be more research before doctors can say with certainty that the benefits outweigh the risks. Because studies have highlighted the risk associated with long-term HT, it seems more sensible to look at other medication if you need treatment for osteoporosis. Many doctors in Europe and the UK recommend it.

Bisphosphonates

The bisphosphonate category contains the well-known medicines *alendronate*, *risedronate* and *ibandronate*. You might recognise them by their trade names, Fosamax, Actonel and Boniva. Bisphosphonates suppress the activity of the osteoclasts so that the breaking down of bone is limited. These medications can be taken daily or weekly, depending on your particular case. Most women who are on them don't seem to suffer from bad side effects, though some complain of stomach upsets and irritation of the oesophagus, others of aching joints, or both. Alendronate and risedronate increase bone density in the spine and hip in postmenopausal women and decrease the risk of fracture. Bisphosphonates don't work as well in postmenopausal women who don't have osteoporosis. Another bisphosphonate called *zoledronic acid* (Zometa, Reclast, Aclasta) comes in tablet form and is given as an *intravenous infusion* (put through a drip into a vein, generally, in your arm). One of the upsides of this treatment is that it will only be given at 12-month intervals, which would eliminate much of the discomfort associated with daily or weekly doses of bisphosphonate. As far as dosage of bisphosphonates is concerned, the length of time for which you will need to take the medication will depend on your individual case.

Anabolic agents

Teriparatide (Forteo), which is based on parathyroid hormone (PTH), which regulates the amounts of calcium and phosphate in your blood, is an anabolic agent. It is given as a daily injection *subcutaneously* (under the skin) for menopausal women who are at high risk of fracture. Studies have shown a real increase in the bone mass of the women using it. Side effects of this product are rare, but include nausea, muscle cramps and headaches.

I have already written about SERMs in the chapters on hormones and cancers. SERMs are hormones that have a beneficial estrogen effect on certain areas of your body, while blocking unwanted estrogen effects in other parts of your body so that the amount of active estrogen is not increased. The best known SERMs are tamoxifen and the second-generation SERM raloxifene. These SERMs have an estrogenic effect on your bones, controlling the activity of the osteoclasts, which are the cells responsible for breaking down bone material.

In general, tamoxifen would be used primarily to prevent breast cancer but some doctors use raloxifene (Evista) because it decreases bone turnover and fractures, and increases bone mineral density in the spine in women with osteoporosis. Although there are side effects such as muscle cramps, increased risk of blood clots (women who are at high risk of stroke shouldn't use it) and sometimes hot flushes, some women who aren't happy taking bisphosphonates do very well on it. Currently raloxifene is a second-line treatment after bisphosphonates, which are still the gold standard, but further research is needed to understand all its risks and benefits.

Two new third-generation SERMs, *lasofoxifene* and *bazedoxifene*, are now in phase-three trials.

(A short digression here to explain what these different trials mean. All medicines passed by a regulatory body, as I discussed in Chapter 3, must have undergone extensive testing to make sure that the benefits of the drug outweigh the risks, so a drug looks very promising if it reaches **Phase 3 trials**. These trials are both expanded controlled and uncontrolled trials, and are conducted after **Phase 2 trials** have obtained evidence. This suggests that a drug will be effective at an optimally selected dose. Phase 3 trials gather additional information about the safety of the drug to evaluate the overall benefits and risks, and provide adequate information for physician labelling. Phase 3 trials usually include between several hundred and several thousand volunteers.)

These third-generation SERMs could help to treat women with breast cancer who enter early menopause due to chemotherapy and are, as I explained earlier, at high risk for premature bone loss. Lasofoxifene appears to decrease bone loss, increase bone density in the spine, decrease vertebral fracture risk, have favourable effects on blood cholesterol levels and lower the risk of estrogen receptor-positive breast cancer. Bazedoxifene is promising as a treatment for osteoporosis, as trials show that it prevents bone loss and decreases bone turnover, and may have fewer adverse effects on the lining of the womb and fewer vasomotor effects (hot flushes and night sweats) than those SERMs that are currently used in clinical practice. Some recent studies are looking at combining bazedoxifene with estrogen, which will give the benefits of estrogen without the cancer risks, and allow women with wombs not to take a progestogen. The jury is still out and more controlled clinical trial data is needed to confirm these results.

Calcitonin, which I discussed earlier in this chapter, is a hormone normally produced by the thyroid gland. As a medicine, its job is to control the activities of the osteoclasts and prevent overactivity. Its trade name is Miacalcic or Miacalcin and it is given as a nasal spray, which means that among its side effects, which are fairly mild, there may be some nasal irritation. Studies have shown that it is effective in reducing fractures of the spine but not hip fractures, so although it does reduce bone resorption, it is not a first-line treatment like the bisphosphonates.

NEW TREATMENTS FOR OSTEOPOROSIS

In the first edition of this book, some of the medications that I wrote about were still undergoing trials to ensure their efficacy and safety. Today, several have been approved as effective treatments for postmenopausal osteoporosis. One of those is *strontium ranelate* (Protos), approved in many countries but not yet in the USA. It works in a very different way from the two medications I mentioned earlier. Anti-resorptive agents (bisphosphonates) reduce fracture risk by slowing down the breakdown of bone by the osteoclasts (resorption), but because of 'coupling', which I mentioned earlier, they also slow down the formation of the bone by the osteoblasts.

On the other hand, anabolic agents like teriparatide increase the formation of bone but also increase the breakdown of the bone. Strontium ranelate was found to have a different effect. It works by 'uncoupling' this process of bone remodelling so that in a dual action, it simultaneously helps to decrease the breakdown of bone while increasing the process of bone formation. Instead of just strengthening one part of the bone (see the diagram of the structure of bone on page 208) because of its ability to 'uncouple', it improves the structure of trabecular bone and stimulates the formation of cortical bone. The side effects of this medication may include mild nausea and diarrhoea and, in some women, blood clots.

A new treatment recently approved by the FDA is called *denosumab* (Prolia). This works in quite a complicated way, so I'll try to explain it as simply as possible. Earlier I wrote about a connection between the osteoblasts and the osteoclasts called 'coupling'. RANKL is a molecule that is found on the surface of the osteoblasts (cells that replace old bone material). It connects with another molecule called RANK on the osteoclast (cells that remove old bone) and helps to activate the osteoclast. Denosumab is called a 'fully monoclonal antibody' and blocks the interaction of RANKL and RANK, which helps prevent bone resorption (see page 210) by the osteoclasts. Denosumab is given twice a year as an injection, which makes it easier to take than a bisphosphonate oral medication. Studies show it seems to increase bone density at the spine and hip and significantly reduces new vertebral fractures, fractures of the hip and non-vertebral fractures; best of all it didn't appear to have too many side effects, apart from eczema and cellulitis, which is a bacterial skin infection.

EMPOWER YOURSELF

- Living well is a good way to help protect yourself against osteoporosis: eat sensibly and exercise at least five times a week.
- Take adequate calcium and vitamin D in the dosages recommended in this chapter, by the IOM or by your doctor.
- Osteoporosis is a silent disease.
- Know your risk factors for osteoporosis. If you do, you can eliminate any that are within your control and protect yourself against those that aren't, like a family history or a particular medication or illness.
- Check out your FRAX risk score (http://www.shef.ac.uk/FRAX/tool.jsp).
- Don't rely on your GP to diagnose osteoporosis. Proper screening and an examination by a specialist in this field will show whether you are at risk for it.
- These steps may be part of the diagnosis for osteoporosis:
  - A physical examination (is your spine curving and have you lost height over the past year?)
  - DEXA scan of the hip and spine

- – Listing your risk factors, either by using FRAX or another tool
- – In some cases, blood tests to examine your thyroid function, your calcium level, parathyroid levels, 25(OH) vitamin levels and biochemical marker tests of your urine or blood to check how fast you're losing or making bone and if a new treatment is working
- – An X-ray or a vertebral fracture assessment performed on the DEXA machine to see whether you have compression fractures of the spine.
- Treatment for osteoporosis should be carefully discussed and all risks and benefits should be explained by the specialist.
- T-score measurements:

  Normal bone density   = T-score equal to or better than -1.0

  Low bone density   = T-score between -1.0 and -2.5

  Osteoporotic bone density = T-score equal to or less than -2.5

10
Food is my drug of choice: weight and diet in menopause

The workshop had been over for a while but I noticed that Tessa and Stephanie were still deep in conversation. They were discussing diets: the most popular subject among many middle-aged women.

Tessa must have been very pretty when she was younger; her eyes sparkle and her hair shines, but she is very overweight; as she heaved herself up she was breathing heavily and though the room was not particularly warm, there was a fine sheen of moisture on her skin. Stephanie was reasonably slim, though some unwanted kilos had obviously settled themselves on her hips. Although she and Tessa were the same age, she moved lightly and easily and seemed full of energy.

'I don't know why you're complaining, you look great!' Tessa exclaimed. Stephanie shook her head. 'I don't mean to sound like I'm looking for compliments but since I've started menopause, I don't know what's wrong with me. I've never had a problem with weight but suddenly I've picked up four kilos. I have always exercised and I haven't started eating more or anything but it's really hard to lose. It doesn't matter what I do, it keeps coming back. I'm fed up!'

'You don't know how lucky you are. I think I've been dieting all my life,' said Tessa. 'There isn't a diet I haven't tried. I've always thought there must be something wrong with me. Yesterday I saw a new nutritionist and she said I may have something called met ... meta ...?'

'Metabolic syndrome?' I interrupted.

'That's right,' Tessa responded. 'She says that is why I'm not losing weight, but she's told me there's a medicine that will fix it and help me to lose weight as well. I can't wait.'

> *'That's funny,' said Stephanie, 'my GP was also telling me about it but he said that he thought I was insulin resistant. He took some blood and said he would see if my insulin levels were up and would then give me this great medication. I think it's called Glucophage.'*

I thought, as I listened to them, that one of the most difficult aspects of menopause is weight gain. Because it is such a loaded topic there is a lot of confusion around it. Tessa's nutritionist was quite wrong when she said that Tessa couldn't lose weight if she had metabolic syndrome – a change in lifestyle, diet and exercise is far better than taking a drug.

How often, while watching the Oscars, have we stared in horror as a star of decades past who we once idolised lumbers on stage to receive an award, beautifully coiffed and made up, but fat. What has happened to the object of all that teenage envy? I used to be shocked when I saw them, but I know better now. It is a fact of life that when you become peri- or postmenopausal you will put on some weight. The most important thing is to find out how to remain reasonably slim while at the same time living happily and well.

My aim in this chapter is not to bombard you with scientific information that will confuse you, or to give you advice that you find unpalatable and hard to follow. In any case, every woman is different and has her own way of handling things, so the cookie-cutter approach won't work here any more than it does with any of the other problems of menopause. I won't give you any diets to follow; what I will do is explain basic biochemistry relating to weight and hormones; information that you have probably been given during your peri- and postmenopausal years and that may have confused you.

I will also share some suggestions that may work for you. As you read this chapter, many of the isolated facts that you have learnt in the preceding chapters come together. You've read that being fat puts you at risk for various illnesses and increases menopausal symptoms; that exercise is beneficial in protecting your body and helping you to lose weight; and that eating correctly optimises your health, so you will understand why being an appropriate weight for your age in peri- and postmenopause is essential if you are going to live to a happy and healthy old age.

There are several things to notice about Tessa and Stephanie's conversation. Stephanie complains that since she has become menopausal she has put on weight, which she is battling to lose. Like most women, unless you are unusual, you will put on a couple of kilos during and after menopause.

There may be several reasons for this. As your hormone levels begin to change in menopause, they affect the way your body fat is distributed so that it moves away from your legs and arms and seems to settle around your stomach and thighs. This would account for the phrase 'middle-aged spread', which strikes

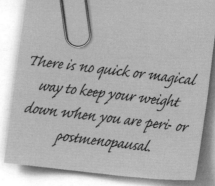

There is no quick or magical way to keep your weight down when you are peri- or postmenopausal.

fear into so many hearts. In addition to causing discomfort – that awful tight waistband and the resulting red ring – increased waist circumference has some serious health implications for middle-aged women, as you will read below.

The theory is that the body knows that its levels of estrogen are dropping and, as I explained in Chapter 2, estrogen is produced both in your ovaries, which are now slowing down, and in your fatty tissues. In an effort to conserve estrogen, your body may want to retain or even encourage more fat storage, so it seems that the metabolism slows and the fat is redistributed to the areas where it produces the most estrogen – waist, bottom, hips and thighs!

Quite apart from that, when you age your metabolism slows as certain hormone levels drop, your thyroid is not as efficient and you become less active. The sad fact is that you can't continue to live as you did when you were 20. Once your doctor has ruled out any hormonal imbalances or illnesses, you are going to have to change your lifestyle if you don't want to get too fat. A very large study done over a period of four-and-a-half years showed that women who made an effort to change their lifestyles did not gain weight; in fact, some actually lost it. A control group of women who had not been on a low-fat, calorie-reduced diet with increased physical activity gained an average of 2.5 kg. These results clearly show that you don't have to get fat after menopause. You can stay reasonably slim or maintain your weight.

The first point is that there is no quick or magical way to keep your weight down when you are peri- or postmenopausal. Stephanie hadn't actually started eating more, but her metabolism had begun to slow down and her body had redistributed fat, adding it to her hips, stomach and thighs. This redistribution of her fat mass began to compromise her muscle mass. Since she was already exercising, Stephanie needed to look at the amount she was eating and to cut down on quantity because her slower metabolism couldn't deal with the amount of calories she was consuming. It is thought that in order to lose weight peri- and postmenopausal women should cut out 3 000 to 4 000 kilojoules a day (for those of you who prefer to think in calories, that's about 700 to 950 calories; 1 calorie = 4.2 kilojoules).

Stephanie also needed to reassess the type of food she was eating. If you have always been slim in spite of the fact that your favourite snack is four slices of chocolate cake washed down with a fizzy drink and you never exercise seriously, it's hard to face the reality of ageing and the changes it brings. As you will read below, certain changes will take place in your body when you start to gain weight that make it even harder to lose it. The fact that Stephanie had always exercised was in her favour and if she is careful, it seems unlikely that apart from those few kilos about which she is sensitive, she will put on more weight.

When I married I weighed 52 kg. I can't believe I ever fitted into my wedding dress and I have kept just one glamorous outfit as a bittersweet memory. Menopause, too little exercise and too much of the 'wrong' foods have taken their toll. Often clients bring photos of themselves when they come to talk about menopause and I sympathise, but the reality is we are no longer 18 and our bodies are changing inexorably as we get older. So instead of mourning the changes, we need to learn to deal with them.

There are serious health implications of gaining too much weight in middle age – breast cancer, heart disease, diabetes and high blood pressure. There are many benefits to staying slim. A new study shows there is a strong link between increased body mass index (BMI) in midlife and the risk of developing postmenopausal breast cancer, compared with those women who maintain a healthy BMI over the years. Another benefit to watching your weight during midlife may be that if you're obese or overweight and troubled with hot flushes, these may improve when you lose weight. In any case, I think it's important to feel good about yourself, to be able to exercise without puffing and panting, to feel not only light-hearted but light-footed and to be happy in the knowledge that you really are looking after yourself, so that your menopausal years are happy and healthy.

INSULIN RESISTANCE

Before I discuss various diet options and the kind of exercise programme that may suit you, I would like to get the serious stuff about weight gain out of the way. In the past 10 years or so, a new catchphrase has come into play: insulin resistance. The moment Stephanie mentioned to her doctor that she couldn't lose the weight she had gained, he immediately suggested that she was insulin resistant. I meet many menopausal women who blame their weight gain on insulin resistance, but the fact is it is not the insulin resistance that made you fat in the first place, it is the weight you gained that caused you to become insulin resistant.

This may be a good place to explain how your body digests food and breaks it down into various components. The major component is glucose, the sugar that is vital for energy production in the cells. Insulin, which is a hormone secreted by the pancreas, plays an extremely important role in maintaining the steady levels of glucose in your body's cells by regulating the process whereby the sugars and, to a lesser extent, the fats and proteins you eat are properly broken down and used to make new tissue. Insulin ensures that the broken-down foods are used as *efficiently* as possible and that the food energy that is not needed is properly stored and released when it is needed. It also controls the way fat is stored in the body. However, all sorts of problems can be triggered by raised insulin levels and many women who gain weight in midlife may start to experience these.

Remember that your body is a very complex and delicate machine. In Chapter 1, I described how the pituitary pumps higher and higher levels of follicle stimulating hormone (FSH) when the ovaries don't respond to normal amounts of FSH. The same principle applies to insulin. When you are overweight, eat the wrong foods and/or don't exercise, your insulin doesn't work as well as it should (insulin resistance). When the cells in your body don't respond to insulin, the pancreas goes into overdrive and pumps out more insulin, which is still not properly used because of the insulin resistance. If the relevant cells don't respond to insulin they cannot process the glucose. So, because glucose isn't being used and stored properly, after a while – and this can take years – it begins to build up in the blood, which can eventually cause diabetes.

Once you understand how your body becomes insulin resistant, it is not terribly difficult to correct the problem, as long as you remember that insulin resistance does not initially cause weight gain: it is a direct result of being overweight. So, don't let your doctor tell you that you are fat because you are insulin resistant – you are insulin resistant because you are fat!

Simply, if you have become insulin resistant because you have gained too much weight, you need to get back into shape and lose the weight that is causing the problem. Basically, one of insulin's jobs is to promote the proper use and storage of fat and to ensure that it is effectively used (burnt) by the muscles to release energy. In a very complex process, when you become fat, the excess fat interferes with the way the muscles metabolise fat.

If you are insulin resistant you need to do something about it. There is no reason for you to take medication at this point but you must bring your weight down and start to exercise. The best and most effective medicine for insulin resistance is the correct amount of exercise and weight loss. Research has shown that exercise increases your body's response to insulin; it improves insulin sensitivity.

TYPE 2 DIABETES

If you ignore the diagnosis of insulin resistance and continue with your old lifestyle – eating too much, drinking heavily and not exercising – the symptom of insulin resistance could lead to type 2 diabetes. This is different from type 1 diabetes, which usually happens in childhood or adolescence and is due to the self-destruction of the beta cells (insulin-making cells) in the pancreas. In type 2 diabetes, your pancreas produces higher and higher amounts of insulin as it responds to cells that seem to be 'ignoring' the insulin. Finally the pancreas 'runs out of steam' and is unable to make enough insulin to control the levels of glucose in your blood. The blood glucose levels then start to rise and type 2 diabetes develops.

Sometimes type 2 diabetes goes undiagnosed for quite a long time. Some of the typical symptoms for this include tiredness, memory loss and poor concentration. Your blood pressure may be raised and even though you aren't dieting you may start to lose weight. The diagnosis for type 2 diabetes is not based on levels of fasting insulin but on levels of fasting glucose. If your doctor suspects you have type 2 diabetes, you will be asked to have a fasting blood glucose test, and sometimes an oral glucose tolerance test to check your levels. As with cholesterol tests, you fast before the test so that the results are as accurate as possible.

If type 2 diabetes is not treated, you could be at risk for all sorts of serious illnesses, including heart disease, damage to your eyes and kidney disease.

METABOLIC SYNDROME

Another danger of insulin resistance is metabolic syndrome. Metabolic comes from the word metabolism, which is the way your body breaks down or synthesises food to keep it functioning. Syndrome is the medical term for a disease that can be diagnosed because you have a number of symptoms that characterise it.

Metabolic syndrome is diagnosed if you have three of the following: increased waist circumference (greater than 80 cm), high blood pressure (130/85 or more), high levels of triglycerides, elevated blood glucose levels and low levels of good cholesterol (HDL). However, there are different guidelines from several health organisations and their criteria may vary a bit. The guidelines listed below apply to women and may differ depending on ethnicity. There are women, however, who may be neither obese nor have an increased waist circumference but who still suffer from metabolic syndrome. The biggest issue in relation to this syndrome is that if you have it, you are at serious risk for cardiovascular disease, so it should be treated and carefully monitored.

Diagnosis for metabolic syndrome in women
- Waist larger than 80 cm (35 in)
- Triglycerides measure more than 1.7 mmol/L (150 mg/dL)
- HDL (good cholesterol) lower than 0.9 mmol/L (50 mg/dL)
- Blood pressure higher than 129/84 mm Hg
- Fasting blood sugar higher than 5.6 mmol/L (99 mg/dL)

Glucose levels
- Between 3.9 and 5.5 mmol/L (70–99 mg/dL) = normal fasting glucose
- Between 5.6 and 6.9 mmol/L (100–125 mg/L) = impaired fasting glucose
- Greater than 7.0 mmol/L (>129 mg/dL) for more than one test = diabetes

MANAGING INSULIN RESISTANCE AND ITS CONSEQUENCES

This may all sound very frightening but the good news is that insulin resistance can be reversed and type 2 diabetes can be well managed. Some excellent research has shown that you can improve insulin resistance with medication like Glucophage, which increases insulin sensitivity throughout your body, though this should not be prescribed if your fasting glucose levels are within the normal range (see above) **or** you can help improve it by losing weight and exercising properly. There is some excellent research that shows that by seriously modifying their lifestyles, women with metabolic syndrome actually reduce their chances of getting diabetes, and – here's the really interesting part – the group that was on medication did less well than the group that dieted and exercised. Tessa told Stephanie that she had been diagnosed with metabolic syndrome and it is clear that the 'medicine' her doctor was prescribing would help her, but she also needed to put in the effort to lose weight and to exercise.

BODY MASS INDEX (BMI)

Having said all that, I think it's time to get back to reality, which is that most of us will put on a couple of kilograms at menopause, but if we look after ourselves our weight will remain more or less stable. One of the things we need to pay attention to is body mass index (BMI). BMI is the ratio of your weight to your height and shows a healthcare professional whether you are underweight, just right, overweight or obese. The way to work it out is like this: Calculate your mass (frequently referred to as 'weight') in kilograms and divide it by your height in metres squared. The equation looks like this:

$$\frac{\text{mass in kilograms}}{(\text{height in metres})^2}$$

For example, if you weigh 60 kg and your height is 1.65 m, the calculation would be 60 divided by 2.72 (which is 1.65 squared), giving an answer of 22, which means your body weight is normal (see the chart below for the normal range). Your doctor will keep an eye on your BMI as you move towards menopause and see that it does not increase too much. You may think it's only a couple of points but in terms of weight gain it can be a lot. For example, if you are 163 cm (5 ft 4 in.) and your BMI increases by five points it means you have gained 13.64 kg (30 lb).

If you don't feel like working your BMI out yourself, the following website from the US Department of Health and Human Services can help using either standard or metric measurements: http://www.nhlbsupport.com/bmi/bmi-m.htm

Here is a table to guide you about your BMI:

Body mass index (BMI)	What the numbers mean
Below 18.5	Underweight
18.5–24.9	Normal
25.0–29.9	Overweight
30 and above	Obese

CARBOHYDRATES

Carbohydrates are compounds made up of sugars, starches, cellulose and gums. They are an extremely important source of energy and play a vital role in fat production in our diets. *Simple carbohydrates* are things like cane sugar, beet sugar, lactose (which comes from milk) and fructose; these are natural sugars. Sucrose, like ordinary white sugar, is refined. Your body absorbs simple carbohydrates very quickly, which is why if you eat a sweet or drink a sugary drink when you feel in need of a boost you suddenly feel better. The big problem is that you will quickly need another sugar 'fix' because this energy high doesn't last very long. These rapidly absorbed sugars, which release glucose quickly into the bloodstream, have a high glycaemic index (GI). (The glycaemic index measures the effect of carbohydrates on blood sugar levels.) *Complex carbohydrates* – bread, potatoes, pasta and rice, as well as wholegrains – are composed mainly of starches. Other complex carbohydrates, for instance vegetables and fruits, are composed of starch and dietary fibre. The good news about complex carbohydrates is that they take longer to absorb and the glucose reaction to them is not as rapid and doesn't end as fast, so you feel more satisfied and don't feel hungry quite as quickly again. These foods are said to have a low GI.

More about sugars and fructose

Because sugars play such an important part in our lives, I'd like to unpack some of the above information a little further. A lot of research is focusing on the danger of consuming large amounts of sugar, especially refined sugar, which is very high in calories and has almost no nutrient value. Just as eating the wrong fats can cause the cholesterol levels in your body to change, a new study finds that the same thing happens when we eat too much sugar; our levels of triglycerides rise and levels of HDL drop. The amount of sugar we eat in the twenty-first century is far greater than in our grandparents' day. The reason is that there are so many added sugars or sweeteners in our food, both processed and prepared, because we believe it tastes better. Some people may have as many as 46 teaspoons of sugar daily. This sounds crazy but when you work out that a can of soft drink can contain 12 teaspoons of sugar and a piece of iced cake as much as 25 teaspoons, it's not too difficult to work out just how quickly you can reach that level. You probably need only about a teaspoon of sugar a day to meet dietary needs, though for women the American Heart Association says no more than 6 teaspoons daily, about 2 tablespoons.

There are certain sugars that are found in foods such as fruits and milk. The amount of fructose found in fruit is small compared with the levels found in fructose-sweetened soft drinks, and eating fruit has many benefits due to its natural vitamins, antioxidants and fibre, and is extremely healthy. The use of the word fructose can be confusing and many women believe that all fructose is natural and does not have the same effect on blood glucose levels as refined sugar. This just isn't true. As I explained earlier the fructose found in fruit is not the same as high fructose corn syrup. The latter is a combination of fructose and table sugar. Fructose that is added to sweeten foods is usually in much higher amounts than that found naturally in fruits and vegetables. Research found that fructose in high amounts causes weight gain and propels you towards diabetes. Fructose, as in high fructose corn syrup, which is found in many of the foods and drinks we consume, is more rapidly absorbed, allowing large amounts of it to be released into the bloodstream, contributing to a high GI load.

Be alert; research shows that sugar-sweetened drinks, including soft drinks, fruit drinks, sports drinks, energy and vitamin waters, sweetened iced tea, punch, cordials, squashes and lemonade, contribute to rapid weight gain and elevated triglyceride levels in your blood, leading to increased risk for type 2 diabetes and heart disease. These are drinks sweetened primarily with sucrose, high fructose corn syrup or fruit juice concentrates. Incidentally, women who only had one or two of these sugar-sweetened drinks a month were found to be much healthier than those women who had one or more daily.

So don't fool yourself: when sweeteners (including brown sugar, which is often touted as healthier than white sugar) are added either independently or to processed foods, they are generally bad for us. Try to check for hidden sugars in the foods you eat by reading the labels carefully and seeing whether sugar, in one form or another, is listed first or second on the list of ingredients. Limit sweet foods and substitute a piece of cake with a piece of fruit if you're longing for something sweet. Moderation is the key. The jury is still out as far as the long-term effects of artificially sweetened drinks are concerned, but it is probably sensible to drink water (the best health option of all) or coffee and tea, unsweetened.

FATS

Your body needs fat to function optimally. There are 'good' and 'bad' fats, and there are different fats. The three main kinds of fats are *saturated fats*, which include animal fats, dairy fats, and coconut and palm oil. The fats in avocado, olive oil, canola oil and peanut oil are known as *mono-unsaturated* fats and the vegetable oils like corn and sunflower oil, as well as fish oils, flaxseed oils, sesame and walnut oil, are called *polyunsaturated fats*. In small quantities polyunsaturated fats are fine for us; it's only when the vegetable oils have been heated at a very high heat followed by bubbling hydrogen through it (which is the way margarine is made) that they become the very unhealthy *hydrogenated fat* or *trans fats*. Beware of these. They have a very unhealthy effect on your bad cholesterol (LDL).

Animal fats have small amounts of trans fats, which is why dieticians recommend low-fat milk and lean red meat. A bit of butter now and then doesn't hurt anyone, just watch the quantities and don't slather it onto your toast (a pity, because there are few things as delicious as hot buttered toast, though if you're into lifestyle change the toast had better be made from rye bread!). Essential fatty acids like the omega-3 and omega-6 fatty acids are all quite healthy and, in some cases, flaxseed and fish oil for instance, are beneficial in small to moderate quantities and it's fine to add olive oil to your diet. However, rather than just adding these supplements, eat enough oily fish, which is particularly good for you. You should eat this at least three to four times a week because it is very rich in omega-3 fatty acids and has been shown to help reduce your risk of heart disease. Remember to remove the skin before you eat it to reduce the risk of contaminating agents such as mercury, which are now polluting our seas. You know enough to stay away from deep-fried foods and foods like cakes and biscuits, ice-cream and hamburgers, sausages, salami and bacon, which are rich in fat. The problem is that they taste great, but we know that they are harmful and not doing our middle-aged metabolism any favours.

WEIGHT LOSS AND 'MIRACLES'

Before I discuss dieting, I would like to write about weight loss medication and so-called weight loss experts who give women all sorts of 'miracle cures' and supplements to help them lose weight. Here are two cases which show that they don't work and are not good for your health.

> *At 63, Maria was extremely overweight and had tried every diet available. She lost weight quickly and then gained it when the regimes she tried were too stringent to stick to on a long-term*

basis. As was to be expected from someone who was 45 kg overweight, she had certain health problems: type 2 diabetes, high blood pressure and an underactive thyroid, though these conditions were under control with the appropriate medication. However, her doctor was concerned about her weight and repeatedly warned her that her health would really suffer if she didn't lose weight and keep it off.

Maria had heard via the grapevine of a woman who got 'miraculous' results in her patients with a so-called miracle weight loss programme. In desperation she decided to make an appointment. The woman assured her that if she came off all her medications and strictly followed the instructions for her special programme, which included a drastic diet of only 800 calories daily and a special tea supplement to be drunk six times a day, her weight problems would be over.

Two weeks later, Maria saw her GP because she was feeling so dreadful. Not only had she barely lost any weight, but she had terrible headaches, felt weak, nauseous and was very depressed and weepy. Shocked that she had been advised to stop all her medications, the GP did some blood tests and found to her horror that Maria had a very low thyroid level, which meant that she was suffering from some symptoms described in Chapter 2. In addition, Maria's blood pressure, which had been controlled when she was taking her medicine, was very high again. Her doctor advised her to stop the programme immediately and go back onto her medications. Once her health was stabilised she advised Maria to see a registered dietician, who helped her slowly but surely to lose the weight in a controlled way over a year, taking into account Maria's food preferences, so that she was encouraged to stay on her eating plan.

The moral of this story is that there are no magic cures when it comes to losing weight. Often women are so desperate to lose weight that they will become seriously ill in order to do so. No woman should stop her chronic medication without first discussing it with her doctor. There are unscrupulous people with no clinical expertise in the area of weight loss or endocrinology who play on the emotions of overweight women. They take huge risks with the health of the desperate clients who seek their help as the following story shows.

Denise was a very pretty, slightly overweight woman. Newly divorced, at 54, she had just entered into a relationship with a slightly younger man with whom she was very much in love. They planned to go on a romantic seaside holiday and she was very anxious about how he would judge her when she put on a swimsuit – she felt fat and unattractive when she was with him. She decided that she needed to lose at least 10 kg and went to see a doctor who styled himself as a weight loss expert. He prescribed a thyroid medication, thyroxine, usually prescribed for an underactive thyroid, which she had never been diagnosed with, and a medication called Reductil (sibutramine). He did not do any of the relevant blood tests or bother to take her blood pressure which, if it was raised, may have alerted him to any risk factors that might have been present.

Sibutramine is an appetite suppressant that is usually given to obese women and has now been suspended across Europe and the UK. It has been withdrawn from the USA market at the request of the FDA following the results of a very large randomised, double-blind placebo-controlled study, the Sibutramine Cardiovascular Outcomes Trial (SCOUT), which showed that the cardiovascular risks outweighed the modest weight loss seen with use of the drug, particularly in women with raised blood pressure and heart disease risk.

Thrilled that she was losing weight, Denise continued with these medications for many months. At no time did the so-called weight loss expert monitor her blood pressure or check her blood results; he just glibly wrote out a script after each of the expensive visits. One evening she suddenly had all the symptoms of a heart attack and was rushed to the emergency room, where she was diagnosed with severe heart damage and cardiomyopathy, a very serious disease where the heart muscle becomes damaged and doesn't work properly. Her cardiologist didn't understand why someone who had been relatively healthy a few months earlier should have become so desperately ill and questioned her closely. When he discovered the medications she was taking, he was appalled and stopped them immediately. He could not understand why she had been prescribed these medications as she had neither an underactive thyroid, nor was she obese.

Denise has now recovered without permanent heart damage, but she was lucky.

There are many cases of women on thyroid medication supposedly to increase their thyroid function when they have normal thyroid levels. No one should take thyroid medication without proper testing. There is no magic bullet when it comes to weight. All of us would prefer a quick and easy way where we wouldn't have to give up the unhealthy food we love. Medicines that may help us lose weight have a chequered history. It's been found that women who are on weight loss drugs often don't lose more than a moderate amount of weight and once they are off the meds, quickly gain weight again. Many weight loss drugs are associated with health risks as you can see from Denise's story, and the perfect weight loss drug hasn't been found yet, though it's clear that it will be a gold mine for the pharmaceutical company who solves this particular problem! Medical scientists are still looking for a medicine that helps us lose weight, isn't costly and that has benefits outweighing the risks. There are new products in the pipeline, but I honestly believe that a healthy lifestyle is the best way to go. If you are set on taking medication or a so-called miracle drug, it's a case of buyer beware; there is no quick and easy way to lose weight without consequences.

DIETS

If you are like most women, you will have tried an amazing number of diets in your lifetime. Who can forget the Grapefruit Diet, the Drinking Man's Diet or the Scarsdale Diet; who of us hasn't been to Weigh-Less or Weight Watchers or Sure Slim? Today, flavours of the month include the X Diet, the Cabbage Soup Diet, the Zone, the Atkins Diet, the South Beach Diet and the Dukan diet. As with everything in our world, there is a plethora of choice.

Basically diets fall into two broad categories: low carbohydrate and high protein, or high carbohydrate and low fat. I will describe the basics of both and you can make your choice based on the information, selecting the one that will best encourage a long-term healthy lifestyle.

Very low carbohydrate, high protein

This category is best represented by the Atkins Diet. It comprises a very low carbohydrate load, where only 25 per cent of the diet is carbohydrates, and 75 per cent is protein and fats.

The diet works on the theory that when you don't eat a lot of carbohydrates your insulin levels will be reduced, which will encourage your body first to burn its stored carbohydrates and then, when they are depleted, to use the energy stored in fat cells and to burn fat for energy. The process where your body burns fat (fat oxidisation) leads to ketosis: the release of ketones into the blood. Your body may also lose essential stores of water when you diet this way. The problem is that you may be eating more protein and fat than is good for you and not enough grains and fruits, which are complex carbohydrates that are highly recommended for protection against various cancers and contain essential antioxidants that may guard against raised levels of C-reactive protein and homocysteine.

People who are on an extreme form of this type of diet have bad breath and often feel queasy or giddy and have very bad headaches. Although weight loss is quick and effective, if you decide to take this route you need to have your cholesterol levels monitored because you are probably eating more saturated fats than are good for you. As with most extreme diets there is hot debate about the efficacy and safety of the Atkins Diet. What has emerged from studies is that although the diet is effective, at the end of a year people on more traditional, moderately low carbohydrate diets had lost more weight or stuck to their diet better, which is probably no surprise to most of us who find ourselves becoming bored and fed-up after a lengthy period on any one diet.

Another problem is that very high protein levels can be associated with the loss of essential minerals and calcium from your bones, putting you at greater risk for osteoporosis. Also, some carbohydrates like vegetables, fruits, wholegrains and legumes are really good for your health and contain important vitamins, minerals and fibre. Extra protein just won't fill the gap left by excluding them. So, though the Atkins Diet does recommend a variety of leafy, green vegetables, some experts think that the selection isn't varied enough to compensate for the variety of complex carbohydrates missing from the diet.

High carbohydrate, low fat

The Pritikin Diet, an example of this type of diet, assumes that 63 per cent of your food intake will be carbohydrates, 20 per cent fats and 17 per cent proteins. The theory is that by increasing your intake of carbohydrates your body will speed up the mechanism whereby it metabolises carbohydrates so the excess carbohydrates will not be stored as fat. Proponents of the high carbohydrate diet believe that your body will know that you have had enough carbohydrates and won't demand as many.

The other advantage of a high carbohydrate, low fat diet is that you limit your fat intake, but there are downsides. The first is that our bodies need appropriate amounts of fat to function properly – hormones, cell function, brain, central nervous system, skin and tissues all benefit from the correct amounts and types of fat. The other problem with high carbohydrate diets is that people may think any carbohydrate, like white bread, marshmallows and cakes, will be fine, instead of better carbohydrates like fruits, vegetables and wholegrains.

Also, if you are consuming huge amounts of carbohydrates your body is programmed to react by pumping out higher quantities of insulin and glucose, and I have already discussed how these high levels can lead to heart disease. Finally, spiking glucose plays havoc with your appetite and leaves you feeling hungry instead of comfortably satisfied after a meal.

Here's a little tip: if you are offered a 'low-fat' drink look at the ingredients carefully. Something is making it taste better and something is needed to take up the space left by the fat that has been removed; it may be sugar, which will add to your calorie intake. (See the section on sugar and fructose above for more information.)

The moderate carbohydrate diet

This is probably the most sensible diet for perimenopausal and menopausal women. It includes a moderate amount of carbohydrates, about 45 per cent, about 35 per cent proteins and 20 per cent of mainly healthy fats like olive oil and avocado. After years of yo-yo dieting it seems to me that the main 'trick' to losing weight and maintaining the weight loss is a lifestyle change, which is ultimately more effective than a diet that helps you lose weight quickly but is not sustainable. I have also found that if I lose weight too quickly, I regain it quickly.

Many middle-aged women diet for special occasions, because they need the motivation to look good, but if they do succeed, ten to one the weight will be back within months of the wedding, or the 21st, that special birthday celebration or exotic trip. My advice, from bitter experience, is to change the way you eat on a daily basis. If you eat a varied diet that has the right amount of healthy carbohydrates, fats and protein there is always room for some of the luxury foods, like a glass of wine, a chocolate or a luscious dessert.

All the research that I have done has given a clear message: portion control and reduced calories. So wave goodbye to a diet that says eat only four pieces of chocolate cake a day. You will lose weight because you will have restricted your food intake, but ultimately it won't be sustainable because you will die of boredom and because the calories in a piece of chocolate cake are actually quite high because of the fat content. In general, if you want to lose weight stick to lots of fruit and vegetables; fish, especially oily fish like salmon, but really any fish; wholegrains and rye bread or a rye bagel, if you need some toast or bread; and see that your food is poached, grilled, steamed or boiled. If you roast anything keep the oil to a minimum.

FOODS THAT MAKE SENSE

Like most peri- and postmenopausal women you are probably a walking encyclopaedia of the foods that are good for you, but here's a quick overview to jog your memory or to confirm that you've been right all along.

Protein

Lean meat, fish (eat a lot of this, especially oily fish; its benefits are amazing); chicken without the skin (though I always eat the wing and I'm not stopping now – don't be fanatical, if you want a bit of skin now and then, it's not going to kill you); legumes; eggs; beans; unsalted nuts; soy products; and low-fat dairy products.

Vegetables and fruits

Each of these has its own special benefits. Go easy on the potatoes and bananas, but see that you have at least five or more servings of a variety of vegetables and fruits a day. Choose those that are strongly coloured like spinach, carrots, berries and tomatoes because these contain more micronutrients. Fruit juice is not as healthy as whole fruit because the fibre content is lower and it is not as filling.

Healthy fats

Fish oils, avocado, nuts, olive oil, canola oil and flaxseed oil.

Wholegrains

These are grains like wholewheat, barley, oats, cracked wheat, whole cornmeal and brown rice that have not been refined, so much of the goodness in them, like the fibre and the germ of the grain, is retained. Replace refined grains with wholegrains whenever you can.

Dark chocolate

In **moderation** this may be good for you! Some research has shown that it may increase HDL ('good' cholesterol) levels and improve endothelial (the cells that line the blood vessels) function in healthy adults. Recently, however, other research has shown that it might not be as healthy for us as we thought and different brands of chocolate and dark chocolate may affect us differently, so we live in hope for some definitive results.

Stay away from these

Processed foods; greasy foods; fast foods; highly refined foods; cakes; rich desserts; carbonated, sugary drinks; foods that are high in salt; solid fats; sweet, milky drinks; sweet alcoholic after-dinner drinks; alcohol in general; sweets and milk chocolate. Though everything in moderation, so eat what you want occasionally but in small amounts.

As you saw earlier, sugar-sweetened drinks aren't good for you. If you are hooked on them, your risk for type 2 diabetes and metabolic syndrome is higher; basically they make you fatter. Try water; in fact it's really good for you to drink at least four glasses of water daily. Studies have shown that when women are thirsty they often mistake it for hunger. Here is more bad news about these sugar-sweetened drinks. The International Study of Macro/ Micronutrients and Blood Pressure (INTERMAP) showed there is a strong connection between blood pressure and fructose and glucose intake, so drinking these sugar-sweetened drinks increases both systolic and diastolic blood pressure. Worse still, if you like to combine these soft drinks with salty foods full of sodium (potato chips, for example), these risks are even greater.

As far as alcohol is concerned, women should not have more than one drink a day – 250 ml of wine or about 100 ml of spirits like vodka. A glass of wine or a tot of spirits contains roughly the same amount of alcohol. If you are at a party, dilute your wine with sparkling mineral water, have plenty of water and don't mix your alcoholic beverages with sugary cold drinks. Cocktails may taste wonderful but they are very high in calories.

EXERCISE AND WEIGHT

As I explained early on in this chapter the dice are loaded against menopausal women when it comes to weight gain. Various factors related to age and hormone changes make it harder to lose weight. Throughout this book I have stressed the benefits of exercise in protecting you against chronic diseases including heart disease, type 2 diabetes, high blood pressure, cancers, osteoporosis and depression. But women are often distressed to find that regular exercise does not guarantee they will lose weight. I know this can be very discouraging but don't despair. The good news is that middle-aged women who exercise regularly do much, much better on the weight front than those who are sedentary. Literally hundreds of pieces of research have shown that no matter how fat you are, physical exercise is great for your health and vital if you want to lose or maintain weight. Women who exercise have smaller waists, which means they are at lower risk for insulin resistance and type 2 diabetes, and have lower levels of bad cholesterol. Regular exercise also helps to maintain your weight loss.

What is important is the amount of exercise you do. A gentle stroll around the garden or the mall does not constitute serious exercise. The current recommendation is 30 minutes at least five times a week; enough to *work up a sweat*. But if you are trying to lose weight it will obviously be helpful to increase your daily physical activity to 60 minutes.

You need to make a commitment to an exercise regimen and stick to it, which means that you should apply some careful time management. Women often tell me that they are too busy to exercise. But if you cut back on the time you spend sitting at the computer, watching television or other unnecessary – although pleasant – sedentary activities, you will find that there is plenty of time to exercise. Try to walk whenever possible; park further away; take the stairs rather than the escalator or the lift; spend time gardening.

When I wrote about osteoporosis in Chapter 9, I recommended brisk aerobic exercise, resistance training and Pilates or yoga as forms of exercise that will contribute to maintaining your bones. New research indicates that you should include some kind of resistance training at least twice weekly. When you decide to make exercise part of your lifestyle you shouldn't stick to one type only. Apart from the boredom factor, you need to challenge your body. The moment you reach a comfort zone, the benefits of exercise are not as great. You need to work on all aspects: cardiovascular, muscle tone, flexibility, suppleness and good posture. This doesn't mean that you have to go overboard and become an exercise fanatic. In fact, if you overexercise, apart from the injuries you could inflict on your body, if you're too lean you could be depleting your already low levels of estrogen and you also won't look great. Every middle-aged woman needs a bit of fat to plump out her skin. Find an expert and work out an exercise regimen that will fit in with your lifestyle and really work for you. Decide when you have adequate time to exercise, see whether you can be flexible and whether you have the discipline to go it alone day in and day out.

If you are like me and would rather be lying on your bed with a novel and a bar of chocolate than working up a sweat, exercise with a trainer, or work out or walk with a friend. It's less easy to skive off that way. There is a lot of choice available. Some women do well with personal trainers, others like to work out at a gym with a predesigned programme, still others prefer to walk and exercise with a friend or their partners. As long as you have a varied programme that encompasses some aerobic work, some resistance training and some flexibility and stretching, you are doing the right thing. For some the bad news is that you must exercise five days a week and when you exercise your breathing should change and your heart rate increase. To lose weight the 30 minutes should be increased to 60 minutes and some suggest that this

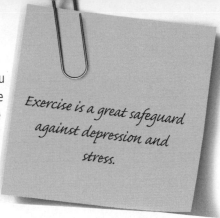

Exercise is a great safeguard against depression and stress.

increased time should be adhered to on a daily basis to maintain weight loss.

Recent research in a huge study of over 39 000 midlife women, following them over 11 years, showed that brisk walking lowered the risk of stroke. Other studies show that when you increase your aerobic activity it helps to improve your metabolism. I have become a convert to the idea of walking briskly at least three times a week. There are several advantages to this. You can just get up and go, you can wear almost anything as long you have good training shoes – cross-trainers are good (and a hat and sunscreen depending on the climate), no gym membership is required, and it's good to get out and enjoy the neighbourhood. My daughter recently gave me an iPod nano; loaded onto it was a pedometer, which after an extensive explanation and lesson from her, I have come to love using. You enter your own personal information and it will count the steps you take, the average speed you walk at and the distance you go. It records the distance you have walked the whole week (no cheating), the calories you have burnt and the feeling of achievement is wonderful, plus the rewards are enormous.

The good news is that all exercise programmes say that you must rest your body, so you can enjoy your days off. In any case the benefits of exercise are wonderful. Exercise is a great safeguard against depression and stress. Many of us have found that when we feel down, food is our first comfort stop, but studies have shown that if you exercise you are less likely to be depressed and to turn to food to cheer yourself up.

EATING FOR COMFORT

Some time ago I had a bad year. I was depressed and felt that my life was out of control. But there was one area where I convinced myself I was in charge: eating. Whenever I had that empty, sinking feeling, I went to the fridge or cupboard and tried to make myself feel better. I say I tried because for a few moments it worked, but moments later I would feel more depressed than ever. The brief high that the comfort food had given me wore off very quickly and I found myself in that cycle of eating that starts with something savoury, say a packet of chips, then goes on to a chocolate, then a fizzy drink, then a piece of chicken, followed by something else. I was guilty but defiant, and tired all the time because I felt too down and listless to exercise, and when I didn't exercise I felt even more angry and depressed.

At night I would lie in bed and touch the roll of fat round my hips and remember how none of my clothes fitted me anymore and how I didn't want to look at myself naked and feel really miserable, but the next day, in spite of the stern lecture I had given myself, I would be back at it again. Food had become my drug of choice.

Many middle-aged women will know what I'm talking about. Food can become as much of an addiction as alcohol and drugs. The problem is that you need to eat in order to live, which is why, when you decide to lose weight and keep it off you need a serious lifestyle change. It's very clear that eating something with lots of refined sugar (a simple carbohydrate) does give us that quick boost, but it's not sustained and we probably find ourselves craving some more chocolate or cake or whatever is at hand to get that energy back. Insulin levels go higher, blood sugar levels rise higher than they should, then drop quickly and we need an energy boost.

It is a medical fact that the feel-good neurotransmitter serotonin regulates not only mood and sleepiness (which is why we often feel sluggish after a meal high in carbohydrates), but also our appetite and desire to eat. Research shows that there is a relationship between insulin and serotonin levels. It's a very complex biochemical procedure. It seems that high levels of carbohydrates increase levels of *tryptophan*, which is one of the things that triggers the production of serotonin. (See Chapter 6.)

So, if you eat a meal that has a lot of carbohydrates in it, tryptophan levels will rise and trigger a greater production of serotonin. Much more research needs to be carried out to clearly understand this association, as well as the role of another neurotransmitter, *dopamine*, and the part it plays in appetite satisfaction. The other side of this coin is that foods rich in protein seem to inhibit serotonin production, which is why many women on very restricted diets, or diets very low in carbohydrates and very rich in proteins, may feel down and depressed

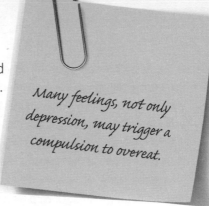

Many feelings, not only depression, may trigger a compulsion to overeat.

or moody and start craving Chelsea buns. It's also well known that certain carbohydrates seem to increase serotonin levels more quickly than others, especially simple carbohydrates, so it's quite logical that our brains, knowing that our serotonin levels are low, would encourage us to pick up a bun, or something else that is starchy, to help us feel better.

The food fix is different for different individuals because our biochemistry is different. I'm sure you've heard women talking among themselves about the different foods that make them feel better when they're down. Many middle-aged women battle with depression, as I will explain in Chapter 13, but going on an eating binge isn't the answer – talking to a therapist to help you over your rocky patch may be a solution. But many feelings, not only depression, may trigger a compulsion to overeat. Don't act out your feelings by raiding the fridge. Eat when you are hungry. Ask yourself what you are feeling when you start eating compulsively, crave something sweet or eat throughout the day. Don't try to submerge your feelings of anxiety, sadness, loneliness, fear or anger with food. Ask yourself what you are feeling when you make for the fridge. For example, if you are anxious, acknowledge that feeling and just sit with it for a while.

Some women find it helpful to write about their feelings; others discover that when they deal with them by seeing a therapist or working through them in a group, their need to overeat disappears. There are several good groups and books that deal with the issue of food when it seems to have taken control of our lives. The age of perimenopause can be a time of many conflicting emotions and feelings, and it is important to recognise and deal with them constructively. Some women, who during this time have become obsessed with food, their weight and dieting, find that joining Overeaters Anonymous (OA) helps. For some this is a gentle, non-threatening way to deal with food and weight issues. You can access your nearest branch through the Internet.

Some women find that taking antidepressants during the perimenopausal period helps them, while others discover that eating correctly and exercising is the answer. Once again, it depends on your individual context. I found that eating sensibly actually stopped the sugar cravings because my glucose levels were balanced rather than spiking, and when I was eating properly and exercising, I no longer felt out of control. I also found it helped me to eat mindfully and to identify feelings of real hunger. I learnt to deal with my emotional issues so that I wasn't using food to fill up the empty spaces in my life. I learnt not to eat when I was distracted either by reading or watching TV. You can get back on track with a proper lifestyle programme, but the slippery path to overeating and not exercising is steep.

Many women have found that it is very helpful to go to a dietician when they have decided to re-examine their lifestyles and eat healthily. A sensible, sympathetic ear really works in this area because you can check your weight and often find out why something is or isn't working. You can get a meal plan that will be individually tailored to your food likes and dislikes. It's pointless going on a diet that includes most of the foods you hate. You may lose weight in the beginning but you will soon give up.

Studies have shown that women who are monitored on a one-on-one programme maintain weight loss better than those who do it alone. You will probably begin your weight loss programme by seeing your dietician once a week and, as you lose the weight and get the hang of sensible eating, your visits will be fewer, but still regular. Some women who have kept their weight down for more than five years go biannually and always have the option of increasing the number of appointments if they are worried about their weight. Others find it works to go to group weigh-ins and lose weight and keep it off that way, but if you can afford it, I think that the individual attention really helps. Other ways to maintain weight loss are to exercise regularly, have breakfast, stick to a sensible eating plan, and weigh yourself on a regular basis. In the past I have said that your clothes will tell you when you are putting on weight. While this is true, research has shown that if you weigh yourself once a week, you can't fool yourself about the weight that has started to creep up; this self-monitoring may help to bring you back to your healthy lifestyle if you've been going a bit crazy or eating too much 'comfort' food. However, I am a firm believer in not only losing weight but also dealing with the issues (there may be many and they may have been around for much of your life as a woman) that made food your drug of choice in the first place.

Now that you've had a little reality check, let's look at how you can manage your weight in menopause and still enjoy your life. The rules below are what I have learnt over the years as I have struggled to lose my middle-aged spread.

- There is no such thing as a painless way to lose weight. By this I mean that there will be some things you will have to give up, like second helpings and fast food (or at least not eat it more than three times a year). If you decide to try one of the hundreds of diet pills that are on the market, be careful. They usually don't work, so you'll have wasted your money and when they do work they can often have serious side effects.

- Stay away from fad diets. They may work well at first but the weight you lose quickly may be mostly water and lean muscle mass instead of fat; you'll gain it back, perhaps even more than before, and it will be harder to lose. Lose weight on a sensible meal plan at a sensible rate: not more than 2–4 kg (4.5–9 pounds) a month.

- No second helpings. This really works. Look at your slim friends. At a dinner party they seldom have a second helping or they take a tiny bit to start and may have a minuscule second taste.

- Watch your portions. Look at a fat woman helping herself to food at a buffet. The chances are her plate is laden. Most research concludes that in the matter of losing weight and maintaining it, it doesn't matter what the diet is – once the portions and calories are restricted, people lose weight.

- Watch your calories. It's no good having small portions of high calorie food. Well, it's better than having large portions of high calorie food, but it's not sensible. That's why dieticians often suggest that rather than ordering a huge plate of pasta with a rich cheesy sauce you have a big green salad with your meal. It takes up space, it's healthy and it's low in calories. My suggestion is that when you eat a salad you dress it with something tasty, interesting and low fat. Feeling deprived and bored when you eat is the quickest route I know to a trip to the sweet cupboard.

- If you know you're going to a dinner party or will be eating dinner at a special restaurant, pace yourself during the day. Certain slim women who seem to eat huge quantities at night often leave out lunch or breakfast. Obviously this isn't the healthiest way to do things, but it gives you a bit of room to manoeuvre.

- Some women do better when they eat every couple of hours. So you may have breakfast at 8 am, a snack at 10 am, lunch at 1 pm, a snack at 4 pm and dinner at 7 pm, with a snack at about 9 pm. If the food you eat is sensible, you will keep balanced levels of insulin and won't have uncontrollable food cravings.

- Get your family involved; helping them to eat wisely is doing them a favour too.
- Learn to know what true hunger feels like. Don't eat out of habit, boredom or for comfort and don't wait until you're ravenous before you eat. When I was overeating I felt hungry, or at least in need of food, all the time. I had forgotten what proper hunger felt like and only remembered it when I started to eat properly and felt satisfied for the periods between meals.
- Vary your diet. As I have emphasised, to lose or maintain weight requires a lifestyle change and there's no point in dieting frantically for two weeks for a special occasion and then putting it all back on. It's too depressing. There really are plenty of choices out there. You don't have to sit glumly over an endless array of cottage cheese and plain lettuce. Ask your dietician to help you find a way to include the foods you like in a meal plan. You'll be surprised at how many things you can eat and still lose weight.
- Don't eat when you're distracted. Sit down at a table and use a plate.
- Find someone to monitor you. It's sensible when you start your new lifestyle regimen to get help from a professional who can help you through the bad bits and explain why you aren't losing weight when you could have sworn that you had stuck to your meal plan. Professionals understand how your metabolism works and can give you lots of helpful hints. Research has clearly shown that women who had support when they were on diet and then went onto a weight maintenance programme did much better than those who had to go it alone.
- Don't eat out of depression or boredom and don't eat to suppress your feelings. There's a moment of triumph and defiance, and then reality bites. Learn to recognise when you are anxious or angry and develop mechanisms to deal with those feelings. Read Geneen Roth's books. I have found them very helpful in this regard. Overeaters Anonymous may also be helpful in enabling you to recognise why you are eating compulsively.
- Watch the amount of alcohol you consume. There's no problem with a glass or two of wine, but it can play havoc with the levels of glucose in your blood, which can make you very hungry. Also, when you drink too much your willpower falters.

- Don't fall into despair if you've pigged out. And don't make it an excuse to go on a binge. Say to yourself: 'I ate exactly what I wanted last night. It was delicious and I enjoyed every mouthful. It made no difference and today I'll resume my eating plan and my exercise.' Take everything one day, or even one meal, at a time.
- Treat yourself occasionally and do it guilt-free. There's no reason not to have the hot-buttered toast (as long as it's rye toast!) or the piece of cheesecake or the Christmas pudding. Just don't go mad, and watch your portions. If you're eating mindfully and savouring your food it's amazing how a little goes a long way.
- Exercise for at least 30 minutes five times a week. See that you have a varied exercise programme and always work up a sweat.
- Ensure that you drink enough, but not too much, water. Six to eight glasses a day will stop that hungry feeling you may get when you're dehydrated. Those women who drink more than two litres of water a day may have mineral imbalances and often have urinary tract infections and urinary problems, a situation that doesn't help women who already have vaginal dryness and urinary incontinence.
- You are not a 'bad girl' when your diet goes awry or you diverge from your meal plan. What you've done may not be great for your health, but that's it. Take the emotion out of eating once and for all. When you eat well and exercise you're being kind to and looking after yourself. A middle-aged woman doesn't need to be bullied and bossed about her weight or judged on it. It's no one's business but your own. Do it for your health's sake and the rest will follow.
- Some women are very disciplined in their eating habits from Monday to Friday and then eat more or less what they want at the weekend. Others are generally disciplined all week but eat luxury foods and have a drink or two when the need arises: a dinner party, a meal at a restaurant, or a special occasion. It depends on what suits you best.
- Here are the six easy guidelines to healthy eating from the US Department of Agriculture (USDA) (http://www.choosemyplate.gov/): Enjoy your food, but eat less; avoid oversized portions; make half of your plate fruits and vegetables; switch to fat-free or low-fat milk; compare sodium in foods like soup, bread and frozen meals, and choose the foods with lower numbers; drink water instead of sugary drinks.
- TAKE CONTROL. What you eat should NEVER control you. Don't give your power away to a bar of chocolate or a piece of cake!

11
Looking good, feeling better: body image in menopause

BODY APPEARANCE

> *'The problem,' says Amy, 'is that I hate the way I look. My boobs hang, my hips are wide and my skin is mottled and not smooth any more. I've got a double chin and no matter how much I exercise, I just don't feel firm. I don't feel sexy, in fact, when I look at myself I'm "turned off", although the weird thing is that Rob tells me I'm gorgeous and he loves my body and he is always eager to make love.'*

Amy is blonde and extremely pretty and although she's no longer slim, she glows with vitality and is beautifully groomed. From what she has just told me, her husband agrees with this assessment, but she can't accept her middle-aged self. Many of us hold in our minds a picture of ourselves at 18 and it's very hard to accept that gravity and life have altered us. We are going to continue to age, no matter how much time and energy we put into preserving ourselves, and one day we're going to be old. This is a fact of life. It doesn't mean that we can't be sexy and attractive in midlife because we are no longer young and firm.

> *Take Sue and her younger lover, who I write about in Chapter 12: 'I love the way I feel,' she says. 'I work out and my body is as good as it's going to get, but that's okay because I feel healthy and good about myself. I like looking good, but I've accepted that I can't wear things like tight midriff tops. So I buy clothes that suit me and get vicarious pleasure from shopping for my daughter. It may sound like a rationalisation, but I don't think the faces of young girls are as interesting as the faces of my friends. Those lines add character; they tell a story of lives well lived, full of happiness and sorrow and laughter.'*

I know that the ruling message in the media today is that young is better, but we don't have to accept this. If we feel great and take care of our health, both emotional and physical, we can look and feel wonderful. When a woman feels good about herself, it's amazing how few people judge her physical appearance. So don't regret the passing years but spend some time working out how to live as well as you can: exercise and eat sensibly, get rid of bad habits like smoking and drinking too much, take care of your skin, dress appropriately but with enjoyment, and find time to groom yourself so that you look healthy, fit and glowing and feel wonderful.

YOUR MENOPAUSAL SKIN

Exercise and a sensible lifestyle should help you maintain a reasonable body and good health, but there's no doubt that the skin is a major indicator of age. We've all looked into the mirror and seen the fine lines, wrinkles, sunspots, uneven pigmentation and the larger pores that are signs of an ageing skin. Obviously many of these signs are, as Sue says, testament to the long, fulfilled lives we have led, but there are things we can avoid and others we can pay attention to so we can keep our skins looking younger.

Smoking and your skin

Here I am again, going on about smoking. You've worked out by now that I am somewhat obsessed with it. But it is clear that when women smoke they look older and it certainly affects their appearance. There is no doubt from all the available data that smoking definitely causes premature ageing and wrinkles. You've probably noticed that women who don't smoke have younger-looking skin than those who do. One of the major culprits in this is the nicotine in cigarettes. It causes the tiny blood vessels in the outer layers of your skin to narrow, which interferes with the flow of blood to these areas. When this blood flow is impaired your skin won't get enough nutrients like vitamin A, or the vital oxygen it needs. Other reasons include the damage caused to the collagen and elastin in your skin (the connective tissues and fibres in the skin that contribute to its strength and elasticity) by the chemicals in the cigarette smoke. These chemicals also increase the damaging amounts of free radicals and your face loses that glowing, healthy look we associate with being young. Your skin usually ages prematurely when you smoke, although it is difficult to see this early skin damage, which often only becomes apparent about 10 years after you've started smoking. If you are a heavy smoker this effect is likely to be even more severe. The wrinkling caused by smoking also appears on your body; look at your inner arms if you've been smoking for a long time and see what this habit has caused. You can't reverse these wrinkles without some cosmetic surgery but you can certainly stop them from becoming worse if you quit smoking now.

The changes that smoking causes on a smoker's face were graphically described in a recent medical journal article I read. I have tried to summarise them here: Lines or wrinkles come out from the upper and lower lips and the corners of the eyes; deep lines on the cheeks or hundreds of fine lines both on the cheek and lower jaw. The features of the face seem to be slightly gaunt and cheekbones often look more prominent (due to the damage to collagen and elastin). The skin looks dry and has a slightly greyish colour, and in certain areas, such as the cheeks, it looks red and blotchy. Smokers may also have blackish or yellow bumps or blocked pores on their skin. Their nails are often yellowish, as are their teeth, and their gums are also discoloured. Going grey earlier and hair loss have been associated with smoking, though there is not definitive research about this as yet.

Other things about smoking increase these woes. The heat from the cigarette and the flow of smoke upwards causes smokers to squint to avoid the smoke; imagine doing this several hundred times a day. In addition, check out how you purse your lips when you stick the cigarette in your mouth and inhale, then go to the mirror and see what happens to the tiny lines around your mouth when you do this – they deepen. In addition, new research has shown that if you smoke and are exposed to the sun's ultraviolet rays, the sun damage will be worse.

Just some facts about why smoking is implicated in so many diseases. There is a mixture of well over 4 500 chemicals in cigarettes and about 250 substances, which are toxic. At least 43 of these are carcinogenic, in other words known to cause cancer. I am quite sure you'd never voluntarily ingest these: nail polish remover, arsenic, wood varnish, industrial solvent, rat poison, insect poison, nicotine, tar, paint stripper, lighter fuel, rocket fuel and toilet cleaner. Perhaps being aware of the presence of these entering your system whenever you inhale deeply may put you off smoking.

Some of you may wonder why there is so much about smoking in a book about menopause. It is because apart from the health risks and the less serious but upsetting effects on appearance, research shows that women are more likely to become addicted to cigarettes than men and find it harder to stop. It seems that when women smoke they feel less stressed; they say they can concentrate better and feel more alert. Remember Kim in Chapter 8, who had been diagnosed with cancer and was battling terribly with both breast and cervical cancer, both associated with smoking, and still couldn't quit. Many women I have spoken to say they are frightened of gaining weight and use smoking as an 'appetite suppressant'. As we discussed in Chapter 10 you may eat to deal with emotional issues, so it makes sense that if you smoke for the same reasons and give it up, you will probably need to binge. But you can get help with this. If you are aware of this possibility, you can deal with it; a kilo or two seems slightly less important than the serious disease risks that come with smoking.

There is a mixture of well over 4 500 chemicals in cigarettes and about 250 substances, which are toxic.

The American Heart Association explains that if you exercise when you stop smoking (and you'll be able to exercise more easily if you're not smoking) and eat healthy foods full of good nutrients and antioxidants, you may not even gain weight at all. If smoking helped you to stay calm, then exercise, which has been shown to reduce stress and increase mood-enhancing chemicals (*endorphins*), is a great substitute for a cigarette.

It's hard to stop smoking alone, though many women have done so; find an organisation or counsellor who can help. There are also medications that can help you over the worst part of quitting, like *bupropion* (Wellbutrin, Zyban), but you must speak to your doctor first and discuss all the risks and benefits of this drug, as side effects include dizziness, sleepiness, insomnia, restlessness, headaches, dry mouth and vomiting. A new medication called *varenicline* (Chantix) has been approved as an anti-smoking treatment in the USA. It seems to help because it stops the good feelings you get when you smoke and reduces severe withdrawal symptoms. Side effects associated with it include strange dreams, bloating and gas, constipation and vomiting. There may be other more serious side effects like seizures and depression, so you should **only** take it under the care of a specialist who is well informed about this drug. Nicotine patches, gums and lozenges may help to reduce your craving for nicotine. There are also alternative treatments that might help, such as acupuncture, relaxation techniques, hypnosis and some herbal supplements. Whatever route you take – and you may find a combination of the above is best for you – discuss the options with your healthcare practitioner and remember that your mental attitude and determination are crucial to your success.

The sun and your skin

If you have worshipped the sun all your life it's bad luck, because nothing, except perhaps smoking, is more ageing. When I was young I couldn't wait for a sunny day because all I wanted was a tan. We knew nothing about the damage the sun could cause and couldn't wait to get really brown tan. On the first day of my holidays I would rush down to the beach, wearing the briefest of bikinis, and slather my skin in baby oil or coconut butter; some of my friends used cooking oil, which was quite appropriate. We would then sunbathe for hours, turning ourselves like chickens on a spit and basting ourselves occasionally with our favourite potions in the hottest sun – midday was the best time. I would come home bright red, tender and not feeling great as I would usually have mild sunstroke, but happy, knowing that sooner or later the red would turn to golden brown and I would look like the models in the magazines I loved to read; *Seventeen* and *Cosmopolitan*. I had absolutely no idea about the damage I was causing or that it would only appear years later in the form of brown spots and pigmentation marks and, in some of my friends, as the dreaded skin cancer.

Perhaps it's too little too late, but for the past 20 years I've been rigorous about the following rules. Try not to be on the beach at midday (dermatologists recommend you stay out of the sun when the rays are strongest, approximately from 11 am to 3 pm) but if you are, wear a sunscreen with an SP factor of at least 30 (don't forget your lips and the delicate area around your eyes) and try to cover up. If you need to be outdoors, always wear a sunscreen on exposed areas and use a moisturiser that contains one. Always wear a broad-brimmed hat or if you are on the beach stay under an umbrella if you can. Fair-skinned women are at greater risk for skin cancer from sun damage so be careful if you're blonde. I believe that to minimise age spots, you should wear a sunscreen on your hands as well. Look at the hand that is nearest the window when you drive to see why. If age spots get too bad, they can be burnt off.

Before I describe the products and treatments that are available to help our ageing skins, a quick word about skin cancer. We all have little moles all over our bodies, some of us more than others, but you should go to a dermatologist for a yearly check-up to monitor any of them that may have changed and check out signs of sun damage as they appear. Watch for suspicious skin patches and ulcers that may be caused on your lips by sunburn. You are at risk for skin cancer if you have a **family history** of it, are **fair skinned**, have **red or fair hair**, and have had many **years of sun exposure** or any **unusual or changing moles**. Skin cancer can appear anywhere on your body, not only on those areas that have had the highest exposure to the sun. Be aware of any changes in the moles on your body or the appearance of new ones.

Melanoma is the deadliest skin cancer and it can occur anywhere on the body. When found early, before it penetrates deeply into the skin, melanoma is completely curable, so it is important to have it diagnosed early. See the ABCDE of skin cancer in the Empowerment Points at the end of this chapter. Be alert for a mole that suddenly changes colour, gets darker or bigger, or seems to be composed of more than one colour. If a mole is itchy, inflamed or painful, or if the skin is broken and it bleeds, you should alert your doctor. Melanoma is a sun-related cancer, though it **often occurs in areas of minimal exposure**, such as the back of the leg. Red areas that bleed easily in sun-exposed skin should also be checked because this might indicate a cancer known as *basal* or *squamous cell carcinoma*. While rarely fatal, these cancers can grow rapidly and become severely disfiguring. Basal and squamous cell carcinomas typically do occur in sun-exposed areas such as the face.

If something on your skin looks suspicious, the dermatologist or surgeon will do a biopsy to remove as much of it as possible and send this section of cells and tissues to the laboratory to see if it's cancerous. Many doctors like to get two opinions when a melanoma is found because it is difficult to diagnose. If the diagnosis is positive the specialist will do a series of tests to check how far the cancer has progressed. Once this has been determined they will devise a treatment plan that centres on the complete removal of the cancer. New research has shown that **not even** indoor tanning machines are safe.

'Anti-ageing' skin care

There are certain things that you can do to prevent your skin from ageing too quickly. Of course, if you've got good genes, that's first prize. My mother was well into her eighties and had the skin of a 40-year-old woman. She always cared for her skin. I can remember watching her having facials from the time I was a little girl, but ultimately, I think that her genes determined the way her skin looked. Exercise is excellent for waking up your skin and helping it glow, but if you're walking always wear a sunscreen and a hat and see that your lips and all exposed areas of your body are protected. Deal with your stress levels and try to get enough sleep. I believe that you should be hydrated inside and out so drink at least six glasses of water daily, as well as using a good moisturiser.

Some women suddenly develop acne as they transition into menopause which is often due to the changes in the ratio of androgen to estrogen in their bodies, as I explained in Chapter 3. And it is often those who had acne during their teenage years who seem to have the problem. It is important to see a dermatologist if this happens to you, as it can be very upsetting. Certain women in early perimenopause may find relief from this problem if they use a low-dose combined oral contraceptive, as I discussed in Chapter 4.

As you know to your cost and from the crowded shelves in your bathroom, there are thousands of skincare products in the marketplace that promise you a glowing skin, a finer skin, a youthful skin and a radiant skin. The problem is that these creams and potions may be beautifully packaged and look and feel wonderful, but they may not work. Because the baby boomers are now ready to spend a lot of money on their appearance, new and exciting research is being done on skincare products to try to find the 'magic' anti-ageing formula.

The issue is whether you should buy prescription products that have been seen to work but are often costly and complicated to use, or trust the over-the-counter products that promise us so much. As you get older, the collagen, which is a fibrous tissue found throughout your body, and the elastin, which are the fibres that make the skin elastic, begin to age with wear and tear so that your skin looks less plump and supple. In addition, exposure to the sun, the build-up of dead skin cells on the surface of the skin, fine lines and wrinkles, and the thinning appearance of the skin make us look older.

Anti-ageing products play several roles in the rejuvenation of the skin: they exfoliate (slough off) the dead layers; they help build up the collagen and elastin; and they thicken the skin so that it looks firmer and more glowing. Below is a list of ingredients that appear time and again in anti-ageing creams. Read the labels of products carefully and buy those that contain the appropriate ingredients. And sometimes just pamper yourself with a wonderfully scented product that will be good for your soul, even if it doesn't do much for your skin.

Glycolic acid is found in green fruit and young plants. It is also made from sugarcane. It is the most powerful of the a*lpha hydroxy acids*, or the fruit acids, and stimulates the surface of the skin to peel by a chemical action, which helps to reduce the build-up of dead skin cells. It is used as a skin peel, which means that it exfoliates the dead cells of the epidermis or surface layer of the skin. This means that when you use it, your skin should look younger and more glowing. Another of its functions is to trigger the production of collagen, which may make your skin look plumper. If you see either of the above ingredients listed on your product, you are probably on the right track.

Retinol or *retinoids* are derived from vitamin A. Because one of the main functions of vitamin A is to preserve the skin's elasticity and prevent excessive wrinkling and accelerated ageing, vitamin A derivatives seem to be an ideal anti-ageing ingredient. If you see any of the following: *retinol, retinyl palmitate, retinyl linoleate* or *retinyl acetate* on the label of a product you know that you are dealing with an anti-ageing product. It is thought that retinoids or retinol can correct the damage caused to the skin by the sun and strengthen the epidermis (the outer layer of the skin) by thickening it, which helps to prevent sun damage. Retinoids are natural exfoliators. *Retin A* is a stronger version of the retinoids and is used under a doctor's supervision rather than sold over the counter.

The following ingredients are often found in over-the-counter anti-ageing skincare products, but a great deal more scientific research, using well-designed trials, needs to be carried out to prove whether any of them are really effective in reversing the ageing process:

Vitamin E (α-tocopherol) may act as an antioxidant on the epidermis and help to repair damage by preventing the actions of free radicals that cause ageing, helping the skin to become smoother and refining fine lines and wrinkles. It also seems to have an effect on plumping out the skin.

Vitamin C (L-ascorbic acid) is another ingredient you will find in many over-the-counter skincare products. It appears to help lighten the skin, improves skin pigmentation and sun damage, and may also act as an antioxidant, which helps to prevent the damage caused by free radicals.

Coenzyme Q10 (ubiquinone) antioxidants, as I explained earlier, may help prevent skin damage and play a role in repairing the skin. Some researchers have reported that CoQ10 levels decrease in our skin as we age and believe that by adding this ingredient to our skincare regimen we may reverse some sun damage, smooth out some wrinkles and increase the collagen levels.

Soy isoflavones are also popular ingredients in the new spate of anti-ageing products directed at postmenopausal women. One of the reasons for this is that they are plant estrogens, as you saw in Chapter 5, which suggests that they might have a beneficial effect on the estrogen receptors in the skin and contribute to the reversal of age-related damage.

There are some very powerful new anti-ageing agents available called *cosmeceuticals*, some of which I describe below, but these should only be used by an expert dermatologist or plastic surgeon. It would be very unwise to buy them in over-the-counter products. If you find a 'miracle' anti-ageing cream that contains them, ask your dermatologist about it and only use it under strict supervision.

Kinetin (or cytokinin), a plant hormone that regulates cell growth, is one of the newest, most powerful anti-ageing products. It is thought to reduce fine lines and wrinkles, smooth out the skin and diminish skin mottling and pigmentation. It appears to be used very effectively in combination with *retinol palmitate*, but should only be used under medical supervision.

Hydroquinone is a very powerful skin-lightening agent, or bleach. Like kinetin, it should only be used under a doctor's supervision. It can cause extreme sensitivity and should be used with caution. It can be applied in combination with *glycolic acid* to refine and smooth an ageing, sun-damaged skin.

There are a variety of skin care treatments that may work in conjunction with a good skin care product regimen. A physician who has aesthetic care experience may be able recommend the ones that may be most useful. Microdermabrasion uses small beads like grains of sand to exfoliate the superficial skin layer, giving the skin a nice glow while removing ageing skin cells. Intense pulsed light (IPL) treatments use high energy light pulses to heat the skin and target visible brown and red discolorations or unwanted hair growth. Lasers have more focused energy than IPL and may be more effective for larger or denser, visible blood vessels in the skin or fine wrinkles.

PLASTIC SURGERY

Many postmenopausal women who feel that the available products do not work quickly or dramatically enough turn to plastic surgery to help them recover a much younger-looking skin or face. Several procedures, which used to be extremely costly and difficult, have been refined and can be performed in an outpatient situation in the plastic surgeon's rooms. You should make extensive enquiries before you commit yourself to any of the following treatments and make sure that the practitioner is very well trained and well versed in these procedures.

Some women are very happy with the lines on their faces and, like Sue, who I quote at the beginning of this chapter, think they add interest and character. However, this is a very personal choice and the decision must be yours alone. Do not allow anyone to judge you, or label you frivolous. If it feels right to you, go ahead.

You can improve the texture of your skin by means of botox injections. Botox is a poison (*botulinum toxin*) that is injected in tiny amounts into the skin and helps to smooth out wrinkles and frown lines by temporarily paralysing the tiny facial muscles. It relaxes the muscles on each side of the wrinkle and flattens it out. The problem is that this procedure wears off in four or five months, so that you may need to make frequent visits to maintain the effect.

Some women want a lighter, smoother skin and want to refine the fine lines and wrinkles. For this they would have a chemical peel, where a strong exfoliating product is applied to the skin to remove the damaged layer or layers and unsightly bumps and pigmentation. The strength of the peel depends on the extent of the damage. The time the skin takes to heal and stop looking sensitive depends on the strength of the peel. The peel also causes the skin to regenerate while it is healing, giving you a smoother, younger-looking skin.

The same type of result may be obtained through laser treatments, where the imperfections of the skin are burnt off using a very fine, high-intensity beam of light. Some laser and peel treatments are very mild or superficial and need to be repeated monthly for four to six months before changes can be seen. The recovery time is rapid, with some skin redness for only 24 hours.

Other treatments are more aggressive or deeper and result in more noticeable changes in skin texture and pigment. The recovery time is longer, more in the order of a few days to a week of skin redness or sensitivity. Deeper lines can be plumped out using injections of one of the many available 'fillers' like fat, collagen or *hyaluronic acid*, which may last a year or more.

Finally, you can investigate the possibility of a facelift, the only effective treatment for the excess hanging skin in the neck, jowl and cheek areas. The latest procedure in this type of surgery has gone beyond 'pull and tuck'. Surgeons now operate in such a way that they reposition the face and fill it out. If you don't want anything as drastic as a facelift, you can have surgery to remove the bags above or under your eyes.

BRIGHT EYES IN MIDLIFE

Talking about eyes, many women really battle with dry, red, itchy and blurred eyes when they reach menopause; the blurring is caused by the fact that the eye no longer has a smooth film over it. Apart from the fact that red, blurry eyes don't look great, these symptoms can make you feel very tired at the end of a day because when clear vision is compromised and you are struggling to see clearly, it can be exhausting. Other eye-related problems that can beset us at menopause are sensitivity to light and increased tearing. As with the other complaints in midlife, I would recommend that you have an annual check-up. Certain illnesses, like diabetes, can impact on your eye health. Some of the symptoms listed above may be caused by Sjörgren's syndrome (an autoimmune disease) or rheumatoid arthritis. Medications such as antidepressants or allergies can cause some of the above problems too.

Less serious factors can be air conditioning, pollution and hours spent in front of your computer.

Here's a tip: don't wait until your eyes are dry all the time. When you reach perimenopause, start to use eye drops that have the same composition as natural tears to keep your eyes moist. You can use them several times a day (hourly or once every two hours) and they really help. There is also a tear gel that mimics the moisturising action of your tears, coating the surface of the eye and protecting it from the drying effects – the dose depends on what works for you. At night you can try a special lubricating eye ointment to help your eyes stay moist. You should keep these natural tears with you at all times, even next to your bed. Many of us sleep with our eyes a tiny bit open, so the surface of the eye becomes dryer. If you wake during the night to go to the bathroom, use the drops.

If your eyes are very dry, don't smoke, don't have the air conditioner on in your car, drink a lot of water and use a humidifier at night if you have a heater or air conditioner on in your bedroom or if you live in a very dry climate. There is a new product, *cyclosporine ophthalmic emulsion* (Restasis), which may be helpful in treating a severe dry eye problem. If the drops, gels or ointments are not at all helpful, there is a procedure that may relieve the dryness. The ophthalmologist will insert punctal plugs into your eyes. The *punctum* is a tiny duct that drains tears from your eyes into the nose. It is situated in the lower part of your eye, near your nose. The plug is a mechanical blockage and helps whatever tears you have left in your eye to stay there and not drain out.

You should get your eyes checked annually for age-related problems such as *cataracts* and *glaucoma*. Cataracts are a clouding of the lenses and happen slowly as we age, but can be easily and safely removed if they become opaque. You should also be monitored for glaucoma as you get older, especially if your parents had this condition. Glaucoma is an increase in pressure behind the eye as a result of fluid build-up. Glaucoma can be well controlled if it is diagnosed early and treated. You've probably already noticed that your eyesight has changed in middle age, so you must have regular eye examinations. A lot of headaches are caused by impaired vision.

Earlier when I talked about sun damage, I didn't mention the problems that very bright sunlight and UV exposure can cause to your eyes. It can contribute to tissue growth, which look like little cloudy bumps that you may see on the surface of your eye if you look closely in the mirror. Sunlight can also increase cataract development and *macular degeneration*, a disease that causes the cells in your *macula* (the area in your retina responsible for central vision including facial recognition, reading and detailed work) to die and in the process destroys your sharp central vision, so you need to protect your eyes from the sun. Always wear sunglasses when the sun is brightest or when you go out because the sun's rays can pass through the clouds too. Wear wraparound sunglasses or those with a wide arm so that the sun cannot come in from the exposed sides. Your sunglasses should block at last 95 per cent of harmful UVA and UVB rays.

Some experts believe that the omega-3 fatty acids that I discussed in Chapter 5 should be part of your diet, either in supplement form or by eating oily fish at least twice a week, and recent research suggests that they may help lower the risk of macular degeneration. Eating healthily impacts on your eyes as it does every other part of your body, so always have plenty of fruits, nuts and vegetables. Dark green, leafy vegetables like spinach contain an antioxidant called lutein that may also protect against cataracts and macular degeneration.

YOUR TEETH

One of the most telling areas in our appearance as we age is our teeth. They've served us very well for years and years and it shows. If we have osteoporosis we may be at risk for tooth loss, another reason to know your status in this area. Falling levels of estrogen in some perimenopausal women may cause gum issues and sometimes inflammation or increased sensitivity. There are midlife women who experience an unpleasant condition, which is not associated with menopause, called burning mouth syndrome. This is present even when there are no obvious signs in the mouth or medical reasons for it. This may be caused by nerve damage in the nerve cells that carry taste signals, and is very distressing.

You should be vigilant about caring for your teeth, have regular dental appointments and floss and brush regularly. It is very important to keep your teeth clean and if you feel you are not doing a thorough enough job, see a dental hygienist a couple of times a year.

Some women find the appearance of their yellowing and discoloured teeth distressing and there is the option of having them whitened. In my opinion a dental specialist should do this. Each person should be assessed individually to exclude those with gum disease or other related problems; the procedure should be carefully explained, and the potential success and any risks frankly discussed. Stains caused by antibiotics may be harder to whiten, for example. The process is generally safe, though more research is needed to say this definitively, and there should be few side effects. It usually takes about two hours; a special gel that is activated by a blue light (not containing harmful UV rays) is used during the process.

EXERCISE MAKES YOU LOOK AND FEEL WONDERFUL

I have written about exercise throughout the book and extolled its benefits. I am convinced that it is a vital tool in helping us to look healthy and glowing. Here once again are compelling reasons to exercise: it reduces the risk of heart disease by improving blood circulation throughout the body; it keeps weight under control, improves blood cholesterol levels, prevents and manages high blood pressure, helps prevent bone loss, boosts energy levels, helps manage stress and releases tension, improves the ability to fall asleep quickly and sleep well, improves self-image, counters anxiety and depression, increasing enthusiasm and optimism, and increases muscle strength, increasing the ability to do other physical activities. In other words, movement is medicine.

Women who exercise regularly but sensibly look better in general. You should exercise five days a week for a minimum of 30 minutes – you need to move so your breathing changes and your heart rate increases. Find an exercise you enjoy and that doesn't exhaust you. Exercise is meant to energise you, not whack you to the wall. Don't just think of it as a grim period of reps and sets; integrate different kinds of exercise, including aerobic, stretching and moderate weight bearing.

Use your whole body so you have mobility, flexibility and stability. Try to make exercise a habit, but be flexible. If you miss your exercise one day there's no problem in working an activity into your day another way. Many committed exercisers I know exercise to music to keep them moving and inspired. Choose songs you love and make an exercise mix on your iPod.

Exercise should also translate into the way you move in your daily life. It should help you stand straighter and move with confidence so you look great. Don't just slump around when you're doing a task; be aware of how you're moving. Hold your head high and dance your way through your days.

EATING DISORDERS

I spent a whole chapter discussing the problems related to being overweight in menopause but I think I should also mention that not only are there problems with being too thin at midlife, as at other stages in the reproductive cycle (for example, bone fragility increases), but being too thin does your looks no good. Have you ever noticed what happens when a woman loses too much weight?

Unless she's told us she's on a drastic diet we assume with some anxiety that she's ill. The first place we notice it is on her face, because no matter how great her body looks we all need a little extra plumpness on our faces. Her neck may get a stringy appearance and her hands may also look much older because the skin may have become loose, as may the skin on her upper arms. Many of us are obsessed with looking younger but the sad truth is though we can look great in midlife, there's no way, short of a time machine, that we can become young again. Sadly, there is an increase in women with eating disorders because they fear weight gain or are deeply dissatisfied with their body image. None of us wants to be fat but it is normal to carry a few more kilos into middle age and a kilo or two shouldn't cause too much concern.

GROOMING

We may not be able to erase the years, but we can have healthy, well-toned bodies, glowing skins and hair, and dress well. We can look groomed and attractive without being ridiculous and accept that mini skirts won't look as good on us as they do on our daughters. We can't like we did at 18 but we can embrace our older selves and still wear clothes that are fashionable, chic and glamorous. I meet countless women who look fabulous as they age. I watch world experts as they give talks at international conferences. They may be slim and toned if they're watching their health, or they may carry some extra weight. They are well turned out and confident; these are the women I aspire to look like. I am not looking for the girls in the fashion magazines to be my role models. I am inspired by women on the world stage who are using their midlife years to achieve some incredible goals. I look at women in business and women in government, those who are medical scientists, engineers, economists, journalists, or who fight for human rights. Look at Hilary Clinton, who at 63 is not the slimmest or best dressed but is one of the most powerful women in the world, or Christine Lagard (55), who looks fabulous and is the head of the International Monetary Fund. I am sure if you look around your own world you will be able to pick out those of your friends who are confident and content with their lives, who look their age but always look wonderful and who, in their own way, are making a difference and enhancing the lives of those around them.

- Know the **ABCDE** of skin cancer. Have your moles checked out by a dermatologist if you have any of the signs below:
  ○ **A**symmetry – one half of a mole doesn't match the other.
  ○ **B**order – the edges or borders of the mole are irregular, blurry or raggedy.
  ○ **C**olour – normal moles are usually one shade of colour. It's a red flag if there are different colours in the mole: tan, browns, black, white or red or a bluish shade. Another warning sign is when the mole becomes lighter or darker.
  ○ **D**iameter – the diameter of the mole changes; a mole shouldn't be bigger than 6 mm ($^1/_4$ in.).
  ○ **E**levation or **E**volving – the mole becomes raised or bumpy or changes shape.
- Other changes include itchiness or tenderness, or if a mole doesn't heal and has a red area around it.
- Check your body once a month – changes may happen to your skin in midlife – and see a dermatologist for a check-up annually.
- If you are a swimmer, rinse your skin well after your swim and moisturise it.
- Don't smoke. You know all about the dangers of smoking by now but it's also very bad for your skin.
- Eat a healthy, balanced diet and don't drink too much alcohol.
- Keep yourself hydrated. If you are drinking enough water, it will be reflected in your skin tone.
- Protect your skin during the day with a moisturiser and a sunscreen or a good base containing a sunscreen.
- At night you must clean your skin well. At your age, you should be using treatments that not only moisturise but also exfoliate.
- Dress with enjoyment and embrace the way you look.
- Glowing skin, shining hair and a toned body are not age-dependent.
- Choose your skincare products carefully. The fact that something smells and feels good is no guarantee that it will benefit your skin.
- Be glad of your smile lines – they are a testament to a life well lived.

12

'The dreaded pole in the back in the middle of the night': sex and menopause

Alexandra sipped her coffee reflectively. 'It's the dreaded pole in the back in the middle of the night,' she said. 'I don't know if other menopausal women feel like me, but sex has become a bore. I mean he hasn't talked to me all day except to ask if I've collected the package from the post office. During dinner he's exhausted and afterwards he slumps in front of the TV with a whisky in his hand and drops off to sleep. He falls into bed still without saying a word; he snores loudly and suddenly in the middle of the night he grabs me. I couldn't feel less like sex by that time.'

'How do I feel about sex?' Sue grinned. 'I love it. I'm in my mid-fifties and he's quite a bit younger but he makes me feel great. I love his energy and, to be frank, his body. We talk for hours in bed and laugh a lot. He makes me feel beautiful.'

'I used to really enjoy sex,' said Connie. 'We've been married a long time and now that the kids are gone, we don't have to worry about someone bursting into the bedroom at the wrong time. I love my husband and I feel like sex, but it's so painful that I don't even let myself get excited any more. John's become anxious about even touching me. It's become a huge worry. I've also been very depressed during this last year, worse than I can ever remember apart from a bad period of postnatal depression after our third child was born.'

'After my hysterectomy, I was really worried about our sex life,' said Vicki. 'My gynaecologist removed my cervix as well as my womb and for a while I didn't feel like going near my husband

because I felt so different. Perhaps it was in my mind. I don't know, but after a while my hormones were sorted out, I started using the estradiol-releasing ring so my vagina didn't feel sore anymore and sex isn't bad at all. I still have an orgasm and I'm not sure if I could tell you whether it feels different or not. In any case I've always felt that Dave liked sex more than I did, he still thinks I'm sexy and wants to make love nearly every night. I decided that if we just made love and I didn't make a big thing about it, it would become easier – like a pleasant habit. In fact it's fine. He's really happy with our sex life and so am I.'

Sexuality in midlife is dependent on many different things – psychological, physical and social. Since all these aspects of our lives are intertwined and since they affect us particularly during the peri- and postmenopausal years, I will discuss all of them in greater or lesser detail. They are intrinsic to the way we feel about ourselves, how we relate to our sex lives, our psyche and the way we look during menopause.

One of the biggest issues for menopausal women is sex. In Chapters 2 and 4, I mentioned that many perimenopausal women suffer from a low level or even a lack of sexual desire, and I wrote that this might be the result of lowered levels of testosterone, but I also wrote that I had a lot of thoughts on the subject. I don't think that the only solution to women's lowered libido is to add testosterone. Women are very complex and there may be myriad reasons why they don't have the same level of sexual desire and energy that they had when they were young.

The problem is that many doctors are uncomfortable about discussing sexual issues with their patients and, to do them justice, many of their patients, especially the older and more conservative women, are embarrassed about the subject. In my ideal world a discussion around sex and all related issues would be an integral part of the annual gynaecological examination. I once gave a workshop and the organiser, a woman in her seventies who had been at a previous talk, asked me not to bring up the subject of sex or vaginal dryness. But I took a deep breath, disregarded her wishes and at the appropriate place in the workshop, tactfully began to discuss the issue. Many of the women present were in their seventies and eighties and I was fascinated by the lively discussion that ensued. At the end of the talk, a woman came up to thank me. She said she was in her eighties and wished with all her heart that the subject had been as openly discussed when she was going through the menopause transition, as she had really suffered for many years. However, I understand that this is something that often takes time and patience to unpack and the annual gynaecological check-up appointment is not long enough to deal with it satisfactorily. Your healthcare practitioner should bring up this topic and that of vaginal dryness at the beginning of the appointment. If they don't, you need to ask about it and don't wait until you're going out the door. If you're uncomfortable discussing this with a male doctor for any reason, you may need to switch to a female gynaecologist. You may also ask for a longer appointment if you need to take time to discuss this.

Each of the women I have quoted above has a different take on her sex life. Alexandra's husband is a farmer who gets up early and is exhausted at night. He doesn't bother to talk to her anymore; she feels that he doesn't even 'see' her, and for him sex has become a mechanical exercise. While Alexandra doesn't find sex painful, like many menopausal women she's lost interest, and with good reason! She feels like a call girl and there is no intimacy in their relationship. If Alexandra were confronted with a loving man who appreciated her, she might be surprised at how sexy she felt.

Sue is lucky; after a painful divorce she found someone who thinks she's gorgeous and has the energy and stamina to make sex fun. He's made her change her mindset and she has no sense that she shouldn't be enjoying sex in middle age.

Connie is suffering from painful intercourse – *dyspareunia*. It's very common in menopause when estrogen levels drop and a woman's vagina becomes dryer because the cells lining the vagina have less estrogen. She is also suffering from depression, which is also very common in peri- and postmenopausal women, especially when they've had a previous bout of depression, and it is well known for putting a damper on sexual desire.

Unlike Connie, Vicki has dealt with the changes in her body and seems to have moved on to a new and rewarding sexual period in her life. Her hysterectomy didn't seem to affect her ability to have an orgasm and though she doesn't describe sex as an earth-shattering experience, it is pleasant and comfortable.

Lack of sexual desire and painful sex mean that many midlife women are unhappy with sex and often stop having sex at this time. This creates several problems in long-term, stable relationships and creates huge anxiety as women worry that their partners will not understand and may seek satisfaction elsewhere. Many women find it as hard to discuss this issue with their partners as they do with their doctors. The emotional results of this can badly affect a relationship but much of the latest research shows that this can be dealt with and if a woman seeks help, the problem may be resolved.

Dry vagina

When you are a young, reproductive woman or even when you are older but not yet menopausal, your vagina is probably well lubricated and looks, on examination, plump and luscious. As you embark on perimenopause and your estrogen levels start to drop, the endothelial cells that line the vagina become thinner, less elastic, dryer and less estrogenated. This is called *vaginal atrophy*. As with sexual problems, many women are embarrassed to discuss this, and only a small number, about 5 per cent, are comfortable about asking for help for this condition. They also may feel that their healthcare practitioner may judge them if they ask about something they see as sex related. Many women don't feel they are entitled to enjoy sex as they age because it isn't 'proper'. But make no mistake, vaginal health and sexual satisfaction are extremely important, and if your gynaecologist doesn't discuss this during your appointment, be brave and bring it up.

A gynaecologist can see at once whether you have vaginal atrophy, because the walls of your vagina will look pale and dry on examination. The vaginal tissues are now more fragile and often they may tear or bleed more easily. These endothelial cells that line your vagina also line your urinary tract so when they lose estrogen, you may suffer burning during urination, urinary tract infections, urinary incontinence, stress incontinence and vaginal itchiness. Remember to check that the reason for all these symptoms is your dry vaginal and urinary tissue, and not anything else more serious, as I explained in Chapter 8. It never hurts to be sure. When you have vaginal atrophy, the pH level in your vagina changes and may go from the normal acidic pH to alkaline.

Obviously, if you aren't properly lubricated and your vagina is dry, sexual intercourse will be painful. Many menopausal women find that even though they are aroused, it hurts when they are penetrated and during the sexual act. This pain may induce them to fear sex and become uptight and worried, which further inhibits sexual arousal. Most women know that even in the days when their vaginas weren't dry, a lack of sexual desire or the feeling of suddenly being turned off prevented them becoming moist and ready for sex, so when they are menopausal the situation becomes fraught with pitfalls. But even if you do not have regular sexual intercourse you should be aware that you have some vaginal dryness so you can deal with it.

Luckily, the cure for a dry vagina is relatively simple. There are several different local estrogen vaginal products, such as vaginal estrogen creams, that can help to alter the state of your vagina. Most of them have very low levels of estrogen and work excellently. You will not need a progestogen with these products. This type of estrogen is effective locally and because, as I explained in Chapter 4, only very small amounts enter your system, you

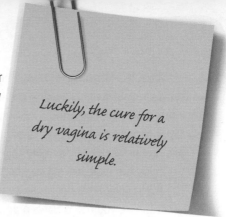

Luckily, the cure for a dry vagina is relatively simple.

generally aren't exposed to any risk. If you decide to use a conjugated equine estrogen (CEE) vaginal cream the effects may not only be local, and if you have a womb, the lining may thicken. It's a question of finding the product that suits you best.

Vicki chose the estradiol-releasing ring, but there are estrogen creams and vaginal tablets (called pessaries, which are oval suppositories inserted into the vagina with a small applicator) that may also help. You can choose what you feel works best for you and what you would be most comfortable to use. If you are battling with a dry vagina, the first time you insert either the ring or the tablet with an applicator, it may hurt a bit, so use a little lubricating cream on your finger to moisten the vaginal entrance and help ease the discomfort. Many women who are on HT find that they don't usually need a vaginal estrogen as well, but some who are on ultra-low doses of estrogen may need some additional help. Often the absorption of vaginal estrogen is higher when you first start to use it but research shows that after you have used it for a while, the levels of estrogen in your blood will become lower again. The problem is that of all the menopause symptoms, the one that continues when the others subside is the dry vagina. It's not going to improve when your hormones settle down after perimenopause. In fact vaginal dryness will probably worsen without estrogen treatment. So you will need to understand that treatment needs to be long term. This can be an issue for women where estrogen is contraindicated, as I discussed in Chapter 8, so you **must** talk this over with your specialist.

If you don't want to use a topical vaginal estrogen, some practitioners suggest a silicone-based vaginal gel before sex. Water-based lubricants also work well and may not be as irritating, but they can dry up while you're making love, so you need to find the type that suits you and your partner best. To increase intimacy, ask your partner to help you apply the lubricant. Interestingly, some research has shown that postmenopausal women who have regular sex have a slower rate of vaginal atrophy or dryness than women who are not sexually active.

There is a difference between vaginal lubricants and vaginal moisturisers. A moisturiser coats the vagina and supplies moisture for between 48 and 72 hours, will last longer than a lubricant and helps to replace and maintain the water content in the vagina. Lubricants help to ease penetration during sex and do not last longer for more than an hour.

If you are experiencing painful sex, I would urge you to find a solution. The psychological element is very strong here. When you are frightened that sex will hurt, you don't want to initiate it or participate in it, so if you don't deal with this problem it can become a vicious circle, which may be difficult to break.

Urinary tract problems

When I described earlier how your vagina starts to change in perimenopause, I mentioned some urinary issues that often beset women in menopause. You may find that you are having occasional, or sometimes frequent, involuntary episodes of leaking, called *urinary incontinence*, when you aren't able to control the flow of urine or when you urinate. This may be as a result of the thinning of the lining of your bladder outlet. But lower levels of estrogen are not the only culprits; as you get older the pelvic muscles surrounding your bladder begin to weaken, increasing the risk of one of the most common types of incontinence, called *stress incontinence*. These weakened pelvic muscles, nerves and ligaments may not necessarily only be due to ageing but to previous damage from natural childbirth. You may leak when you laugh, cough or sneeze, or lift heavy objects. Another type of incontinence is an *overactive bladder*, where you have a sudden overwhelming urge to go to the bathroom and you leak before you can get there. An irritated bladder may cause this. If you have both types of incontinence it is called *mixed incontinence*. The onset of stress incontinence is very common in perimenopause but doesn't usually get worse with age. However, as the years after menopause increase many women battle with overactive bladders.

If you are very overweight you may be incontinent or if you drink too much liquid; more than two litres of water daily. On the other hand, if you don't drink enough water you may find that this can also cause problems as concentrated urine can cause your bladder to become irritated. The nicotine in cigarettes can irritate your bladder, as can spicy foods, citrus fruits, chocolate, sugar, honey, too much coffee, tea or caffeinated drinks, and acidic drinks like tomato or grapefruit juice. Alcohol may also cause an irritated bladder, as do some medications like diuretics.

Many women battle with different types of incontinence but are too embarrassed to discuss it with their doctors. This is a great shame because appropriate treatment may cure it completely and if it can't, it can be treated in order to help lessen the frequency of the leaking. I would strongly suggest that if you have this problem you see a specialist urologist or a urogynaecologist. They will take a complete medical history and often ask you to keep a urinary diary including a record of what, how much and when you drink each day, when you leak and the amount you leak, and what triggers or worsens your problem. Stress incontinence is often helped by practising a series of exercises to strengthen the muscles of the pelvic floor, called *Kegel exercises*. Your specialist may also prescribe medication to treat an overactive bladder.

Because, as I described earlier, low levels of estrogen may affect the healthy acid balance of your vagina, women in menopause may become more prone to urinary infections. Some of these may also contribute to urinary incontinence and can be treated with the appropriate antibiotic medication. Interestingly, in spite of the fact that lower levels of estrogen are associated with incontinence, it has been found that systemic HT sometimes makes stress incontinence worse or even causes it. However, local vaginal estrogen may be helpful for some women with *urge incontinence*, and also in some women who have recurring urinary tract infections after menopause, by helping to restore the normal acid balance, though it has not yet been regulated for this in some countries. Other ways to lessen the risk of urinary tract infections are not to wear jeans that are too tight and the same applies to pantyhose and underwear. Anything that causes a change in your normal vaginal milieu, like highly perfumed bath products or some feminine hygiene products, can cause irritation. Staying well hydrated and remembering to urinate after intercourse may also help. Many women believe that cranberry juice will reduce their risk of urinary tract infection but a recent well-controlled trial showed that this is not the case.

Lack of sexual desire (libido)

A lot of research has focused on whether women enjoy sex less after menopause or hysterectomy. The interesting thing is that for many years it was thought that when your hormone levels, especially your androgen levels (see Chapter 2), dropped, you lost the desire. But as I have written repeatedly, women are complicated and although some women did very well with added testosterone or a combination of estrogen and progesterone, others found that the HT made no difference at all. As I indicated in Chapter 4, women who have had a natural menopause continue to produce amounts of testosterone similar to those they produced prior to menopause, so low libido cannot necessarily be blamed on lower levels of testosterone. In fact, recent research has shown that when testosterone levels were measured using what is known as a gold standard method (the most accurate and sensitive) in two groups of women, those with lowered libido and those whose sex life was just fine, there was no difference.

The *methyltestosterone* implant may have had a good effect, but the studies did not clarify how much of the increased sexual desire was the result of the placebo effect, the idea that sex would be more appealing if there was additional testosterone – women's minds play a big role in their sexuality. Another problem with the implant was that it probably gave women more testosterone than their sensitive adrenal cascades could deal with and many found themselves with all sorts of unwanted side effects like aggressiveness, greasy skin, unwanted facial hair, adult acne and weight gain. They also had raised levels of bad cholesterol.

Newer research has shown that women battling with lowered sexual desire after a surgical menopause had improved sex lives when using a testosterone patch, which gave them a daily dose of 300 mcg of testosterone, in conjunction with transdermal ET. As I discussed in Chapter 4, it may be better to take a hormone through your skin because it seems to create fewer side effects, but there are women who just don't respond to this patch. However, many doctors feel that the treatment option may be the way forward for those women who suffer from low libido.

Some experts strongly advocate supplementing DHEA, which as I wrote in Chapters 2 and 4 is a main precursor hormone of androgens and estrogen. There is ongoing research to establish the efficacy and safety of this hormone. In fact, in the same study where testosterone levels were measured, it was found that levels of DHEA were somewhat lower and levels of DHEA-s were much lower in women who had less desire. So given that the women who had higher levels had less vaginal dryness and fewer symptoms, it may be an important direction to research further. If you decide you want to try DHEA, only take it if you are under the care of an experienced endocrinologist or a doctor who really knows about it. As I explained to a friend of mine, a medical scientist who believes that adding some testosterone may be the answer for women who have low sexual desire, I would accept that added testosterone works if these women are monitored about how they feel about themselves, the way they look and their emotional relationship with their partners at the same time they are using the testosterone.

Very sensitive, tender breasts

Many women going through perimenopause or who are on HT suddenly experience very tender and sensitive breasts. Being sensitive in this case doesn't mean that you become more sexually aroused, it means you can't bear to have your breasts touched, which can be a big problem for someone who finds touching their partner's breasts exciting and for the woman involved, who has always enjoyed this aspect of her sexuality and now finds herself shying away.

Tender breasts can probably be blamed on fluctuating levels of estrogen, though some progestogens can cause your breast tissue to retain water, which can also make the breasts oversensitive. Sometimes balancing your hormone levels with HT can solve this problem, but as with most menopausal symptoms, this one will usually resolve itself. Your best bet is to be frank with your partner and find another part of your body that can be touched and that will give you pleasure, not pain.

Lack of sensation during sex

The bad news is that many women who are well into middle age no longer have the tight, supple vaginas they had in their youth: babies and life have taken their toll. It helps to remember that the vagina is a 'potential' space. This means that the walls of the uterus fold in on themselves and there is no space there, but when something like a tampon or a penis is inserted, or a baby is born, it opens to provide the space needed. Over the years, the tissue and muscles have stretched; the vagina is no longer as elastic as it was when you were younger. During sex these muscles may not be able to tense as they once did. The problem is that many women may not find sex painful, but may have no sensation when they make love.

Some of these women believe that a vaginal reconstruction will be the answer. However, don't follow this route blindly; this surgery is usually performed when there is bad tearing or scarring. For those middle-aged women who have problems when the womb drops into the vagina or the bladder falls down, a hysterectomy would be the surgery of choice. If you don't have any of those problems, the best way to deal with this may be to change your position when you make love, so that you are able to feel your partner's penis.

There are no set rules for this; you'll just have to experiment a bit. Another problem that could compound the situation is that many men no longer have the firm, long-lasting erections they had in their youth. I mention this because it takes two to tango and many middle-aged women blame themselves when sex is no longer as good as it used to be. As you get older, it may take longer to feel pleasurable sensations or build up to a climax than it used to, so you need patience and sometimes a sense of humour; but laugh with each other.

Middle-aged men can suffer from all kinds of potency problems for a variety of reasons – lowered testosterone levels, high blood pressure and other medical problems, stress, performance anxiety and prostate cancer, as well as some of the medications prescribed for these. Prostate cancer in particular can have huge implications for the lives of middle-aged couples, especially in the area of sexual dysfunction. If your partner is battling, talk to an expert. There's no shame in this and there are many ways to deal with the problem or get around it. If you are embarrassed to discuss sex with your partner and explore all your options, this too can become a vicious circle. The same applies to asking for what gives you pleasure and saying what doesn't. Many sexual issues can be resolved with frank and open discussions and mutual respect.

Hysterectomy and sexual functioning

Like Vicki, some women may battle after they've had a hysterectomy. Women may be profoundly attached to their wombs and there may be psychological issues around their own feelings of diminished femininity and a sense of loss. But if they deal with these, the problems are usually short-lived. Most women find that they are functioning quite well six months after their hysterectomy, though for some it may take up to a year to get back to normal.

There has been much discussion about whether the removal of the cervix affects sexual functioning or not. I've done my own anecdotal research and it seems that most women find that they still have orgasms after a hysterectomy, though whether they are the same type or not is open to discussion. That said, some women say that their orgasms feel different, especially if stimulation of their cervix was important to their sexual response. These are women who get pleasure from cervical stimulation, which means that for these women the loss of their cervix may make their orgasms less intense. During sex the uterus contracts, so women who found these contractions pleasurable and noticeable, especially during their orgasms, will no longer feel these after a hysterectomy and will notice a difference in the depth and intensity of their orgasms. Generally, women will still feel the pleasurable vaginal contractions. The good news is that most women experience a clitoral orgasm and since in a normal hysterectomy the clitoris remains, most women find that they can still have a very satisfactory orgasm.

There are two different kinds of orgasm, the *external* orgasm, achieved through stimulation of your clitoris, and the *internal* orgasm – when your G-spot and the area around it are stimulated. We've all heard about the G-spot, which is the region situated in a woman's genital area behind her pubic bone. This area surrounds the urethra. Tiny glands called Skene's glands are found here in the upper wall of the vagina and the lower end of the urethra. The name G-spot is given to the area where the Skene's glands are found. These little glands are like prostate glands in men. Their size differs from one woman to another, and they may not even be present in some women. The theory is that the G-spot is extremely sensitive and if this area is stimulated women can climax. So certain women who have very tiny Skene's glands, or none at all, may not experience an internal orgasm. Other women who still have their cervix experience orgasms when the cervix is stimulated or when there is pressure on the anterior wall of their vagina, or both. Because a woman's orgasm is highly individual, women can have orgasms that combine all three sensations. What this information tells you is not to despair when you have a total hysterectomy, you can still achieve great sexual pleasure.

Sleep deprivation

No woman who is feeling exhausted from lack of sleep is going to feel sexy. The only thing she can think of when she gets into bed is whether she is going to fall asleep and, if she does, for how long the sleep will last. Insomnia is very common in peri- and postmenopausal women. It comes in many forms.

Some women find that they no longer experience a deep, uninterrupted sleep and their nights are disturbed as they transition into menopause, either because they are battling with night sweats and wake several times drenched to the skin or they have troubled dreams, or they sleep so lightly that the slightest sound wakes them. Sleep disturbances are also very common in postmenopause. Other women fall into a deep sleep but wake unusually early, with a panicky feeling or a pounding heart; still others struggle to fall asleep or are wide awake after only an hour's sleep.

Fluctuating hormonal levels are not the only problems that deprive women of sleep; depression, anxiety and stress can also affect sleep patterns. The need to go to the bathroom may wake you several times a night. But since it is well known that we sleep less well as we age, this may also be a factor. Another issue is the loud levels of snoring that may emanate from your ageing partner and may be caused, if not by too many whiskies at bedtime, then as result of sleep apnoea, which is very common in older men. But this may not apply to him alone. Sleep apnoea, which is when your breathing during sleep is interrupted, stopping and starting, has been found to be a common cause of disturbed sleep in midlife women. If a woman battles with this she may have the following symptoms: snoring very loudly, waking abruptly and feeling breathless, waking with a sore throat or dry mouth and a morning headache.

We probably need a bit less sleep as we get older, so don't stress if you are waking up earlier.

This may suddenly emerge or increase after menopause, especially in overweight women. You or your partner should consult a specialist if either of you have this condition as, apart from the other factors mentioned above, in more severe cases it may increase your the risk of high blood pressure and be a red flag for heart disease.

Having a glass of warm milk before bedtime may encourage sleepiness because the milk contains lactose, a carbohydrate that may affect the serotonin pathways (see Chapter 10). Many women who start to take antidepressants (SSRIs) during the perimenopausal stage find they may sleep better, and a new study has shown that this result may be even better when combined with a small dose of *zolpidem*, a nonbenzodiazepine medicine. You may want to ask your doctor for one of the newer, safer and less addictive sleeping pills, which do not have residual effects the next day, to get you back into the habit of uninterrupted sleep. These are called nonbenzodiazepine hypnotic agents such as *zolpidem* (Stilnox, Ambien) and *ezopiclone* (Lunesta). These newer nonbenzodiazepines don't seem to suppress something called slow wave sleep and may even increase it.

Insomnia can often be a self-fulfilling prophecy because you are so worried about not falling asleep that you work yourself up into a frenzy and then there's no way you'll be able to sleep. Certain supplements, such as melatonin, have been recommended for the problem. It is thought to be safe in small doses, but more research needs to be done to determine its efficacy and long-term safety. If you want to try it, consult your doctor first. Calcium and magnesium are thought to help promote sleepiness, but once again, the jury is out until more data is in. Regular exercise can be helpful in promoting sleep, as can eating sensibly and not too heavily at night. Remember not to drink too much: alcohol may help put you to sleep, but you may wake dehydrated and with a pounding headache, and the other risks of alcohol aren't worth it. Research suggests that for the sake of our health we should sleep for between seven and eight hours a night, though not longer, so you should get to bed at a decent hour at least a couple of nights a week.

Exhaustion can lead to raised cortisol levels, an impaired immune system, anxiety, poor cognitive functioning and depression, which are risk factors for other illnesses like heart disease. There are all sorts of behavioural suggestions, like not reading or watching television in bed, creating a calm environment and a darkened room, but I think that each woman knows what suits her best at bedtime. I for one can't fall asleep unless I read for a while. We probably need a bit less sleep as we get older, so don't stress if you are waking up earlier, as long as you wake feeling rested and alert – your body will tell you whether you are getting enough sleep or not. Don't panic if you have one or two sleepless nights, but find help if the situation persists.

Body appearance (you and your partner)

Remember Amy and Sue from Chapter 11? Amy just can't accept her midlife body, even though her husband still finds her attractive. She is turned off by sex because she hates the way she looks and doesn't feel sexy. Sue, on the other hand, feels wonderful about herself; her attitude is an aphrodisiac by itself. It's clear from the way Sue talks that sexual desire for many of us may be conditional upon the way we feel about ourselves.

I was very inspired by a book by Janet Juska called *A Round-Heeled Woman*. Aged 66, she decides she's tired of being celibate and advertises in the *New York Review of Books*: 'BEFORE I TURN 67 – next March – I would like to have lots of sex with a man I like. If you want to talk first Trollope works for me. NYR Box 10307.' I opened the book with some trepidation, as I thought it might contain gratuitous sex and I wasn't sure that I would like or approve of what I read. In fact I was blown away by her courageous and endearing story. It contains a hopeful message for all older women who think their sexy days are over. It also says to single women that there's nothing wrong with wanting a physical relationship and letting the world know it.

We have to stop buying into the mindset foisted on us by the media that young is better. There is nothing more attractive than a good-looking, middle-aged or older woman who is happy with herself and her life. And while we're lamenting our lost looks, let's spare a thought for our partners. Their bodies are no longer firm, a beer belly is often the first thing we come into contact with in bed at night, they have more hair on their chests than on their heads, their skins have reacted to years of sun and weather, and their bodies no longer look the way they did some 30 years ago, when a glance from them made us go weak at the knees.

Their appearance may be a turn-off, but most men don't spend an inordinate amount of time worrying about that. They have absolute confidence that we will still find them sexy and attractive, and that we couldn't ask for more than to make love with them every night. At worst, if your man is not the Adonis he once was, you can close your eyes and fantasise.

WHAT ELSE CAN AFFECT YOUR SEX LIFE?

As I wrote at the beginning of the chapter, there are many things that can affect your sex life. These include chronic illness, and cancers. There is so much going on in our lives at this time, from both an emotional and physical perspective. Illness can play a huge role. If you have cancer you may not have the energy or inclination for sex. You may be concerned about your body image if you have had a mastectomy or chemotherapy, which can cause certain physical problems like hair loss. You may be feeling depressed and anxious, all of which can lower sexual desire. Certain medications that middle-aged women may have to take, such as beta-blockers, antidepressants and corticosteroids, can also cause low levels of libido. It's very important to ask your doctor about the possible side effects when you start taking a new medicine.

Personal issues also come into play. If you are worried about something it is hard to put it aside, and as I discuss in Chapter 13 there may be many problems at this stage of our lives, so it may be difficult to either want or not be distracted during sex. Interpersonal factors are also implicated. Many women in long-term relationships find that they have less sexual desire and like Andrea may have lost emotional contact with their husbands and stopped trying to reinvent or enhance their marriage. As I explained above, men at this stage of their lives have their own issues about sex; they may be taking medicines for high blood pressure or other age-related conditions that may affect their ability to have an erection, and they too may be struggling with many of the life issues that women battle with as they age.

Research has shown consistently that there is a **very** strong relationship between women's low sexual desire and their mental health. Problems from their pasts like physical and sexual abuse that have never been dealt with may come into play as we age, and present issues also have an impact. If we're anxious, worried, sad or depressed our sex lives suffer. I believe these emotions need to be dealt with, as I discuss in detail in Chapter 13, but we also should be able to have a frank and honest discussion with our partners about our sexual feelings and worries. If you find it difficult to do this by yourselves, sometimes talking to a marital counsellor may help, especially as it takes place in a stress-free environment. Many of us find we are more at ease with someone unfamiliar than with our long-term GP or gynaecologist, who may have known us for years.

Sex should be a shared experience, but as I wrote above, as we get older the satisfying sensations take longer to happen. This means that you need to pay attention to foreplay and to try to rekindle the intimacy of your first sexual experiences together. In our busy lives we may need to schedule time for sex; anticipation can be exciting. So try to create a romantic environment that will make this a special time for both you and your partner. You may find that you are not as energetic as you once were and are too tired for sex at night, but there's nothing wrong with weekend afternoons. Take the phone off the hook, be glad that you don't have to worry about the children bursting in, and enjoy yourselves.

EMPOWER YOURSELF

- Know that there are many, many factors that play a part in your level of sexual desire: psychological, physical and social.
- Most menopausal women have vaginal dryness and it can be the cause of painful sex and urinary tract infections. See your doctor and deal with this condition. There are excellent products to help moisturise dry vaginas. Find the one that suits you best.
- Be brave. If you are having a problem with sex, speak frankly and openly to your partner about it. There are ways to deal with it. Good sex in middle age is not only possible, it's good for you.
- Low levels of testosterone are not necessarily associated with low sexual desire – there may be many reasons why you don't feel like sex.
- Neither you nor your partner look like you did at 18, but accepting this and feeling good about yourself as you are today makes a huge psychological difference.
- Having a hysterectomy with the removal of your cervix doesn't mean that you can't have an orgasm. There are several different kinds of orgasm. Experiment to see what positions are best for you and your partner and what turns you on.
- Sort out your sleep problems. It's hard to feel sexy if you're exhausted.

13
Menopause and the mind: memory, depression, anxiety and stress in menopause

Sharon phoned me in tears. She explained that at 49 she had recently become menopausal and at the same time felt very depressed. She has a family history of breast cancer so her doctor said he wasn't keen for her to be on estrogen, though her gynaecologist felt that as it was only her mother's sister who had had breast cancer and she had no other risk factors, he saw no reason why she shouldn't try a low-dose estrogen. Nevertheless she still felt anxious about HT. She had seen a psychiatrist, who put her on a 'cocktail' of antidepressants, but they didn't seem to help and she was having side effects from these medications. She said she was very confused about what she should do.

Stella had recently been divorced at the age of 52, and had still not come to terms with the fact that her husband of 18 years had been unfaithful to her. She explained that she felt very tearful and depressed and in addition was worried that she had become incredibly aggressive, especially with those closest to her, and blamed it on her recent menopause.

Corrie, a busy bank manager, was very anxious that she was losing her memory. She said she often found herself distracted and sometimes forgot where she was going. She was in the early stages of perimenopause with all the attendant symptoms, including some very severe night sweats that kept her awake most of the night. In addition, her beloved sister had recently died in an accident and she could not come to terms with this loss. At 48 she had become afraid that she was getting Alzheimer's disease, though she was managing well at work. She had read that HT therapy was harmful and although no one in her family had had breast cancer, she was frightened to take HT.

Alma's husband had lost his job and so, at 50, she had gone back to work as a secretary. Up until then she seemed to have led a charmed life and never felt depressed or anxious. Both her sons had left home and were doing well. She missed her friends and the fun things she previously always had time for, and found she was arguing continually with her husband. She had recently started HT as her gynae told her that she had low bone density and said that her mood swings were due to low levels of estrogen. She had no menopausal symptoms but listened to her doctor and obediently took the treatment. In spite of the HT, she often felt deeply lonely and sad.

Each of the women in the stories above is battling with a problem that involves her mind; depression, memory loss, anxiety, stress and mood swings. Sharon may find that HT could help her symptoms of depression. However, that said, depression is often an illness that must be treated and Sharon should find a gynaecologist and psychiatrist who are happy to work together to find the right combination of medicines that will help her. She should be aware of the type of HT she is taking. She should be monitored regularly to be reassured about her fear about cancer risk. Because she has a womb she needs to have a progestogen, but be alert to the fact that certain progestins may enhance depression. On the other hand, some studies have shown that estrogen may help to increase the effect of some antidepressants.

Stella blames her mood swings on menopause but I think she has not dealt with her anger about her husband's infidelity and should work through these feelings with a registered counsellor or therapist.

The levels of stress that Corrie is experiencing and her grief over the death of her sister may well be affecting her short-term memory. Lack of sleep and severe menopausal flushes and night sweats may also be culprits. In Corrie's case, since there are no apparent risk factors contraindicating the use of HT, she should have a frank discussion with a gynaecologist about these risks and benefits, since HT has been shown to be very effective in helping severe hot flushes and night sweats. She should be regularly monitored, which will help to allay her fears. There is no harm in her seeing a neurologist to reassure her about her risks for Alzheimer's disease. She may also find that a couple of sessions with a grief counsellor may help her come to terms with her loss.

Alma is obviously angry that she had to give up her comfortable lifestyle and feels that her husband has let her down. She and her husband may want to try some marital therapy to try to work through these issues. Her feelings of sadness and loneliness may be related to her sons' leaving home or to other life events. When problems like this occur in midlife, they may often be rooted in past issues. In her case it doesn't seem that HT is necessary and she should get a second opinion as to whether she should continue to take it.

This chapter is in some sense a summing up of many of the issues I have written about throughout this book. In writing about them, I have a heightened awareness of how complex this time of life is for midlife women and how many factors can affect our brains and mental health. I hope as you read about these you will understand how interrelated they are.

HEADACHES AND MIGRAINE

While on the subject of the brain, I think this is a good time to look at headaches and migraine in peri- and postmenopause. There's no doubt if you think back to the headaches you may have suffered when you had PMS that fluctuating hormone levels can cause these. Many perimenopausal women battle with headaches, even though some of them have had many headache-free years after their adolescent episodes, while others who never had a headache in their lives are suddenly experiencing some real shockers. Some women find their headaches get better in perimenopause, while other long-time migraine sufferers battle as never before.

There are many different kinds of headaches; tension, cluster, sinus and migraine headaches, the latter with and without aura. So it's very important that you and your doctor identify what kind of headache you have and whether it's related to stress or hormonal changes and what may have triggered it.

Usually women with migraines find that they have warning of an attack when they experience an aura. The aura warning of a migraine disturbs your vision with a variety of different light effects. This means either lots of little flashing lights, or a funny zigzag light that cuts your vision in half, or a kind of sparkling at the side of your eye that pursues you when you turn your head. You may also get blurred vision, a funny taste in your mouth, slur your words, feel a tingling on your face and have numb fingertips. These are usually accompanied by a sinking feeling as you prepare for what's in store.

Migraines are usually headaches where an attack lasts between four and 72 hours and may have at least two of the following symptoms: nausea or vomiting, or both; extreme sensitivity to light or noise; a pulsating in the head; moderate to blinding pain; severe disruption to your normal life; they aren't caused by another illness and they are situated in a specific part of your head.

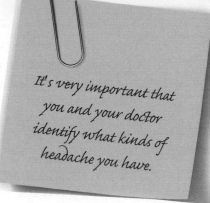

It's very important that you and your doctor identify what kinds of headache you have.

Many women who have in the past had these warning signs before a migraine with the attendant symptoms described above, find suddenly in perimenopause that they just go straight into the migraine. Strangely though, some women whose aura was always followed by migraine just experience the aura, which continues for a short while and then disappears, leaving them without a headache. If you have always suffered from migraines, you shouldn't be too concerned, but if you start to get migraines with an aura, or if you just get the aura, you should have yourself thoroughly checked by a neurologist. In fact, it is a good idea never to take migraines, severe headaches, new headaches or changes in chronic headaches of any kind for granted. Have a neurological check-up and rule out any sinister possibilities, like a risk for stroke.

A new research study has shown that women who have migraines with aura may be at a slightly greater risk for haemorrhagic stroke (where a blood vessel ruptures, causing bleeding in your brain). But the authors of the study say don't panic and rush off to the emergency room because the causes of migraine are extremely complex, but do **pay attention** to what they call *modifiable risk factors* (things in your life you can control) that increase your vascular health, like watching that your blood pressure and bad cholesterol stay low, eating healthily, exercising regularly and not smoking.

A very common type of perimenopausal headache seems to cause a pounding in the head accompanied by the sensation of a vice-like grip at the back of the head. It is thought that fluctuating levels of estrogen may be associated with bad migraines in perimenopausal women, but it's not the temporary high levels of estrogen that cause it but the sudden drop afterwards. The bad news is that if you were the kind of woman who got bad headaches during your period, you will probably find that your sensitivity to fluctuating hormone levels affects you quite badly now.

If you were a migraine sufferer and have had a hysterectomy with an oophorectomy, you might have found that your headaches got worse immediately after your surgical menopause, which is probably the result of the rapid drop in your estrogen level. HT has sometimes helped balance the hormone levels of perimenopausal women with migraines. But be careful: if you were the kind of woman whose hormone fluctuations caused migraines, it may be better for you to take continuous combined rather than sequential HT (first the estrogen and then the progestin) and don't forget, as I explained in Chapter 4, the best method is probably through your skin, using a patch, cream or gel. The good news is that once the hormones have stabilised after the perimenopausal stage, most women stop having migraines or have far fewer episodes. However, a very large study showed that women who use HT are more likely to get migraines, and that the actual risk of getting a migraine is increased in these women whether they use ET or EPT. The problem is that the study could not determine whether using HT causes the headaches or if there is a tendency among menopausal women who suffer from migraines to use hormone therapy. So if you find you are suffering worse migraines since you have been on HT, it would probably be wise to stop until there is clearer evidence.

All postmenopausal women who have battled with headaches or migraines (which are vascular events) should discuss all their options with their doctors with regard to the best dose and type of hormone, and whether or not a transdermal hormone might be better. In general, migraine sufferers should be extremely cautious when deciding whether or not to take HT.

Vanessa laughed ruefully: 'Since I've become perimenopausal, if I have more than one glass of wine, no matter what I do, even drinking several glasses of water before I go to sleep, I wake with a dreadful, pounding headache. I can't stand it. My husband and I are wine fundis and get such pleasure from our wine collection, which we've built up over the years. I'm sure it's connected to menopause because my periods are irregular and I'm now in my fifties, but I'd rather have hot flushes than this!'

As Vanessa's hormone levels have changed, so has something in her body's chemistry that is telling her that her body can no longer tolerate more than one glass of wine at a time. It is highly likely that this problem will resolve itself once she is through the perimenopausal stage, but for the moment she just has to grin and bear it, carefully choosing and savouring the one glass she is able to drink. It's important to look out for other headache triggers too in peri- and postmenopause: dieting excessively (especially the high protein, low carbohydrate diets) or detox programmes; dehydration – not drinking enough water; tension in your back and neck muscles; stress, anxiety or depression; and certain foods that contain MSG or sulphur, or are highly processed.

Treatments for headaches

Some women may find they have increased sinus headaches caused by hormone-related changes in their nasal membranes. Others battle with stress headaches. A healthy diet, a proper exercise regimen, massages, anti-inflammatory medication as prescribed by your doctor, drinking six to eight glasses of water daily, dealing with your problems in a constructive way and learning to relax should help prevent bad headaches if you are prone to them.

Certain medications may help, such as beta-blockers, anti-epileptics like Topamax (topiramate) which are taken daily to prevent migraines, tricyclic antidepressants, some calcium channel blockers and selected painkillers and anti-inflammatory medication, prescribed by a specialist physician or a neurologist. Some of these have not been specifically approved for migraines but are used off-label (page 295). Triptans (serotonin receptor agonists) are a group of medications (including Maxalt, Zomig, Axert, Imitrex) that may be prescribed to treat migraine headaches. Since a migraine is a disorder thought to be caused by swelling of the blood vessels of the head due to on and off activation and inflammation of nerve cells in the brain, triptans work by constricting these swollen blood vessels and reducing the inflammation, relieving the headache pain, the light and noise sensitivity and the symptoms of nausea and vomiting that accompany migraine. They usually work best if taken as the headache starts and are generally well tolerated, though some people may experience side effects including dizziness, a tingling sensation, flushing and drowsiness.

Some doctors recommend supplements like magnesium for headaches, but they say you shouldn't give up too quickly if it doesn't seem to work immediately; magnesium needs to be taken for at least three months for possible benefits to be felt. Certain antioxidant supplements like coenzyme Q10 may also be helpful, but there is not enough research yet to prove that they are truly effective. The FDA has just approved the use of *onabotulinumtoxinA* (Botox) for women who suffer from chronic severe migraine (more than 15 headaches a month for more than four hours at a time), which seems to reduce the headaches, but this treatment is only for those with the most severe migraines.

As I said earlier, there are things you can change in your life that may lessen your risk of getting bad headaches. These include exercising regularly, eating regular meals, lowering your stress (I write about some ways to do this later on in this chapter), and avoiding bright flashing lights or glare. Wear glasses that are coated with antiglare if you are subjected to areas with bright or flickering fluorescent lights and make sure that your sunglasses are polaroid. Identify any other migraine triggers, such as certain foods you know can cause a migraine.

Some of the more common food triggers include products that are fermented, pickled or marinated, contain nitrates or higher levels of tyramine, which is formed from the breakdown of protein as foods age, like aged cheese, some aged, cured and processed meats, red wine, sherry, beer and often canned foods, certain types of beans (broad, lima, fava and garbanzo, for example), figs or raisins and overripe avocados or bananas, chocolate and coffee (excessive caffeine or caffeine withdrawal too), as well as cultured dairy products like sour cream and buttermilk. These may be different for different people, so keeping a headache diary to see what triggers your headaches may be a good idea.

Rebound headaches may cause huge problems for many peri- and postmenopausal women. The supplement fanatic Laurie, quoted in Chapter 5, was addicted to painkillers. Many of these drugs have a twofold effect because they have a type of sedative in them, which make a woman feel good, and they also contain a painkiller. The problem arises when you take them for more than three days because once you are hooked on them, not taking them will initiate a headache that will only get better when you treat it with the same medication.

You would be surprised how common rebound headaches are among middle-aged women. You need to see a headache specialist if you are getting these kind of headaches and wean yourself off the painkiller medication, although some specialists may suggest that you go 'cold turkey' and get some kind of anti-inflammatory medicine to help you deal with the pain. If you are really addicted to painkillers, you will find the withdrawal period very hard, but it's worth the anguish, and about five weeks after stopping these drugs you should be either headache-free or much improved.

COGNITIVE FUNCTION – IS YOUR MIND WORKING PROPERLY?

Cognitive problems and memory loss are paramount concerns for many menopausal women.

One of our great fears is the thought that if we go against some healthcare practitioners' advice and decide not to use HT we might be candidates for diminished cognitive ability and, most frightening of all, Alzheimer's disease, which is the most common type of dementia. Dementia means a gradual decline in cognitive functioning as a result of damage or disease in the brain beyond what we expect in normal cognitive ageing. Dementia is a term encompassing a group of symptoms that interfere with daily life such as memory loss, problems communicating and reasoning, and mood changes. There are several kinds of dementia, some of them better known, like Alzheimer's disease or fronto-temporal dementia, which can damage the brain and cause these changes, or vascular dementia caused when the oxygen supply to the brain is compromised either by a stroke or a series of small strokes. Dementia is a progressive disease, which means that the symptoms become worse depending on the type of dementia we have and our individual profile. Dementia can affect both men and women and its likelihood increases with age.

Our worry about getting dementia if we decide not to take HT is further compounded by the fact that we now know that in some women the risks of HT may outweigh the benefits. But many women and their healthcare practitioners have been confused and often unnecessarily worried by some research that suggested that women who were not on long-term HT might be at risk for dementia and damaged cognitive functioning, meaning that they might suffer from poor memory and lose certain intellectual skills. According to the experts, cognition includes all kinds of brain functions like memory, the ability to learn, facility with language and the way you solve problems. We become afraid that if we are prone to severe hot flushes we may be putting ourselves at risk. I think that this kind of anxiety and fear can be very damaging because it can drive women to make emotional decisions without really understanding the facts. In Chapter 6, I described the mechanism of a hot flush but I didn't explain that the brain regulates its own blood supply, so that it is not affected by changes in core body temperature. So even if you feel that you're going to burst into flames during a hot flush, your brain is taking care of itself.

Much of the early research seemed to indicate that menopausal women would do better intellectually if they took estrogen, but after the Women's Health Initiative (WHI), an intensive study into the risks and benefits of HT, the results of which were published in 2002 (discussed at length in Chapter 3), these ideas were turned upside down. Although the experts agree that estrogen may have a protective effect on the brain, there is no adequate clinical proof that this information is valid. Recent studies continue to show that there is no clear relationship between hormone therapy and your cognitive skills, but the research is not yet definitive and trials continue to try to determine the effects of estrogen and testosterone on the brain.

How to look after your cognitive health

So what can we do? There are obviously genetic conditions that can put us at greater risk for these illnesses in spite of a healthy lifestyle, but there are many things we can do to lower our risk of these. One of the reasons for cognitive problems in ageing women is vascular – problems with blood flow to the brain preventing oxygen and nutrition from reaching the cells in the brain. In Chapter 7, I discussed stroke, where the blood supply to a large area of the brain is interrupted with devastating effects. In addition, some women may have a series of small strokes, which block smaller blood vessels and may deprive certain areas of the brain of oxygen and vital nutrients over time. It makes sense that if we pay attention to our health as far as heart disease and strokes are concerned, it may help to decrease our risk for cognitive decline.

A new study has shown that very heavy smokers in midlife are at a greatly increased risk of dementias 20 years on, which is logical since smoking is so strongly associated with so many diseases, including stroke. Another meta-analysis showed that if you don't smoke you have a 30 per cent lower risk of dementia than those who do.

Another practical thing that you can easily do to maintain your cognitive health is regular physical activity. I have sounded the trumpet for the benefits of exercising throughout the book and many medical studies show that regular exercise, from moderate to vigorous, such as brisk walking, jogging and cycling, is the way to go. Eating sensibly is also important and several places in this book spell out the healthiest foods. As I explained in Chapter 5, eating mindfully and well is better for you than many supplements that manufacturers promise can prevent cognitive decline and memory loss.

MEMORY LOSS

Much has been written about memory loss in perimenopause and once again there are many studies explaining the role of estrogen and extolling its importance, while just as many others say it has no effect. It is clear that when you are battling with hot flushes, distress and high levels of anxiety, your memory may be affected. It is also thought that fluctuating levels of estrogen in naturally menopausal women produce those memory lapses we so fear. But it has also been found that once your hormones level out and stabilise in postmenopause, your memory is generally fine. On the whole, large observational studies on women with natural menopause show no strong evidence that there are significant midlife cognitive changes during the transition from peri- to postmenopause and if there are, these levels will usually return to those experienced in premenopause once the transition is ended. More research needs to be conducted to determine whether some mental abilities may be affected.

It is logical to assume that in perimenopause factors other than lowered levels of estrogen can affect memory and cognitive performance, for instance depression, anxiety, sleep deprivation and an unhealthy lifestyle. However, when some postmenopausal women complain about memory loss, doctors may take these complaints very seriously, because as I explained above, memory lapses experienced by women during the transition into menopause usually improve post the transition period, when estrogen levels have stabilised and no longer fluctuate. So though memory problems in postmenopausal women may simply be a result of ageing, they may, in other cases, be a sign of early dementia. But as far as the terror of dementia is concerned, if you are not taking HT, research shows that there is no real evidence that HT reduces the risk of dementia in older menopausal women; in fact, as the results from the Women's Health Initiative Memory Study (WHIMS) showed, it may put them at greater risk.

Recent research looked into whether there was a difference between mental performance in pre-, peri- and postmenopausal women. The study investigated whether there was a relationship between the amount of estrogen in the blood of these different women and their mental abilities. This research found that once the effects of getting older were taken into account, there was no difference between the three groups in relation to: long-term memory, which includes episodic memory (storage of facts and personal experiences that belong to particular places and times); semantic memory (facts, ideas, words, problem solving); ease in using spoken or written language; visuospatial ability (an ability to understand the way objects work together in a space, like doing a jigsaw puzzle); or in the ability to recognise faces. In addition, there was no relationship between the amount of estrogen in the blood of each group of women and the way they performed in these tests. Two longitudinal studies (studies that follow subjects over a period of time, documenting changes) found that being menopausal did not relate to the women's cognitive decline.

The Women's Health Initiative Memory Study (WHIMS) found that contrary to previous beliefs, the memories of women who had gone through the perimenopausal transition were no worse than those of any other women, nor was there a decline in the speed with which they calculated problems; and, guess what, they actually improved slightly in these areas over time!

Once again, the results of many of the previous studies were influenced by the fact that the women in the trials who had decided to take HT were usually better educated, younger and healthier, so it was highly likely that they were going to do well in cognitive tests.

Several large clinical trials show that HT in women older than 65 does not improve either memory or certain cognitive functioning. Another study showed that the risk of dementia increased in older women (65–79) who used HT. Thus far, research shows that estrogen probably does not slow the progression of Alzheimer's disease or improve its symptoms. However, proponents of the timing hypothesis believe that more research is needed to establish whether the age at which women have HT, or if they start HT at the onset of menopause, will reduce the risk of dementia.

As I described in Chapter 3, newer research seems to be tending towards the timing hypothesis. (Remember, the hypothesis is that when healthy younger women who are starting menopause take HT it may lessen their risk as far as certain illnesses are concerned.) Simply, this means that HT taken at the appropriate time may lower the risk of dementia risk **but**, again, much more research needs to be done on when HT should be given, the length of time a woman can safely take it, the route of administration (transdermal versus oral estrogen) and the type of HT (for instance, ET versus EPT and whether different types of progestogens cause different effects). Each woman should be counselled individually about this and should understand all the risks and benefits. There are many subtle and complex issues to be unpacked here and the debate continues as to whether estrogen does or doesn't protect our brains.

As I discussed in Chapter 4, women with early or premature menopause may be at greater risk if they are estrogen deficient. Research has shown that sudden and dramatic falls in estrogen in younger women who have had an abrupt surgical menopause may affect brain function, so those women may want to have HT, subject to the advice of their doctors. For those who cannot take HT there is comfort in the fact that a healthy lifestyle is exceptionally important in lowering the risk of dementias, and regular moderate exercise is a vital component.

LIVING MINDFULLY

Here are my thoughts, which are based on my reading and the recommendations of international menopause societies.
- **The role of HT.** HT should not be given at any age to prevent or reduce the risk of dementia and protect your cognitive health. HT when started in

older women may contribute to stroke risk and seems to worsen the risk of dementia. The available research does not show whether HT taken soon after menopause will increase or decrease the risk of dementia. The way you lead your life will certainly impact on your risk and it is essential that you take responsibility for your health.

- **Diet and exercise.** Ensure that you live sensibly and control the amount of saturated fats in your diet so that you lower your risk of developing atherosclerosis, which could cause the arteries in your brain to get clogged up with plaque, affecting the blood supply to the brain and causing cognitive damage. Be aware of the many things I have written about that can protect the health of your blood vessels. There is ongoing research investigating the protective and anti-inflammatory effect of estrogen on the brain, but in the meantime it seems sensible to consider revisiting the old adage 'healthy body, healthy mind' and keep your bad cholesterol levels low. Monitor your blood pressure (see Chapter 7) and live healthily. Be careful what you eat (see Chapter 10) because you also need to keep your blood sugar levels stable, since both too much and too little glucose can affect brain function. A heart-healthy diet will improve your blood pressure and, as physical fitness is key to good brain health, regular exercise is a must. It's also wise to drink in moderation.

- **Be well informed.** Don't get too hung up on all the conflicting information you read or every scary newspaper article. If you have a family history of dementia or Alzheimer's disease, or any of the other risk factors that I have mentioned above, get expert help from a good neurologist or endocrinologist. See that you keep an open mind about all the available treatment options and never be afraid to ask questions and get answers that you understand. This will enable you to make careful, informed decisions about your cognitive functioning. Your doctor should be staying abreast of all the current research in this area, and there are robust, ongoing studies that may shed some light on the role estrogen plays in the brain.

- **Use it or lose it.** I think it's very important that middle-aged women don't just 'veg out' but exercise their brains as thoroughly as they do their bodies. If you don't have a career or an interesting job, find an intellectual pursuit. Perhaps join a book club that demands a written report on the books you have read. Learn a language, play bridge, join a music appreciation group. Study something new. Go back to university and get a second (or first) degree. Start becoming involved in politics or world issues and stretch your mind by reading widely. Some midlife women develop a fascination with share portfolios and investments. Others find that they have time to 'give something back' and become involved in community work; donate your skills and time to a community initiative or a charity. Apart from filling the spaces that may have been left by the 'empty nest' I discuss below, it's a great way of using a whole range of cognitive, organisational skills and has the additional benefit of making you feeling happy and useful too. Once you start using your brain, you'll be amazed at just how well it works.

DEPRESSION

Depression is an umbrella term that can encompass quite a few of the emotional symptoms of menopause. Several symptoms of perimenopause are mood-related and you will probably recognise many of them – mood swings, panic attacks, a lack of positive feeling or the absence of your usual cheerfulness, weepiness, anxiety, impatience, a short temper, grumpiness, lowered tolerance, unwarranted anger at what you feel to be invasions of your space, tension, jumpiness or restlessness, a sense of worthlessness and hopelessness. As you can see from the stories of the group of women quoted at the beginning of the chapter, they experienced a wide spectrum of these.

Many trials have been dedicated to determining whether depression in peri- and postmenopausal women is related to estrogen levels and whether the transition into menopause will make us more vulnerable to depression. More women suffer from depression than men and it is linked to hormonal and psychosocial factors that are specific to women. Women are very vulnerable to hormone changes throughout their reproductive cycles, and different stages will usually affect us. Some research shows that certain women who battled with symptoms won't experience depression in perimenopause, while other women with the same level of symptoms will suffer badly from it.

One interesting finding was that once women had gone through the perimenopausal years and become fully menopausal, levels of depression dropped, which means that the depression can be blamed on **fluctuating** rather than **low** levels of estrogen, since women who have bad hot flushes and/or night sweats seem to become more depressed. This may also be related to the discomfort and lack of sleep caused by these symptoms, or to other issues that crop up at this stage of your life. Other studies showed that women who battled with PMS had worse depression in perimenopause, as did those who were depressed even before they started the transition into menopause.

An interesting study showed that although taking HT didn't reduce depression, women who stopped taking it were more likely to become depressed within a couple of years. Perhaps they found their symptoms had begun again, as I explained in Chapter 4, as sometimes when a woman stops HT and the symptoms return, they may be more severe. As you know by now there are no simple answers and the risks of long-term estrogen therapy may well outweigh the benefits. HT is not an antidepressant and should not be prescribed as such.

Medical research has shown that menopausal women may suffer from bad hot flushes as a result of reduced serotonin levels, which are probably caused by lowered levels of estrogen. In Chapter 6, I discussed the use of various selective serotonin reuptake inhibitors (SSRIs) –venlafaxine, fluoxetine, paroxetine, sertraline and citalopram – which appear to alleviate hot flushes. This is known as *off-label* use, which is the legal use of a prescription medicine to treat a disease or condition for which the medicine has not been approved by medicine regulatory boards.

It may be logical to use these same antidepressants to treat depression in perimenopausal women. Depression is a very common and debilitating illness, yet many women are ashamed that they feel depressed, subscribing to the old notion that it's 'all in their heads' and if they just 'pulled themselves together', they would feel better. This just isn't so, and even if many of the contributing factors are psychological, once you are not well it makes sense to get the appropriate medication so that you can cope better. It is often hard to know when your depression is bad enough to be treated. The rule is that if you only feel sad and down for a couple of days and it passes, there is no need for concern. However, if these feelings continue and grow and you find that you can't get up in the morning, your quality of life is affected and you are causing pain to those closest to you, you should see a doctor because you may be diagnosed with something called depressive disorder and you will probably need treatment to get better.

Some women try complementary medicines during this time, but there isn't enough evidence to show that these are safe and effective in the long run. I find it strange that people have no problem taking medication for diabetes or for bad headaches but baulk at antidepressants. This is a pity, because they may be very helpful for some women.

Many psychiatrists may suggest medication for a short time, between six months and a year. If you're feeling depressed ask your doctor to refer you to a psychiatrist and have a proper assessment. If you decide to take an antidepressant, be warned that it might aggravate any libido problems you may have, but since depression dampens sexual desire in any case, it may be okay just to feel better, so that you can have pleasant sex. For some women antidepressants may have other side effects, such as weight gain or loss, but usually women are so relieved to feel better that these are not problematic.

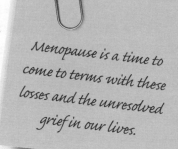

Menopause is a time to come to terms with these losses and the unresolved grief in our lives.

There are other ways to deal with depression. A very interesting study showed that a group of depressed women who were assigned to a regular exercise programme did much better than the control group who didn't exercise. In another study, women who exercised regularly were much better psychologically two years after they began than when they started the programme, because among other things they felt so much better physically. So one solution is to exercise at least five times a week. There is a plethora of literature showing that mood improves with a good workout or a brisk walk. Many women say that they notice that their mood worsens when they don't exercise and they definitely feel more depressed.

In my experience, many women become depressed during perimenopause for reasons other than fluctuating levels of estrogen. These include debilitating menopause symptoms that affect our quality of life and disturb our sleep (and insomnia plays a big part in feeling depressed), we gain weight and lose our libido and on the rare occasions we have sex, it may be painful. There are other very painful emotional issues. When you reach midlife, you may be dealing with many losses. Although many women find it fun to be alone with their partners when their children leave home, some may find that the reason for their existence has been taken away and, more frightening, that they are no longer needed as their children make their way in the world. At the same time though, the demands of their children may have been replaced by the demands of elderly and infirm parents.

When the house is empty, many women are forced to interact on a one-on-one basis with their partners for the first time in many years and the experience may not fill their souls. Some may realise that their marriage is empty or a sham, or that in the intervening years they and their partner have grown apart and are no longer in love. Those women who have given up their identities and careers to look after their families may feel unfulfilled, as though they have wasted their lives. Their partners may still be busy and occupied, while they have a lot of empty time on their hands. There are women who are content with the status quo, but others find themselves unaccountably sad as they examine lost opportunities or missed chances. The world we live in does not usually value ageing women, which may underline feelings of disempowerment and uselessness. We may worry about global issues and fears for our way of life, depending on the country in which we live; economic problems may be overwhelming and we may struggle with poor health. Some women who have never had children and have previously been happy with the fact, suddenly feel bereft when menopause is inexorably upon them. Still others mourn their lost youth and beauty. These feelings of loss may be aggravated by the fact that this is a time in many of our lives when we begin to lose those who have been closest to us – parents, spouses, partners, siblings and friends.

My sense is that menopause is a time to come to terms with these losses and the unresolved grief in our lives. Perhaps we have never had time before to stop and carefully examine our lives. Perhaps we are suddenly aware of the passage of time and the fact that it is running out. We are confronted with elderly parents who are signposts of our own mortality. Is it any surprise that so many middle-aged women suffer from depression? Identifying and working on these issues is vital for your mental health in menopause. Many women judge themselves so harshly that it is no wonder they are depressed. They need to be kinder to themselves, to lose the voice of the critical mother which has played incessantly in their heads since they were little girls, and they may need help to get rid of it.

Often therapy may be a very good idea. There are different types of therapy available and you should choose something that appeals to you personally. It is probably a good idea to work through these issues with a woman, preferably a middle-aged one. This is not because I don't believe there are good male therapists or young therapists available, but because I believe you may need someone who's been there. Menopause is a uniquely feminine and midlife experience. For those women who are suddenly struggling with their relationships, couples' therapy may be a good idea. Although your marriage may be basically sound, certain issues may need to be aired and dealt with. If you feel you can no longer stay in your relationship, you may need help in making the decision to change the situation.

If you can come to terms with your life in menopause, a new phase will open up to you, and there will be all kinds of extraordinary possibilities. Honouring your body and your psyche will help you to be more energised, interested and live better than ever before.

STRESS

One of the biggest health issues for women of all ages is stress. But researchers have found that as women enter menopause they become more stressed, perhaps as a result of the many symptoms that accompany this transition, health-related problems and the many life issues that I have discussed already in this chapter.

Many of us are constantly rushing and running, always tense and anxious. Stress is a physical and emotional reaction we all experience when we face life changes, both big and small. The positive side of stress is that it helps us deal with life's challenges, but when it becomes continuous, it can be negative and impact on our health. Stress is the way our body reacts to changes in the environment – it's our primitive way of dealing with what we see as danger. As adrenaline is secreted, our heart rate increases, our muscles tense and our blood pressure rises, helping us to concentrate better and be physically prepared for what our brain sees as a danger. These instinctive reactions are great in emergencies, such as jumping out of the way of a speeding car. After the challenge is met, our body relaxes and our heart rate and muscle tension return to normal, giving us a chance to calm down. This is obviously good stress. But when these situations are never-ending or we feel they never stop, our bodies don't get a chance to relax, causing a knot in our stomachs and tense muscles. This is called *chronic stress* and if it goes on for too long, it can be very unhealthy. It feels as though your body's on high alert waiting to protect you from danger, when in fact there's no danger at all. Everything that comes into play when there's an actual emergency is now happening to you all the time. Your body is working overtime, with no place to put all the extra energy, which can make you feel anxious, afraid, worried and uptight.

Possible signs of stress include anxiety, back pain, upset stomach – constipation or diarrhoea, depression, fatigue, headaches, high blood pressure, trouble sleeping or sleeplessness, problems with relationships, shortness of breath, a stiff neck or jaw and weight gain or loss. According to the American Institute of Stress, there are over 50 signs and symptoms of stress. If you are continually stressed it will certainly impact on your physical well-being and you may find you can list a number of symptoms, including raised blood pressure, headaches, irritable bowel syndrome, heartburn, panic attacks, a lowered immune system, insomnia, difficulty concentrating, and weight gain or loss. Stress also affects our interpersonal relationships and our quality of life.

Talk to your healthcare practitioner if you think some of your symptoms are caused by stress. As with all symptoms we may experience, it's vital to make sure they aren't caused by other health problems. Any sort of change, whether good or bad, can make us feel stressed. We all know there are major stressful events in life but because we're all unique, different things may stress us, and we need to be aware of what causes us to stress and how we handle these situations.

Dealing with stress

The first step in dealing with stress is to identify what stresses you. Each of us has different stressors. What you might find stressful may not worry someone else at all.

Deal with stress by recognising when you're feeling stressed. Do you clench your hands into fists, feel your jaw muscle tensing, your back and neck going into spasm, your heart racing? Now choose a way to deal with your stress. Sometimes the best way is to avoid the thing that makes you stressed; if you find shopping with your husband stressful, acknowledge it and don't do it. Or if being late for work stresses you out so you drive like a mad person – hooting and yelling, weaving in and out of the traffic, narrowly missing other vehicles, red in the face, drumming your fingers on the steering wheel every time there's a traffic jam – change your routine and arrange your life, assuming there will be holdups, so you have enough extra time to get there.

The real problem comes when we encounter changes or stressors we can't change or avoid. The way to deal with these is to try to change how you react to them. Plan for your major life changes as far as possible, or if you can't and something happens out of the blue, allow yourself to put other things on hold so you can deal appropriately with the challenge. Learn to prioritise. Often we create our own stressors and make life harder for ourselves. Learn to say 'No'. This is incredibly hard for most women and a huge cause of stress. If you say 'Yes' when you mean 'No' you'll be angry at yourself and resentful of the person you agreed to help – leading once again to unnecessary stress. Be honest about your feelings when you can't manage something. Create boundaries that make sense for you. Work to resolve conflicts with other people; don't keep angry feelings in. Learn to discuss them in a quiet and constructive way, rather than pushing them away until they burst out and you have an angry row leading to more stress. Stop worrying about what people think about you, how you look and how you're behaving. We're so busy worrying about how others see us that we may lose sight of our own needs. Don't stress about things you can't control. Try to look at change positively.

Solve the little problems first. This may help you feel you have more control over your life. Prepare for events you know may be stressful, such as a job interview or an important meeting, to the best of your ability.

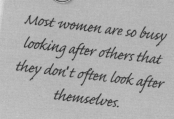

Most women are so busy looking after others that they don't often look after themselves.

If you can't see a way through a problem, discuss it with a friend or family member you trust. They will often see a way through because they aren't so enmeshed in the problem. If problems seem too big or scary and you don't want to share them with someone close to you, talk to a counsellor.

Eat sensibly and don't use food as a comfort; chocolate, though a pleasure in moderation, won't solve your stress in the long term and might even increase your stress as you gain weight and feel distressed about it. Don't drown your sorrows in drink, this can lead to problems in the long run and your 'escape' from reality will only be temporary. Set realistic goals at home and work. Avoid overscheduling. Spoil yourself. It's amazing to me how many women feel guilty doing this. Soaking in a warm, scented bath with a perfumed candle, relaxing with a book or watching a chick flick can do wonders for us. Have a massage, facial or beauty treatment once in a while. Work with your hands, be creative, knit, sew or paint, as long as you can sit quietly when you are doing this. Go to a concert, read a poem, listen to 'golden oldies' that bring back happy memories, walk in your garden or around the neighbourhood and enjoy the world around you. Exercise on a regular basis and get enough sleep.

Learn to have quiet time and meditate or practise slow, deep breathing to still your racing heart. Recently I have become a convert to a type of meditation called mindfulness. In Chapter 6, I wrote about a mindfulness-based stress reduction programme that had helped alleviate severe hot flushes and improved the quality of life in a group of women. I think that in the crazed, anxious lives we lead today some kind of meditation can be very helpful in making us less stressed. If you have a certain personality, it may be very hard to sit still, but if this is really difficult for you and you find your thoughts racing, you may wonder what it's doing to your health. Women are incredibly judgemental both of others and themselves. Mindfulness is trying to live in the present moment in a non-judging and accepting way, to stop frantically trying to analyse the past and control the future, but rather being aware of and appreciating the present moment. Many people have found this a wonderful way to reduce stress, though it may take time to understand the technique. However, I am well aware that different relaxation techniques appeal to different people. Choose one that suits you best, whether it is meditation of any kind, yoga, guided imaging, some spiritual time or prayer, or just sitting quietly and breathing deeply. It doesn't really matter what you do, as long as you commit to something and give the time doing this to yourself as a gift that is vital to your physical and emotional health.

Most women are so busy looking after others that they don't often look after themselves. We are so consumed by the hundreds of things going on in our daily lives that we don't give our partners and ourselves the time we need to nurture our relationships and to enjoy the years that are slipping by so fast. Many years ago I loved watching a TV series called 'Thirty Something'. At one point one of the characters gets divorced; he explains to his friend it wasn't about infidelity but rather that he hadn't been paying attention; he and his wife got so caught up in their jobs, their family and their lives that they'd stopped investing in each other. We all need to pay attention. If you realise your partner barely talks to you, or when you do talk you only discuss problems, if you have no clue what's going on in their daily lives, or when they initiate sex you feel so emotionally exhausted you can't think of anything worse – wake up. Make time for a date night; if you need some space, spend quiet time together. Rediscover the things that made you want to be with that person in the first place. If you find you no longer speak the same language, honestly discuss the problem and, if necessary, get help.

There are many good things about being menopausal in the twenty-first century. We are generally living longer than our mothers and grandmothers; we know so much more about our health that we can be aware of the risks and look after ourselves. Research has shown that women who approach this time of their lives with knowledge and a positive attitude usually have a much easier time than those who dread it. They are less likely to become depressed and live happier, healthier lives. So be aware and know that you do have a say in your mental health – the part you play may make a huge difference to your quality of life and your future health and happiness.

EMPOWER YOURSELF

- Exercise, exercise, exercise, regularly and vigorously. Every time you struggle reluctantly out of your warm bed remember exercise is the key not only to a healthy body but also to a healthy mind: it increases sexual desire, helps you to sleep, protects against depression, cognitive decline and ill health, and makes you look and feel great.
- Exercise your brain as you do your body. Stimulate yourself intellectually.
- Check out all very bad headaches. If you have an aura (visual disturbance) without a migraine or a migraine with an aura, see a doctor to make sure that nothing untoward is happening.
- Get some professional help when you're negotiating the sometimes rocky emotional path of peri- and postmenopause.
- HT is not an antidepressant and should not be prescribed as one.
- Commit to some kind of relaxation technique and make it part of your daily life; this is your gift to yourself.

Conclusion

SPEAKING LOUD AND CLEAR: THE AUTHENTIC VOICE OF MENOPAUSE

When I began to write this book I went to a talk given by Carol Gilligan, a well-known feminist psychologist who taught at Harvard for more than 30 years and is now a university professor at New York University and the author of several books, including the groundbreaking *In a Different Voice*. She suggested that when girls start menstruating, they stop using their 'authentic' voices and use a 'different' voice; one that they and society believe is more appropriate to their new-found sexuality and reproductive role.

The light that went on in my head stayed with me as I wrote, but it is only now as I reach these concluding paragraphs that I truly understand the concept. It seems to me that when women become menopausal and can no longer bear children, they are able to find the authentic voices that many of them lost when they reached puberty, and these voices allow them to be as strong and fearless as they were so many years ago. The stories I have heard and the knowledge I have gained have inspired me. I know now that menopause is not an end, but can be the beginning of a different, exciting and fulfilling time for women. It simply depends on how we decide to live the menopausal years.

The very authentic voice of a famous woman who died at 90, who worked tirelessly for human rights, looked wonderful and partied up a storm until well into her eighties, echoes in my head: 'I'll flirt till the day I die. It might not get the results it used to but it makes me feel great!' Being menopausal didn't stop her, couldn't stop her. She took charge of her life and lived it all as well as possible; both the serious parts and the most light-hearted. If we choose, the final third of our lives will be extraordinary.

If we take responsibility for our health, if we understand what is happening to our bodies and if we determine what is best for us, the fear that menopause heralds the end of our lives and the myth that we will become estrogen-deficient, dried-out, intellectually impaired, sad little old ladies, will be dispelled. We can take charge of ourselves as women and spend the rest of our days living authentically with humour, vitality, wisdom and wit. Strong, powerful, interesting and sexy, we can go forward and make these the best years of our lives.

Even more information …

A COMPREHENSIVE LIST OF SYMPTOMS OF PERI- AND POSTMENOPAUSE

The symptoms listed here are highly individual. You may never experience any of them, you may experience some of them, and very, very rarely will any woman experience all of them. You may just not feel great or you may feel different but not be able to specify why. Because you are not having hot flushes, for example, a friend may say: 'Oh, you can't be having menopause.' Don't listen. Any of the symptoms below may be heralding your menopause.

You may sail through menopause as you did through your menstrual periods, if you never experienced PMS, or your pregnancy, if you didn't have morning sickness. It all depends on your own body's chemistry. These are symptoms that may start only now that you are in middle age, not symptoms that you have experienced for most of your adult life. When you read this list remember that about 76 per cent of women will probably have some kind of hot flush during menopause, while only about 3 per cent will suffer bad headaches or migraines; even if you aren't suffering from hot flushes, the headaches may be a sign that you are menopausal.

Be warned, however, that some of these symptoms may not be related to the menopause transition but may indicate a medical condition, like thyroid dysfunction, so it is always wise to talk to your doctor when you start experiencing symptoms you haven't had before to rule out any more sinister causes. If you are middle-aged and have a constellation of the symptoms that usually indicate changing hormonal levels, they are probably related to perimenopause, but it is always sensible to make sure.

- Hot flushes (there are several types of hot flushes – see Chapter 6)
- Body temperature disturbances
- Night sweats
- Breast swelling and tenderness
- Weight gain, especially around the hips and thighs
- Heavy menstrual periods
- Unusually bad menstrual cramps
- Irregular periods
- Erratic bleeding and spotting
- Loss of libido (sexual desire)
- Vaginal dryness
- Itchiness around the vaginal area

- Painful intercourse
- Changes in urinary function (urinating more frequently, especially at night)
- Greater urgency in the need to urinate
- Leaking
- Urinary infections
- Unusual skin sensations: (prickly or tingling)
- Skin that is highly sensitive to human touch or fabrics
- Dry skin
- Dry eyes
- Heart palpitations
- Headaches and migraine
- Dizzy spells (people sometimes think they have an inner ear infection)
- Sudden bouts of nausea or faintness
- Low-grade fatigue
- Mood swings
- Negative feelings or absence of your usual cheerfulness
- Weepiness
- Generalised anxiety and free-floating anxiety (anxiety not for any clearly identifiable reason)
- Increased anger, impatience, short temper or grumpiness compared to the past
- Less tolerance of things that irritate you
- Forgetfulness
- Confusion
- Depression
- Feelings of worthlessness and hopelessness
- Panic attacks
- Feeling very tense
- Reluctance to be too close to someone
- Unwarranted anger at what you feel to be an 'invasion' of your space
- Jumpiness and restlessness
- Insomnia
- Strange dreams and nightmares
- Altered sleeping patterns
- Disturbed sleep
- Difficulty in falling asleep
- Waking much earlier than usual
- Aching ankles, knees, wrists or shoulders
- Joint pain
- Bleeding gums
- Hairs suddenly appearing on your chin
- Long, silky facial hairs
- Thinning hair
- More frequent flatulence, wind pains and indigestion
- Bloating

MIDLIFE HEALTH CHECKLIST

This list is not meant to be prescriptive in any way. It is simply an aid to jog your memory about some of the tests and evaluations that may help you take responsibility for your health in midlife. These will usually be done annually, but at your doctor's discretion and in consultation with you. Discussing whether or not you should have these tests will improve your partnership with your doctor. They may help you to be aware of whether or not you are being monitored on a regular basis. The clinical evaluations below will depend on your individual medical risk factors and medical history. Your doctor will identify your individual risks and refer you to the appropriate medical specialist for further investigations and tests if necessary.

- Gynaecological examination, including a transvaginal ultrasound of the ovaries and womb, a manual breast examination and a pelvic examination. Vaginal health should be assessed.
- Medical history (including family history, serious illnesses, surgical history, gynaecological history, medication history, psychosocial history and modifiable lifestyle risk factors)
- Pap smear
- Urine check
- Blood pressure (at least annually as part of the check-up, and every time you see your doctor)
- Weight and BMI
- Waist circumference
- Height
- Mammogram (see pages 166–167 for guidelines)
- Eye exam (including monitoring for glaucoma and cataracts)
- Dermatological (skin) check-up
- Dental check-up and six monthly visits to a dental hygienist
- Auditory check-up
- DEXA – Do initially for a baseline and then as your doctor recommends, depending on your bone mineral density measurements. Your fracture risks should also be assessed.
- Sigmoidoscopy – every three to five years. Earlier screening will probably be recommended if you have a strong family history of colon cancer.
- Faecal occult blood test (annually)
- Colonoscopy (family history or unusual symptoms, (see pages 197–200 for guidelines)

Blood tests:
- Thyroid function
- Lipid profile (LDL, HDL, triglycerides)
- Fasting blood glucose
- 25(OH) vitamin D
- Your doctor will recommend other relevant blood tests, depending on your individual needs.

GLOSSARY

Medical terms guaranteed to confuse you when you discuss menopause

Absolute risk – the exact number of people at risk per a specific number

Adenoma – a benign growth that develops in the epithelial tissue

Adipose tissue – fatty tissue

Adjuvant therapy – treatment that is given in addition to the primary treatment or therapy

Adrenal cascade – the order in which the hormones in the body are manufactured from pregnenolone

Adrenal gland – a small gland situated on top of each kidney, which secretes certain sex steroid hormones and cortisol

Amenorrhoea – not having a period when you are still in your reproductive years

Amino acid – a chemical messenger in the body

Antineoplastic drug – a drug that is used to inhibit or control the growth of malignant cells

Antioxidant – a supplement that slows down the rate at which something in the body decays or breaks down because of its interaction with oxygen

Aromatase inhibitors – drugs that block certain tissues from producing estrogen in postmenopausal women

Arteriosclerosis – hardening of the arteries; if you have this you may not have atherosclerosis

Atherosclerosis – hardening of the arteries caused by plaque building up in the arteries; if you have this condition you will have arteriosclerosis

Benign – not life-threatening or dangerous – not malignant

Beta-blocker – a medicine that helps to regulate the heartbeat by calming down specific body responses

Bilateral salpingo-oophorectomy (BSO) – surgery where the womb and both ovaries are removed

Bioavailable – able to be metabolised by the body

Biochemistry – the chemical interactions that take place in the body, from the cells to the major organs; the chemistry of life

Bioidentical – chemically similar or exactly the same as the biological substance

Bisphosphonate – a medicine that controls the activity of the osteoclasts to limit the breaking down of bone

Body mass index (BMI) – the ratio of your weight to your height

Bone mineral density – the amount of bone material that is packed into a certain volume of bone

Bone mineralisation – when bone tissue or material is broken down, releasing calcium and phosphate

Carbohydrates – compounds that are made up of carbon, hydrogen and oxygen, e.g. sugars, starches, cellulose and gums

Cardiomyopathy – weakening of the heart muscle

Cardiovascular disease – disease of the heart and blood vessels

Cataract – cloudiness or opacity of the lens of the eye

Cervix – the opening of the womb; the narrow end of the uterus that leads into the vagina

Chemotherapy – a chemical treatment in either pill or injection form that travels through the bloodstream killing cancer cells in the body

Cholesterol – a fatty substance that is found throughout the body in cells, blood, tissues, the brain, muscles and liver. It is found in proteins like meat, chicken, fish and eggs and in dairy products. The liver produces cholesterol and synthesises it. It is essential for healthy living because it plays a vital role in cell repair and the storage and production of energy. All sex steroid hormones come from cholesterol. LDL is usually called 'bad' cholesterol because if levels of LDL become too high, it may stick to the walls of the blood vessels or arteries and form deposits of the fatty material or plaque that can lead to hardening of the arteries – *atherosclerosis*. HDL is usually called 'good' cholesterol, because it carries cholesterol and triglycerides to the liver, which converts them so that they can be used again in different parts of the body. Higher levels of HDL are 'good' because they help protect the body from excess cholesterol.

Cognitive – intellectual functioning. Cognition is the action of knowing and includes all kinds of brain functions like memory, the ability to learn, facility with language and the way people solve problems.

Collagen – a fibrous tissue found throughout the body

Colonoscopy – a test that allows your doctor to examine your colon and rectum by means of a colonoscope inserted into your rectum

Colposcopy – a procedure whereby the cervix is examined with a high-powered magnifying lens and a light inserted into the vagina

Conjugated equine estrogens (CEE) – a combination of multiple estrogens, isolated from pregnant mares' urine, including estrone, equilin and equilenin. Also called conjugated estrogens (CE)

Core-needle biopsy – a biopsy performed on a breast lump to collect material for examination and analysis

Coronary plaque – fatty material deposited or collected on the artery walls

Corpus luteum – from the Latin meaning 'yellow body'. When the follicle releases the egg by rupturing, it becomes this yellow body.

Cortical bone – very hard bone on the outside of the bone which makes up the shaft of the bones

C-reactive protein (CRP) – a very specific protein that is produced by the liver only when the body is experiencing severe injury, infection or inflammation. High-sensitivity C-reactive protein (hsCRP) may be measured to determine a person's risk for heart disease.

Dementia – a gradual decline in cognitive functioning as a result of damage or disease in the brain beyond what is expected in normal cognitive ageing

DEXA scan – dual energy X-ray absorptiometry. The DEXA measures the amount of bone present in a specific area. Also called DXA.

Diuretic – a medicine or any substance that increases the discharge of urine

Double-blind randomised controlled study/trial – a study or trial in which both the patients and the doctor are 'blinded' to the therapy being given

Ductal carcinoma in situ (DCIS) – a cancer in the breast duct that has not invaded the surrounding tissue

Ducts – tubes or canals; in this book the tubes or canals in the breasts

Elastin – fibres that make the skin elastic

Embolisation of fibroids – an advanced X-ray technique where the blood supply to the fibroid is cut off so that it shrinks

Embolism – the blocking of a blood vessel usually by a blood clot

Endocrine system – the system of glands that controls all the body's hormones

Endocrinologist – a specialist who deals in the complex interaction of hormones

Endogenous estrogen – the estrogen found in the body

Endometrial ablation – the burning away of the lining of the womb

Endometrial hyperplasia – thickening of the lining of the womb

Endometriosis – endometriosis occurs when endometrial cells grow outside the uterus. The endometrial cells can be found in the ovaries, the fallopian tubes and the pelvic cavity.

Endometrium/endometrius – lining of the womb

Endothelium – the thin layer of cells that lines the inside surface of blood vessels. Endothelial cells line the entire circulatory system, from the heart to the smallest capillary.

Enzyme – a protein that helps or causes certain chemical reactions in the body

Epithelial tissue – the cells lining the inside or the surface of an organ

Equilin – estrogen found in pregnant mares

Estrogen agonist/antagonist – a compound with a tissue selective action; it has beneficial estrogenic actions in some tissues but opposes the effects of estrogen on other tissues where estrogen activity may be harmful

Estrogen receptor-negative – a breast cancer tumour that is not sensitive to estrogen; also described as ER-negative

Estrogen receptor-positive – a breast cancer tumour that is sensitive to estrogen; also described as ER-positive or or ER+. Estrogen receptor-positive cancers may be more likely to respond to hormone therapy.

Estrogenic or estrogenated – a state caused by estrogen

Evidence-based medicine – Doctors use the best available evidence from the most current academic research when making a clinical decision.

Exogenous estrogen – estrogen taken or applied to the body

Faecal Occult Blood test – a test that shows, under a microscope, whether there is blood in stools

Fallopian tubes – the two tubes leading from the ovaries to the uterus, down which the egg travels to the womb

False negative result – a diagnosis when you are told that there is no disease or mutation present when it is in fact present

False positive result – a diagnosis which suggests the presence of disease or mutation (a positive result) when everything is in fact normal

Fibroadenoma – a benign lump or growth

Fibroadenosis – used to describe a benign condition of the breast that can cause lumpiness, enlargement, tenderness and sometimes pain

Fibroid – benign growth of muscle and connective tissue in the walls of the uterus

Fine-needle biopsy – a procedure during which the specialist uses an ultrasound and a very fine needle to take a sample of tissue and cells (may be called fine-needle aspiration)

Fluctuating levels – changing levels

Fluid retention – when the body holds excess water

Follicle – a sac-like structure containing the egg

Glaucoma – an increase in pressure behind the eye as a result of fluid build-up

G-spot – the region situated in a woman's genital area, behind her pubic bone. This area surrounds the urethra. Tiny glands called Skene's glands are found here, in the upper wall of the vagina and the lower end of the urethra. The name G-spot is given to the area where the Skene's glands are found.

Haemorrhagic stroke – where a blood vessel ruptures, causing bleeding in the brain

Homocysteine – an amino acid, which can be toxic in high amounts and may be a risk factor in heart disease

Hormones – chemical substances that act as messengers throughout the body

Hydrogenated fats – vegetable oils that have been heated to a very high temperature, then bubbled through with hydrogen

Hypercalcemia – too much calcium

Hypertension – high blood pressure

Hyperthyroidism – an overactive thyroid

Hypocalcemia – too little calcium

Hypothalamus – part of the base of the brain to which the pituitary gland is attached. It regulates many important body functions, memory and emotions.

Hypothyroidism – an underactive thyroid

Hysterectomy – surgical removal of the womb

Hysteroscopy – a procedure whereby an instrument is passed through the mouth of the womb to allow the inside of the womb to be viewed

Immune system – the series of organs and chemical reactions that the body uses to protect itself from disease; it also helps the body fight and control the spread of disease

Insulin resistance – although there is enough insulin available in the system, the cells it regulates do not respond to it

Invasive ductal carcinoma (IDC) – a cancer in the breast duct that has broken through the wall of the milk duct and begun to invade the surrounding tissue

Involuted breast – a breast that has collapsed inward so the fatty tissue is not too dense

Ischaemic stroke – where a clot blocks the blood flow to the brain

Isoflavone – a plant estrogen found in soy

Laparoscopy – a procedure whereby a surgeon inserts a small instrument (laparoscope) through the navel into the abdomen for inspection

Laparotomy – a technique whereby a surgeon makes a cut (incision) through any part of the abdomen

Lesion – a local abnormality or change in tissues or an organ due to injury or disease. It can be benign or malignant. There are many different types of lesions.

Libido – sexual desire

Lignans – plant estrogens

Lobes – sections – in this book, specifically sections of the breast

Lobules – smaller lobes

Lumpectomy – a surgical procedure to remove a lump from the breast that raises concern

Lymph nodes – small areas throughout the body, including in the armpits, neck area, near the collarbone and in the groin and chest, where lymph fluid collects. These help the white blood cells fight infection.

Lymph vessels – these vessels carry a clear fluid called lymph that cleans the tissues throughout the body

Lymphatic system – the system that helps guard the body against infection

Malignant – life-threatening, virulent. The word refers to a growth that tends to spread and recur and so proves fatal.

Mammogram – special X-ray of the breast

Melanoma – a type of skin cancer

Melatonin – a hormone secreted by a small gland in the brain called the pineal gland, which is associated with sleep and biological rhythms

Menopause – the last day of a woman's last period

Menstrual cycle – the cyclical changes that occur in the lining of the womb in preparation for accepting a fertilised egg. If there is no fertilised egg the lining is shed, causing a bleed, which is called a period (menstruation).

Metabolic syndrome – a group of symptoms that can cause insulin resistance, leading to glucose intolerance, type 2 diabetes or risk of heart disease

Metabolises – breaks down or builds up

Metastasis – when a group of cancer cells starts to travel and damages other organs or tissues or forms other secondary growths

Mineral – a natural inorganic substance with a specific chemical make-up that is vital for healthy body function

Modifiable risk factors – risk factors (such as smoking) that you can control

Mono-unsaturated fat – found in avocado, olive oil, canola oil and peanut oil

MRI – magnetic resonance imaging; a specialised medical technique using magnetic resonance rather than X-rays to produce pictures of the inside of the body

Myocardial infarction – heart attack

Myomectomy – a procedure during which a fibroid is surgically removed. Frequently the chosen treatment for premenopausal women because it usually helps to preserve fertility.

Neoplasm – a new and abnormal growth of tissue in some part of the body, where the cells multiply more rapidly than normal. Neoplasms may be either benign or malignant.

Neurotransmitter – a chemical that allows the transmission of impulses along the nerves

Norepinephrine – a chemical involved with the sympathetic nervous system

Nutraceuticals – products taken from foods, which are said to have proven medical benefits, especially in the prevention of heart disease

Off-label – using medicines to treat a symptom or illness for which it has not been approved by a medicines control board

Omega-3 and omega-6 fatty acids – vital fats, crucial for the efficient functioning and maintenance of every single cell in the body

Oophorectomy – removal of the ovaries

Osteoblasts – special cells in the bone that build new bone tissue

Osteoclasts – special cells in the bones that break down old bone tissue

Osteocytes – cells in the bone that send out `messages' to the body that a specific area of bone needs to be remodelled

Ovary – one of two structures in the female body, about the size of an almond, containing all the eggs of a woman's reproductive life

Ovulation – the process whereby the egg is developed and released from the ovary

Ovum – an egg in the ovary

Pancreas – a long gland situated behind and below the stomach, which produces insulin and digestive juices

Perimenopause – the time before; around and just after the actual moment of menopause

Pessary – a small oval suppository that is inserted into the vagina with a small applicator

pH balance – the normal, health acid balance; in this case, of the vagina

Physiological – the normal function of living things

Phytoestrogens – estrogens that are found in plants

Pituitary gland – the most important gland in the endocrine system, situated at the base of the hypothalamus, which produces and controls the actions of many of the most important hormones in the body

Placebo – an inactive treatment which the people taking it believe to be a specific drug, often used in research studies to determine the effectiveness of a medical drug

Polyp – small, benign growth on the lining of the colon and/or rectum

Polyunsaturated fat – the fat found in vegetable oils, like corn and sunflower oil, as well as fish oils, flaxseed oils, sesame and walnut oil

Postmenopause – after menopause

Precursor – a building block that causes a particular chemical reaction

Radiation – a procedure during which a cancer is blasted with X-rays

Radical hysterectomy – surgery during which the womb, cervix and part of the upper area of the vagina, as well as the ovaries, are removed

Radical mastectomy – where the whole breast is removed together with some pectoral muscles

Receptor – a minute place on the surface of or within a cell that recognises and binds to one specific substance producing a certain physiologic effect

Relative risk – the percentage of people at risk per a given number

Remodelling – in this book, the process whereby bone is broken down and reformed

Resorption – the removal of old bone tissue by the osteoclasts

Segmentectomy – a surgical procedure to remove a more extensive amount of breast tissue than in a lumpectomy

SERM – selective estrogen receptor modulator. These hormones have a beneficial estrogen effect in certain areas of the body and block unwanted estrogen effects in other parts of the body, so that the amount of active estrogen in the body is not increased.

Serotonin – a brain chemical involved with mood, appetite and sleep

Sex-steroid hormones – special hormones that are involved with the growth and functioning of the reproductive organs. They are the hormones that affect male or female sexual characteristics.

Sigmoidoscopy – a procedure that allows a doctor to see inside the sigmoid colon and rectum and helps in the detection of inflamed tissues and abnormal growth

Sleep apnoea – a sleep disorder when breathing during sleep is interrupted by one or more pauses in breathing or shallow breaths. It is usually a chronic condition that disrupts sleep.

SSRI – selective serotonin reuptake inhibitor; a drug that slows the action of the enzyme that destroys excess serotonin and helps a certain amount of serotonin to remain circulating throughout the body, making people feel better. Many antidepressants are SSRIs.

Statins – drugs that act on a certain enzyme in the liver, causing a lowering of cholesterol levels in the blood

Statistics – a method of collecting, analysing and interpreting data

Stress incontinence – leaking when you laugh, cough or sneeze, or lift heavy objects

Synthesised – manufactured

Thromboembolic disease – blood clots

Timing hypothesis – the length of time after menopause that a woman starts on HT

Triple negative breast cancer – when a cancer is neither estrogen receptor nor progesterone receptor-positive and is not HER2

Total hysterectomy – surgery where the uterus and part/all of the cervix are removed

Trabecular bone – spongy and soft bone found at the ends of long bones and in the spine

Transdermal – taken through the skin

Transvaginal ultrasound – an ultrasound performed via the vagina

Tumour – an abnormal swelling or enlargement of tissue in any part of the body (see neoplasm). It can be benign or malignant.

Type 2 diabetes – this occurs when the pancreas produces higher and higher amounts of insulin in response to insulin resistant cells. Eventually the pancreas becomes 'exhausted' and is unable to make enough insulin to control blood glucose levels, which then start to rise.

Ultrasound – high frequency sound that produces an image

Urethra – a thin tube that carries urine from the bladder through the vagina and from there to the outside of the body

Urge incontinence – an overwhelming urge to urinate and then leaking before reaching a lavatory

Urinary tract – all organs that are involved in the production and expulsion of urine from the body

Uterus – womb

Vagina – the passage that leads from the womb to the outside of the body; the area where the penis usually enters the body during intercourse

Vasomotor symptoms – symptoms such as hot flushes and night sweats that women suffer in menopause and which are due to widening or constriction of the blood vessels

Venous thromboembolism – blood clot

Vertebral fracture – a fracture of the vertebrae of the spine, also known as vertebral compression fracture

Vitamins – organic substances that the human body needs in varying but usually small quantities in order to grow; they help break down and use (metabolise) the food we eat in the most efficient way, ensuring that we function healthily

Vulva – external female genitalia (genital parts)

HUGE THANKS ...

Thank you to all my extraordinary friends for their help and encouragement during my long journey. My special gratitude to Bev, who soothed my anxiety, listened to worries, put me back on track when I felt overwhelmed and celebrated with me when the job was done. For their unique contribution, thank you too to Marina, Paula, Naomi and Marilyn. Thanks go to Celia, who helped me clarify the diagrams by drawing them so well.

I am so grateful to all the women whose stories are the hooks on which each chapter is hung and who shared their worries with me. Their names have been changed and some of the anecdotes are composites, but the stories are all true and vivid examples of how women battle to come to terms with menopause. Their stories have made this book infinitely richer.

My work on menopause has been a long journey and countless people have helped me improve and complete my books over the past six years. I thank them all very much.

Huge thanks to all at Bookstorm. This book came into being because of the enthusiastic support and belief of Louise Grantham, publisher, who encouraged me with warmth and humour to keep going, and make this the most comprehensive book on menopause ever. The administrative help of Jane Macduff, project manager, in coordinating all parts of this book was vital. I am very grateful to Terry Morris, Managing Director of Pan Macmillan South Africa, for her faith in this project.

Catherine Murray edited this book with respect and sensitivity. Her insights and intelligent questions were invaluable and she showed grace and humour under extreme pressure. She helped to make the difficult and grinding task of editing this complicated text with all its medical minutiae so much easier.

Thank you to Caroline Molema for helping my life to run smoothly during the hours I spent at my computer.

My daughters Sophie and Elizabeth have strengthened me with their ongoing love and pride in my achievements; they are my most vocal fans. Sophie's incisive editing and witty comments helped me to write the introduction. Her hysterical email on the sin of repetition is a classic! Without Elizabeth's advice on learning – 'question on the front of the card, answer on the back' – I could not have swotted and passed the exam to qualify as a North American Menopause Society Certified Menopause practitioner. My husband Nicholas has encouraged me throughout my career. He supported and calmed me when I was most crazed and did the shopping while I was immersed in this book, oblivious to all. He clarifies my thoughts when I get lost in an idea and is my most valued critic. He has absolute faith in me and in anything I decide to tackle, including my board certification exams. He knows how grateful I am for the many hours he spent testing me. Without his belief in me, my books might never have been written, and I would not have embarked on this long, rewarding journey.

REFERENCE AND RESOURCE LIST

This list of books, journal articles and websites is intended to help those of you who wish to read further and learn more about aspects of the subjects I have covered in the book. With that in mind I have divided the list into the chapters to which these publications and Internet sites relate. They will enable you to show your healthcare practitioner where you got your information.

Chapters 1, 2, 3 and 4

Al-Azzawi, F & Buckler, HM (2003). For the United Kingdom Vaginal Ring Investigator Group. Comparison of a novel vaginal ring delivering estradiol acetate versus oral estradiol for relief of vasomotor menopausal symptoms. *Climacteric* 6(2): 118-27.

Alster, T et al. (2004). *The aging face: More than skin deep*. Discovery Institute of Medical Education.

American Association of Clinical Endocrinologists (AACE) (2006). Menopause Guideline Revision Task Force. AACE medical guidelines for clinical practice for the diagnosis and treatment of menopause. *Endocrinological Practice* 12(3): 315-37.

American Congress of Obstetricians and Gynecologists (ACOG) Committee (2005). Compounded bioidentical hormones. Opinion No. 322. *Obstetrics & Gynecology* 106: 1139-40. Reaffirmed 2007

Angier, N (1999). *Woman: An intimate geography*. London: Virago.

Arana, A et al. (2006). Hormone therapy and cerebrovascular events: A population-based nested control study. *Menopause: The Journal of the North American Menopause Society* 13(5): 730-6.

Archer, DF et al. (2007). Drospirenone, a progestin with added value for added hypertensive postmenopausal women. *Menopause: The Journal of the North American Menopause Society* 14(3): 352-4.

Archer, DF et al. (2007). Endometrial effects of tibolone. *Journal of Clinical Endocrinology & Metabolism* 92: 911-8.

Archer, DF et al. (2009). Bazedoxifene/conjugated estrogens (BZA/CE): Incidence of uterine bleeding in postmenopausal women. *Fertility and Sterility* 92:1039-44.

Archer, DF (2011). The gynecologic effects of lasofoxifene, an estrogen agonist/antagonist, in postmenopausal women. Editorial. *Menopause: The Journal of the North American Menopause Society* 18(1): 6-7.

Australian Government. National Health and Medical Research Council (2004). Available online: http://www.nhmrc.gov.au/publications/pdf/hrtsumm.pdf

Bach, PB (2010). Postmenopausal hormone therapy and breast cancer: An uncertain trade-off. *Journal of the American Medical Association* 304(15): 1719-20.

Balasubramanyam, A (2004). *Disentangling the threads of the metabolic syndrome*. Medscape Conference Coverage based on selected sessions at the ENDO, The Endocrine Society's 86th Annual Meeting. Available online: http://www.medscape.com/viewarticle/494115

Banks, E & Canfell, K (2009). Hormone therapy risks and benefits: The Women's Health Initiative findings and the postmenopausal estrogen timing hypothesis. Invited commentary. *American Journal of Epidemiology* 170(1): 24-8.

Barbaglia, G et al. (2009). Trends in hormone therapy use before and after publication of the Women's Health Initiative trial: 10 years of follow-up. *Menopause: The Journal of the North American Menopause Society* 16: 1061-4.

Barclay, L (2004). NIH stops estrogen-alone arm of WHI: A newsmaker interview with Jacques Roussouw, MD. *Medscape Medical News*. Available online: http://www.medscape.com/px/urlinfo

Barclay, L & Lie, D (2004). Estrogen does not prevent chronic disease in postmenopausal women with hysterectomy. *Medscape Medical News*. Available online: http://www.medscape.com/px/urlinfo

Barton, D (2007). Clinical assessment and management of hot flashes and sexual function. *American Society of Clinical Oncology* 7: 73-7.

Beatty, MN & Blumenthal, PD (2009). The levonorgestrel-releasing intrauterine system: Safety, efficacy, and patient acceptability. *Journal of Therapeutics and Clinical Risk Management* 5: 561-74.

Bell, RJ et al. (2007). Endogenous androgen levels and cardiovascular risk profile in women across the adult life span. *Menopause: The Journal of the North American Menopause Society* 14(4): 630-8.

Bentley, G & Muttukrishna, S (2007). Potential use of biomarkers for analyzing interpopulation and cross-cultural variability in reproductive aging. *Menopause: The Journal of the North American Menopause Society* 14(4): 668-79.

Benster, B et al. (2009). A double-blind placebo-controlled study to evaluate the effect of progestelle progesterone cream on postmenopausal women. *Menopause International* 15(2): 63-9.

Beral, V et al. (2011). Breast cancer risk in relation to the interval between menopause and starting hormone therapy. *Journal of the National Cancer Institute* doi: 10.1093/jnci/djq527.

Bernstein, L (2009). Combined hormone therapy at menopause and breast cancer: A warning – short-term use increases risk. *Journal of Clinical Oncology* 27(31): 5116-9.

Biglia, N et al. (2010). Tibolone in postmenopausal women: A review based on recent randomised controlled clinical trials. *Gynecological Endocrinology* 26(11): 804-14.

Birnbaum, L (2002). The case against relative risk: *Professionalism of Exercise Physiology* 5(2). Available online: http://www.css.edu/users/tboone2/asep/relativeRISK

Boothby, LA & Doering, PL (2008). Bioidentical hormone therapy: A panacea that lacks supportive evidence. *Current Opinion Obstetrics and Gynecology* 20(4): 400-40.

Bosarge, PN (2009). Bioidentical hormones, compounding, and evidence-based medicine: What women's health practitioners need to know. *Journal for Nurse Practitioners* 5(6): 421-7.

British Menopause Society Council (2008). Consensus statement on hormone replacement therapy, 12 February 2008. http://www.thebms.org.uk

Buckler, H & Al-Azzawi, F (2003). The effect of a novel vaginal ring delivering estradiol acetate on the climacteric symptoms in postmenopausal women. *British Journal of Obstetrics and Gynaecology* 110: 753-9.

Burger, H et al. (2004). Practical recommendations for hormone replacement therapy in the peri and post menopause. *Climacteric* 7: 1-7. Available online: http://www.imsociety.org/PDF/news_prac_rec.pdf

Cameron, DR & Braunstein, GD (2004). Androgen replacement therapy in women. *Fertility and Sterility* 82(2): 273-89.

Canonico, M et al. (2010). Activated protein C resistance among postmenopausal women using transdermal estrogens: Importance of progestogen. *Menopause: The Journal of the North American Menopause Society* 17(6): 1122-7.

Canonico, M et al. (2010). Postmenopausal hormone therapy and risk of idiopathic venous thromboembolism: Results from the E3N cohort study. *Arteriosclerosis Thrombosis, and Vascular Biology* 30(2): 340-45.

Chatterton, R (2005). Characteristics of salivary profiles of oestradiol and progesterone in premenopausal women. *Journal of Endocrinology* 186(1): 77-84.

Chatterton, RT (2006). *Validation of hormone testing.* Proceedings from the Postgraduate Course presented prior to the 17th Annual Meeting of the North American Menopause Society.

Chervenak, J (2009). Bioidentical hormones for maturing women. *Maturitas* 64(2): 86-9.

Chlebowski, RT et al. (2010). Estrogen plus progestin and breast cancer incidence and mortality in postmenopausal women. *Journal of the American Medical Association* 304(15): 1684-92.

Cicinelli, E (2007). Bioidentical estradiol gel for hormone therapy in menopause. Expert Review of *Obstetrics & Gynecology* 2(4): 423-30.

Coney, S (1994). *The menopause industry: How the medical establishment exploits women.* Almeda, CA: Hunter House.

Cooper, DS (2003). Hyperthyroidism. *The Lancet* 362(9382): 459-68. Available online: http://www.thelancet.com

Crowther, N (2004). The clinical relevance of fasting serum insulin levels in obese subjects. *South African Medical Journal* 94(7): 519-20.

Cummings, SR (2006). LIFT study is discontinued. *British Menopause Journal* 8(331): 667.

Davey, M (2005). Progestogen use in the menopause. *SAMS Journal* 23(4). Available online: http://www.cmej.org.za/index.php/cmej/article/viewFile/639/436

De Villiers, T et al. (2007). SAMS revised position statement on menopausal hormone therapy. *SAMS News* 4(2), Issue 8.

Dennerstein, L et al. (2007). A cross-cultural approach to understanding women's health experiences: A cross-cultural comparison of women aged 20 to 70 years. *Menopause: The Journal of the North American Menopause Society* 14(4): 688-96.

Dennerstein, L et al. (2007). Modeling women's health during the menopausal transition: A longitudinal analysis. *Menopause: The Journal of the North American Menopause Society* 14(1): 53-62.

Drug Digest (2001). What are tibolone tablets? Available online: http://www.drugdigest.org/DD?PrintablePages/Monograph/07765,8144%.html

Domingues, TS et al. (2010). Tests for ovarian reserve: Reliability and utility. *Current Opinion in Obstetrics & Gynecology* 22(4): 271-6.

Ecker, J (2007). Evidence and opinion: Closing the gap. *Menopause: The Journal of the North American Menopause Society* 14(1): 3-4.

Ettinger, B (2006). When is it appropriate to prescribe postmenopausal hormone therapy?. *Menopause: The Journal of the North American Menopause Society* 13(3): 404-10.

Ettinger, B et al. (2004). Effects of ultra low dose transdermal estradiol on bone mineral density: A randomised clinical trial. *Obstetrics and Gynecology* 104(3): 443-51.

Farquhar, C et al. (2009). Long term hormone therapy for perimenopausal and postmenopausal women. *Cochrane Database Systems Review* CD004143.

Freeman, EW et al. (2011). Efficacy of escitalopram for hot flashes in healthy menopausal women: A randomized controlled trial. *Journal of the American Medical Association* 305(3): 267-74.

Flyckt, RL et al. (2009). Comparison of salivary versus serum testosterone levels in postmenopausal women receiving transdermal testosterone supplementation versus placebo. *Menopause: The Journal of the North American Menopause Society* 16(4): 680-8.

Ganti, AK (2010). Another nail in the coffin for hormone-replacement therapy? *The Lancet* 374(9697):1217-8.

Genazzani, AR & Pluchino, N (2010). DHEA therapy in postmenopausal women: The need to move forward beyond the lack of evidence. *Climacteric* 13(4): 314-6.

Germano, C & Cabot, W (1999). *The osteoporosis solution: New therapies for prevention and treatment.* New York: Kensington Books.

Gilson, GR & Zava, DT (2003). A perspective on HRT for women: Picking up the pieces after the Women's Health Initiative Trial – Part 1. *International Journal of Pharmaceutical Compounding* 7(4): 250-6.

Goldman, JA (2004). The Women's Health Initiative review and critique. *Medscape Ob/Gyn and Women's Health* 6(3). Available online: http://www.medscape.com/px/urlinfo

Goldstein, S (2005). The case for less-than-monthly progestogen in women on HT: Is transvaginal ultrasound the key? *Menopause: The Journal of the North American Menopause Society*12(1): 110-3.

Goldstein, SR & Ashner, L (1998). *Could it be … perimenopause?* Boston, New York, Toronto, London: Little, Brown and Co.

Goldstein, SR & Ashner, L (1998). *The estrogen alternative: What every women needs to know about hormone replacement therapy and SERMs, the new estrogen substitute.* New York: GP Putnam & Sons.

Gompel, A et al. (2007). The EMAS update on clinical recommendations on postmenopausal hormone therapy. *Maturitas* 56: 227-9.

Gruber, C et al. (2002). Productions and actions of estrogens. *New England Journal of Medicine* 346(6): 340-52.

Grundy, SM et al. (2004). Definition of metabolic syndrome: Report of the National Lung and Blood Institute/American Heart Association Conference on scientific issues related to definition. *Circulation* 109(3): 433-8.

Hale, GE et al. (2007). Endocrine features of menstrual cycles in middle and late reproductive age and the menopausal transition classified according to the Staging of Reproductive Aging Workshop (STRAW) staging system. *Journal of Clinical Endocrinology & Metabolism* 92(8): 3060-7.

Harlow, SD et al. (2006). Evaluation of four proposed bleeding criteria for the onset of late menopausal transition. *Journal of Clinical Endocrinology & Metabolism* 91(9): 3432-8.

Haskell, SG et al. (2009). Discontinuing postmenopausal hormone therapy: An observational study of tapering versus quitting cold turkey – is there a difference in recurrence of menopausal symptoms? *Menopause: The Journal of the North American Menopause Society* 16(3): 494-9.

Hedrick, RE et al. (2009). Transdermal estradiol gel 0.1% for the treatment of vasomotor symptoms in postmenopausal women. *Menopause: The Journal of the North American Menopause Society* 16(1): 132-40.

Henrich, JB et al. (2006). Limitations of follicle-stimulating hormone in assessing menopause status: Findings from the National Health and Nutrition Examination Survey (NHANES 1999-2000). *Menopause: The Journal of the North American Menopause Society* 13(2): 171-7.

Herrington, DM (1999). The HERS trial results: Paradigms lost? Heart and Estrogen/Progestin Replacement Study. *Annals of Internal Medicine* 131(6): 463-6.

Ingelsson, E et al. (2010). Hysterectomy and risk of cardiovascular disease: A population based cohort study. *European Heart Journal* doi:10.

International Menopause Society (2009). Consensus statement on aging, menopause, cardiovascular disease and HRT. *Climacteric.* Available online: http://www.imsociety.org/position_papers_and_consensus_statements.php

International Menopause Society (2010). *Estrogen-only menopausal hormone therapy and the reduced incidence of breast cancer.* Press release, 14 December 2010.

International Menopause Society (2010). *Menopause clinicians support findings of new report on menopausal hormone therapy which calls for a rethink on use in younger postmenopausal women.* Press release, 20 July 2010.

Interview with Christiane Northrup MD, FACOG (1998). *International Journal of Pharmaceutical Compounding* 2(1): 12-7.

Jacobs, G et al. (2004). Cognitive behavior therapy should be first line therapy for sleep-onset insomnia. *Archives of Internal Medicine* 164(17): 1888-96.

Jadad, AR & Gagliardi, A (1998). Rating health information on the Internet: Navigating to knowledge or to Babel? *Journal of the American Medical Association* 279(8): 611-4.

Jayaprakasan, K et al. (2010). A prospective, comparative analysis of antimüllerian hormone, inhibin-B, and three-dimensional ultrasound determinants of ovarian reserve in the prediction of poor response to controlled ovarian stimulation. *Fertility and Sterility* 93(3): 855-64.

Jungheim, ES & Colditz, GA (2011). Short-term use of unopposed estrogen. *Menopause: The Journal of the North American Menopause Society* 305(13): 1354-5.

Kenemans, P (2009). Tibolone revisited: Still a good treatment option for healthy, early postmenopausal women. Editorial. *International Society of Gynecological Endocrinology* 26(4): 237-9.

Kharode, Y (2008). The pairing of a selective estrogen receptor modulator, bazedoxifene, with conjugated estrogens as a new paradigm for the treatment of menopausal symptoms and osteoporosis prevention. *Endocrinology* 149(12): 6084-91.

Komm, BS (2008). A new approach to menopausal therapy: The tissue selective estrogen complex. *Reproductive Sciences* 15(10): 984-92.

Kotz, D (2009).Why Suzanne Somers loves bioidentical hormones. http://health.usnews.com/health-news

Kritz-Silverstein, D et al. (2008). Effects of dehydroepiandrosterone supplementation on cognitive function and quality of life: The DHEA and Well-Ness (DAWN) Trial. *Journal of the American Geriatriatrics Society* 56(7): 1292-8.

Labrie, F et al. (2009). Comparable amounts of sex steroids are made outside the gonads in men and women: Strong lesson for hormone therapy of prostate and breast cancer. *Journal of Steroid Biochemistry and Molecular Biology* 113(1-2): 52-6.

Labrie, F et al. (2011). Wide distribution of serum DHEA and sex steroid levels in postmenopausal women: Role of the ovary? *Menopause: The Journal of the North American Menopause Society* 18(1): 30-43.

Lacroix AZ et al. (2011). Health outcomes after stopping conjugated equine estrogens among postmenopausal women with prior hysterectomy: A randomized controlled trial. *Journal of the American Medical Association* 305(13): 1305-14.

Landau, C et al. (1994). *The complete book of menopause*. New York: Perigee.

Larsen, R et al. (Eds) (2003). *Williams textbook of endocrinology*, 10th ed. Philadelphia, PA: WB Saunders.

Lee, H (2011). Antimüllerian hormone as a potential predictor for the late menopausal transition. *Menopause: The Journal of the North American Menopause Society* 18(2): 125-6.

Lobo, RA et al. (2009). Evaluation of bazedoxifene/conjugated estrogens for the treatment of menopausal symptoms and effects on metabolic parameters and overall safety profile. *Fertility and Sterility* 92(3): 1025-38.

Long, C et al. (2006). A randomized comparative study of the effects of oral and topical estrogen therapy on the vaginal vascularization and sexual function in hysterectomized postmenopausal women. *Menopause: The Journal of the North American Menopause Society* 13(5): 737-43.

Love, SM & Lindsay, K (1997). *The hormone dilemma: Should you take HRT?* New York: Random House.

Lundstrom, E et al. (2002). Effects of tibolone and continuous combined hormone replacement therapy on mammographic breast density. *American Journal of Obstetrics and Gynecology* 186(4): 717-22.

Manson, J et al. (2006). Postmenopausal hormone therapy: New questions and the case for new clinical trials. *Menopause: The Journal of the North American Menopause Society* 13(1): 139-47.

Martens, M (2007). Ecology and the health of the menopausal vagina. *Menopause Management* 16(4): 30-6.

McGaugh, JL. Panel: *The science of memory and emotion: How emotions strengthen memory*. Project on the Decade of the Brain, Library of Congress, 1990-2000. Available online: http://www.loc.gov/loc/brain/emotion/Mcgaugh.html

Menon, U et al. (2007). Decline in use of hormone therapy amongst postmenopausal women in the United Kingdom. *Menopause: The Journal of the North American Menopause Society* 14(3): 462-7.

Middleton, LJ et al. (2010). Hysterectomy, endometrial destruction, and levonorgestrel releasing intrauterine system (Mirena) for heavy menstrual bleeding: Systematic review and meta-analysis of data from individual patients. *BMJ* 341: c3929.

Mills, D. Because you're trying to get off HRT, here's the approach we recommend. Available online: http://www.women-to-women.com/chooseoffhrt.asp

Morris, CE (1996). *Psychology: An introduction*, 9th ed. New Jersey: Prentice Hall.

Mueck, AO (2010). Exogenous hormones, the risk of venous thromboembolism, and activated protein C resistance. Editorial. *Menopause: The Journal of the North American Menopause Society* 17(6): 1099-103.

Murray, J (1998). Natural progesterone: What role in women's healthcare? Project Aware. Part 1, September 1998. Available online: http://www.project-aware.org/Resource/articlearchives/Murray_references.shtml

Nachtigall, L (2004). The Forum: Hormone therapy. OB/GYN *Special edition*, Spring.

Nachtigall, LE (2006). *Bioidentical versus non-bioidentical hormones*. Proceedings from the Postgraduate Course presented prior to the 17th Annual Meeting of the North American Menopause Society.

Nappi, RE et al. (2001). Course of primary headaches during hormone replacement therapy. *Maturitas* 38(2): 157-63.

National Women's Health Network (2004). Available online: http://www.nwhn.org/about/index.php

Nauton, M et al. (2006). Estradiol gel: A review of the pharmacology, pharmokinetics, efficacy and safety in menopausal women. *Menopause: The Journal of the North American Menopause Society* 13(3): 517-27.

Newton, K et al. (2010). Hormone therapy discontinuation: Physician practices after the Women's Health Initiative *Menopause: The Journal of the North American Menopause Society*. 17(4): 734-40.

Nijland, EA et al. (2008). Tibolone and transdermal E2/NETA for the treatment of female sexual dysfunction in naturally menopausal women: Results of a randomized active-controlled trial. *Journal of Sexual Medicine* 5(3): 646-56.

North American Menopause Society (2003). Position statement on estrogen and progestogen use in peri- and postmenopausal women. Hormone Therapy Advisory Panel, September 2003. *Menopause: The Journal of the North American Menopause Society* 10(6): 497-506.

North American Menopause Society (2004). Position statement on recommendations for estrogen and progestogen use in peri- and post menopausal women, October 2004. *Menopause: The Journal of the North American Menopause Society* 11(6): 589-600.

North American Menopause Society (2007). Position statement on estrogen and progestogen use in peri- and postmenopausal women, March 2007. *Menopause: The Journal of the North American Menopause Society* 14(2): 168-82.

North American Menopause Society (2007). Position statement on the role of local vaginal estrogen for treatment of vaginal atrophy in postmenopausal women. *Menopause: The Journal of the North American Menopause Society* 14(3): 357-69.

North American Menopause Society (2008). Position statement on estrogen and progestogen use in postmenopausal women, July 2008. *Menopause: The Journal of the North American Menopause Society* 15(4): 584-603.

North American Menopause Society (2010). Position statement on estrogen and progestogen use in postmenopausal women. *Menopause: The Journal of the North American Menopause Society* 17(2): 242-55.

Northrup, C (2001). *The wisdom of menopause*. London: Piatkus.

Northrup, C (2004). *Women to women*. Available online: http://www.womentowomen.com/howitworks.asp

Notelovitz, M & Tonneson, D (1993). *Menopause and midlife health*. New York: T Martins Press.

Olié, V et al. (2011). Hormone therapy and recurrence of venous thromboembolism among postmenopausal women. *Menopause: The Journal of the North American Menopause Society* 118(5): 488-93.

Panjari, M & Davis, SR (2010). DHEA for postmenopausal women: A review of the evidence. *Maturitas* 66(2): 172-9.

Parkin, L et al. (2011). Risk of venous thromboembolism in users of oral contraceptives containing drospirenone or levonorgestrel: nested case control study based on UK practice research database. *BMJ* 342: d2139.

Patching van der Sluijs, C et al. (2007). Women's health during mid-life survey: The use of complementary and alternative medicine by symptomatic women transitioning through menopause in Sydney. *Menopause: The Journal of the North American Menopause Society* 14(3): 397-403.

Peled, Y et al. (2007). Levonorgestrel-releasing intrauterine system as an adjunct to estrogen for the treatment of menopausal symptoms: A review. *Menopause: The Journal of the North American Menopause Society* 14(3): 550-4.

Pfizer (2010). Statement regarding *Journal of the American Medical Association* (JAMA) analysis "Estrogen plus progestin and breast cancer incidence and mortality in postmenopausal women". www.pfizer.com/files/news/jama_prempro_statement_101910.pdf

Pick, M (2004). *Perspective on the risks of HRT*. Available online: http://www.womentowomen.com/LIB-perspectiveonrisks.asp

Pinkerton, JV (2009). Bio identical hormones: What you and (your patient) should know. *Sexuality, Reproduction & Menopause: OBG Management Journal* 21(1): 43-52.

Pinkerton, JV & Goldstein, SR (2010). Endometrial safety: A key hurdle for selective estrogen receptor modulators in development. *Menopause: The Journal of the North American Menopause Society* 17(3): 642-53.

Prentice RL et al. (2009). Benefits and risks of postmenopausal hormone therapy when it is initiated soon after menopause. *American Journal of Epidemiology* 170(1): 12-23.

Power, ML et al. (2007). Evolving practice and attitudes toward hormone therapy of obstetrician-gynecologists. *Menopause: The Journal of the North American Menopause Society* 14(1): 20-8.

Prentice, RL et al. (2009). Benefits and risks of postmenopausal hormone therapy when it is initiated soon after menopause. *American Journal of Epidemiology* 170(1): 12-23.

Preston, R et al. (2007). Randomized, placebo-controlled trial of the effects of drospirenone-estradiol on blood pressure and potassium balance in hypertensive postmenopausal women receiving hydrochlorothiazide. *Menopause: The Journal of the North American Menopause Society* 14(3): 408-14.

Pritchard, K (2004). Debating the issues: Should we bury tamoxifen? Should we disclose positive data early? *Medscape Ob/Gyn and Women's Health.* Available online: http://www.medscape.com/viewarticle/47405?

ProjectAware (2002). Association of Women for the Advancement of Research and Education. *About progesterone.* Available online: http://www.project-aware.org/Managing/Hrt/progesterone.shtml

Redmond, G (1995). *The good news about women's hormones: Complete information and proven solutions for the most common hormonal problems.* New York: Warner Books.

Rees, M (2010). Emerging facade of menopausal hormone therapy. *Seminars in Reproductive Medicine* 28(5): 351-9.

Renoux, C et al. (2010). Transdermal and oral hormone replacement therapy and the risk of stroke: A nested case-control study. *BMJ* 340: c2519.

Rigby, A et al. (2007). Women's awareness and knowledge of hormone therapy post-Women's Health Initiative. *Menopause: The Journal of the North American Menopause Society* 14(5): 853-8.

Rivera, CM et al. (2009). Increased cardiovascular mortality after early bilateral oophorectomy. *Menopause: The Journal of the North American Menopause Society* 16(1): 15-2.

Roberts, CGP & Laderson, PW (2004). Hypothyroidism. *The Lancet* 363: 793-803. Available online: http://www.thelancet.com

Robertson, DM et al. (2008). A proposed classification system for menstrual cycles in the menopause transition based on changes in serum hormone profiles. *Menopause* 15(6): 1139-44.

Rolnick, SJ et al. (2007). Provider management of menopause after the findings of the Women's Health Initiative. *Menopause: The Journal of the North American Menopause Society* 14(3): 441-9.

Rosenthal, MS (2008). Ethical problems with bioidentical hormone therapy. *International Journal Impotence Research* 20(1): 45-52.

Rossouw, JE (2008). Postmenopausal hormone therapy for disease prevention: Have we learned any lessons from the past? *Clinical Pharmacology & Therapeutics* 83(4): 14-6.

Salpeter, SR (2009). Bayesian meta-analysis of hormone therapy and mortality in younger postmenopausal women. *American Journal of Medicine* 122(11): 1016-22.

Samsioe, G et al. (2006). Hormone replacement therapy: The agents. *Women's Health Medicine,* 3(5): 213-6.

Santoro, N et al. (2007). Helping midlife women predict the onset of the final menses: SWAN, the Study of Women's Health Across the Nation. *Menopause: The Journal of the North American Menopause Society* 14(3): 415-24.

Sarkar, NN (2003). Low-dose intravaginal estradiol delivery using a silastic vaginal ring for estrogen replacement therapy in postmenopausal women: A review. *European Journal of Contraception and Reproductive Health Care* 8(4): 217-24.

Shakir, Y et al. (2004). Combined hormone therapy in postmenopausal women with features of metabolic syndrome. Results from a population-based study of Swedish women: Women's Health in the Lund Area study. *Menopause: The Journal of the North American Menopause Society* 11(5): 549-55.

Shifren, JL et al. (2006). Testosterone patch for the treatment of hypoactive sexual desire disorder in naturally menopausal women: Results from the INTIMATE NM1 study. *Menopause: The Journal of the North American Menopause Society* 13(5): 770-9.

Shulman, LP (2010). In search of a middle ground: Hormone therapy and its role in modern *menopause management. Menopause: The Journal of the North American Menopause Society* 17(5): 898-9.

Shuster, LT et al. (2010). Premature menopause or early menopause: Long-term health consequences. *Maturitas* 65(2): 161-6.

Simon, JA et al. (2006). A clinical review and discussion of the efficacy and safety of a new transdermal form of hormone therapy. *Women's Health Update.*

Simon, JA et al. (2006). *Understanding the controversy: Hormone testing and bioidentical hormones.* Proceedings from the Postgraduate Course presented prior to the 17th Annual Meeting of the North American Menopause Society.

Slater, CC et al. (2001). Markedly elevated levels of estrone sulfate after long-term oral, but not transdermal, administration of estradiol in postmenopausal women. *Menopause: The Journal of the North American Menopause Society* 8(3): 200-3.

Somers, S (2004). *The sexy years.* New York: Crown, Random House.

Sood, R et al. (2011). Counseling postmenopausal women about bioidentical hormones: Ten discussion points for practicing physicians. Clinical review. *Journal of the American Board of Family Medicine* 24(2): 202-10.

Soules, MR (2001). Executive summary, Stages of Reproductive Aging Workshop (STRAW), Park City, Utah, July 2001. *Menopause: The Journal of the North American Menopause Society* 8(6): 402-7.

Speroff, L (2003). Efficacy and tolerability of a novel estradiol vaginal ring for relief of menopausal symptoms. *Obstetrics and Gynecology* 102(4): 823-34.

Speroff, L et al. (2006). Efficacy of a new oral estradiol acetate formulation for relief of menopausal symptoms. *Menopause: The Journal of the North American Menopause Society* 13(3): 442-50.

Stanosz, S et al. (2009). Influence of modified transdermal hormone replacement therapy on the concentrations of hormones, growth factors, and bone mineral density in women with osteopenia. *Metabolism* 58(1): 1-7.

Stovall, DW & Pinkerton, JV (2008). Estrogen agonists/antagonists in combination with estrogen for prevention and treatment of menopause-associated signs and symptoms. *Women's Health* 4(3): 257-68.

Stram, DO et al. (2011). Age-specific effects of hormone therapy use on overall mortality and ischemic heart disease mortality among women in the California Teachers' Study. *Menopause: The Journal of the North American Menopause Society* 18(3): 253-61.

Sturdee, DW et al. (2004). The acceptability of a small intrauterine progestogen-releasing system for continuous combined hormone therapy in early postmenopausal women. *Climacteric* 7(4): 404-11.

Tan, O et al. (2010). What can we learn from design faults in the Women's Health Initiative randomized clinical trial? *Bulletin/Hospital for Joint Diseases* 67(2): 226-9.

Templeton, A (Ed.) (1998). *Evidence based fertility treatment.* London: RCOG Press.

The Endocrine Society (2006). *Position statement on bioidentical hormones.* Available online: http://www.endo-society.org/advocacy/policy/upload/BH_position_Statement_final_10_25_06_w_Header.pdf

The Endocrine Society (2010). Postmenopausal hormone therapy: An Endocrine Society scientific statement, July 2010. *Journal of Clinical Endocrinology & Metabolism* 95(1 Suppl.): S1-66.

Toh, S et al. (2010). Coronary heart disease in postmenopausal recipients of estrogen plus progestin therapy: Does the increased risk ever disappear? A randomized trial. *Annals of Internal Medicine* 152(4): 211-7.

US Department of Health and Human Services (2005). *Women's Health Initiative: WHI background and overview.* Available online: http://www.nhlbi.nih.gov/whi/background.htm

US Food and Drug Administration (FDA). *Consumer health information. Bio-identicals: Sorting myths from facts.* Available online: http://www.fda.gov/consumer/updates/bioidenticals010908.html; accessed 26 March 2008.

US Food and Drug Administration (FDA). FDA takes action against compounded menopause hormone therapy drugs. *FDA News.* Available online: http://www.fda.gov/bbs/topics/NEWS/2008/NEW01772.html; accessed 26 March 2008.

US Food and Drug Administration. *Obtaining an IND for estriol.* Center for Drug Evaluation and Research. Available online: http://www.fda.gov/cder/pharmcomp/estriol.htm; accessed 13 January 2009.

US National Library of Health and the National Institutes of Health (2004). Cortisol level. *Medline Plus Medical Encyclopaedia.* Available online: http://www.uptodate.com

US Pharmacopeial Convention. *White paper: A model system to promote access to good quality compounded medicines.* Council of the Convention Section on the Quality of Compounded Medicine. Available online: http://www.usp.org/pdf/EN/members/goodMedicine.pdf; accessed 18 January 2011.

Utian, W (2004). Development and clinical application of guidelines, consensus opinions, and position statements: The need for clinical judgement beyond the evidence. *Menopause: The Journal of the North American Menopause Society* 11(6): 583-4.

Vogel, JJ (2006). Selecting bioidentical hormone therapy. Proceedings from the Postgraduate Course presented prior to the 17th Annual Meeting of the North American Menopause Society.

Vogel, VG (2009). Altering the propensity for density: The benefits and risks of selective estrogen receptor modulators. Editorial. *Menopause: The Journal of the North American Menopause Society* 16(6): 1079-82.

Vongpatanasin, W (2003). Differential effects of oral versus transdermal estrogen replacement therapy on C-reactive protein in postmenopausal women. *Journal of American Cardiology* 41(8): 1358-63.

Waknine, Y (2004). Testosterone patch can improve sexual function in women. *Medscape Medical News.* Medscape NAMS 15th Annual Meeting. Abstracts S-3 and S-11 presented 8 October 2004. Available online: http://www.medscape.com/px/urlinfo

Weisberg, E et al. (2005). Endometrial and vaginal effects of low dose estradiol delivered by vaginal ring or vaginal tablet. *Climacteric* 8(1): 83-92.

Wilson, R (1966). *Feminine forever.* New York: Evans & Company.

Woods, NF et al. (2006). Increased urinary cortisol levels during the menopausal transition. *Menopause: The Journal of the North American Menopause Society* 13(2): 212-21.

Wylie-Rosett, J (2005). Menopause, micronutrients and hormone therapy. *American Journal of Clinical Nutrition* 81(s5): 1223s-31s.

Ziel, HK & Finkle, WD (1975). Increased risk of endometrial carcinoma among users of conjugated estrogens. *New England Journal of Medicine* 293(23): 1167-70.

Available online

http://health.msn.com/women's-health/articlepage.aspx?cp-documentid=100217890
http://my.athernet/~nrsprng/stpindex.html
http://www.brainyencyclopedia.com/encyclopedia/a/at/atherosclerosis.html
http://www.brainyencyclopedia.com/encyclopedia/e/en/endothelium.html
http://www.cancer.org
http://www.cushings-help.com/definitions.htm
http://www.drugsdigest.com/MMX/Estrone.html
http://www.healthscout.com/ency/68/352/main.html
http://www.healthywomen.org/content.cfm?L1=3&L2=52
http://www.mayoclinic.com
http://www.nlm.gov/medlineplus/ency/article/003456.htm
http://www.quackwatch.com

Chapter 5

Allen, LV et al. (2000). *A healthcare professionals guide to evaluating dietary supplements.* American Dietetic Association and American Pharmaceutical Association Special Report, from the Joint Working Group on Dietary Supplements. Available online: http://www.pharmacist.com/pdf/dietary_supplements.pdf

Amato, P & Christophe, S (2002). Estrogenic activity of herbs commonly used as remedies for menopausal symptoms. *Menopause: The Journal of the North American Menopause Society* 9(2): 145-50.

Atkinson, C et al. (2000). *The effects of isoflavone phytoestrogens on bone: Preliminary results from a large randomized, controlled trial.* The Endocrine Society's 82nd Annual Meeting, Toronto, Canada, 21-4 June.

Atkinson, C et al. (2004). Red clover-derived isoflavones and mammographic breast density: A double-blind, randomized, placebo-controlled trial. *Breast Cancer Research* 6(3): R170-9.

Atkinson, C et al. (2004). The effects of phytoestrogen isoflavones on bone density in women: A double-blind, randomized, placebo-controlled trial. *American Journal of Clinical Nutrition* 79(2): 326-33.

Atmaca, A (2008). Soy isoflavones in the management of postmenopausal osteoporosis. *Menopause: The Journal of the North American Menopause Society* 15(4): 748-57.

Barrett, S (2010). Glucosamine and chondroitin for arthritis: Benefit is unlikely. *Quackwatch.* Reviewed 22 July 2010.

Bejelakovic, G et al. (2007). Mortality in randomized trials of antioxidant supplements for primary and secondary prevention: Systematic review and meta-analysis. *Menopause: The Journal of the North American Menopause Society* 297(8): 842-57.

Berkow, R & Beers, M (1999). *The Merck manual of diagnosis and therapy,* 17th ed. USA: Merck & Co.

Bisseker, C (2002). Homeopathic and legal. *Financial Mail.* Available online: http://secure.nancialmail.co.za/indexfront. html

Bodinet, C & Freudenstein, J (2004). Influence of marketed herbal menopause preparations on MCF-7 cell proliferation. *Menopause: The Journal of the North American Menopause Society* 11(3): 281-9.

Booth, NL et al. (2006). Clinical studies of red clover (Trifolium pratense) dietary supplements in menopause: A literature review. *Menopause: The Journal of the North American Menopause Society* 13(2): 251-64.

Boothby, LA et al. (2004). Bioidentical hormone therapy: A review. *Menopause: The Journal of the North American Menopause Society* 11(3): 356-67.

Brett, K et al. (2007). Complementary and alternative medicine use among midlife women for reasons including menopause in the United States. *Menopause: The Journal of the North American Menopause Society* 14(2): 300-7.

Bruyere, O et al. (2004). Glucosamine sulfate reduces osteoarthritis progression in postmenopausal women with knee osteoarthritis: Evidence from two 3-year studies. *Menopause: The Journal of the North American Menopause Society* 11(2): 138-43.

Chen, Y et al. (2004). Beneficial effects of soy isoflavones on bone mineral content was modified by years since menopause, body weight and calcium intake: A double-blind randomised, controlled trial. *Menopause: The Journal of the North American Menopause Society* 11(3): 246-54, 290-8.

Chertow, B (2004). Advances in diabetes for the millennium: Vitamins and oxidant stress in diabetes and its complications. *Medscape CME Activity*. Available online: http://www.medscape.com/viewarticle/490306

Cho, YA et al. (2010). Effect of dietary soy intake on breast cancer risk according to menopause and hormone receptor status. *European Journal of Clinical Nutrition* 64(9): 924-32.

Clarkson, TB et al. (2011). The role of soy isoflavones in menopausal health: Report of the North American Menopause Society/Wulf H. Utian Translational Science Symposium in Chicago, IL, October 2010. *Menopause: The Journal of the North American Menopause Society* 18(7): 732-53.

Coghlan, A (2004). Special report: A health fad that's hard to swallow. *New Scientist*. Available online: http://www.newscientist.com/article.ns?id=dn4853

Coghlan, A (2004). Special report: Big errors in herbal remedy labels revealed. *New Scientist*. Available online: http://www.newscientist.com/article.ns?id=dn4665

Cohen, MH (2003). Complementary and integrative medical therapies, the FDA, and the NIH: Definitions and regulation. *Dermatologic Therapy* 16(2): 77.

Cunnae, S et al. (1993). High alpha-linolenic acid flaxseed (Linum usitatissimum): Some nutritional properties in humans. *British Journal of Nutrition* 69(2): 443-53.

Danna, R et al. (2007). Effects of the phytoestrogen genestein on hot flashes, endometrium and vaginal epithelium in postmenopausal women: A 1-year randomized, double-blind placebo-controlled study. *Menopause: The Journal of the North American Menopause Society* 14(4): 648-55.

Daost, J et al. (2006). Prevalence of natural health product use in healthy postmenopausal women. *Menopause: The Journal of the North American Menopause Society* 13(2): 241-50.

Davis, VL et al. (2008). Black cohosh increases metastatic mammary cancer in transgenic mice expressing c-erbB2. *Cancer Research* 69(20): 8377-83.

Dietary Reference Intakes (DRIs) (1997, 1998, 2000, 2001, 2003). Various. National Academies Press, Washington.

Dodin, S et al. (2005). The effects of flaxseed dietary supplement on lipid profile, bone mineral density, and symptoms in menopausal women: A randomized, double-blind, wheat germ placebo-controlled clinical trial. *Journal of Clinical Endocrinology & Metabolism* 90(3): 1390-7.

Ernst, E (2006). *The desktop guide to complementary and alternative medicine: An evidence based approach*. Mosby, Elsevier.

Gallagher, JC et al. (2004). The effect of soy protein isolate on bone metabolism. *Menopause: The Journal of the North American Menopause Society* 11(3): 290-8.

Geller, S et al. (2009). Safety and efficacy of black cohosh and red clover for the management of vasomotor symptoms: A randomized controlled trial. *Menopause: The Journal of the North American Menopause Society* 16(6): 1156-66.

Geller, SE & Studee, L (2007). Botanical and dietary supplements for mood and anxiety in menopausal women. *Menopause: The Journal of the North American Menopause Society* 14(3): 541-49.

Gold, E et al. (2007). Cross-sectional analysis of specific complementary and alternative medicine (CAM) use by racial/ethnic group and menopausal status: The Study of Women's Health across the Nation (SWAN). *Menopause: The Journal of the North American Menopause Society* 14(4): 612-23.

Gompel, A et al. (2008). The EMAS 2008 update on clinical recommendations on postmenopausal hormone replacement therapy. *Maturitas* 61(3): 227-32.

Griffin, MD et al. (2006). Effects of altering the ratio of dietary n-6 to n-3 fatty acids on insulin sensitivity, lipoprotein size, and postprandial lipemia in men and postmenopausal women aged 45-70: The OPTLIP Study. *American Journal of Clinical Nutrition* 84(6): 1290-8.

Haan, MN (2003). Can vitamin supplements prevent cognitive decline and dementia in old age? *American Journal of Clinical Nutrition* 77(4): 762-3.

Hasler, CM (2000). *Functional foods: Their role in disease prevention and health promotion*. A publication of the Institute of Food Technologists Expert Panel on Food Safety and Nutrition. Available online: http://www.nutriwatch.org/04Foods/ff.html

Hercberg, S et al. (2004). The SU.VI.MAX Study: A randomized, placebo-controlled trial of the health effects of antioxidant vitamins and minerals. *Archives of Internal Medicine* 164(21): 2335-42.

Herrero-Beaumont, G et al. (2007). Glucosamine sulfate in the treatment of knee osteoarthritis symptoms: A randomized, double-blind, placebo-controlled study using acetaminophen as a side comparator. *Arthritis & Rheumatism* 56(2): 555-67.

Hodgson, JM et al. (2004). Supplementation with bioflavonoid phytoestrogens does not alter serum lipid concentrations: A randomized controlled trial in humans. *Fertility and Sterility* 12(1 Pt 1): 145-8.

Hodis, H & Mack, W (2007). Postmenopausal hormone therapy in clinical perspective. *Menopause: The Journal of the North American Menopause Society* 14(5): 944-57.

Holick, MF et al. (2011). Evaluation, treatment, and prevention of vitamin D deficiency: An Endocrine Society clinical practice guideline. *Journal of Clinical Endocrinology & Metabolism* 6 June 2011, jc.2011-0385 [Epub ahead of print].

Huber, J et al. (2010). Effects of soy protein and isoflavones on circulating hormone concentrations in pre- and post menopausal women: A systematic review and meta-analysis. *Human Reproductive Update* 16(1): 110-1.

Huntley, A & Ernst, EA (2003). Systematic review of herbal medicinal products for the treatment of menopausal symptoms. *Menopause: The Journal of the North American Menopause Society* 10(3): 465-76.

Jenks, B et al. (2010). Abstract P-22: *Efficacy and safety of natural S-equol supplement in US postmenopausal women*. 21st Annual Meeting of the North American Menopause Society.

Kaszkin-Bettag, M et al. (2007). The special extract Err 731 of the roots of Rheum rhaponticum decreases anxiety and improves health state and general well-being in perimenopausal women. *Menopause: The Journal of the North American Menopause Society* 14(2): 270-83.

Kazlauskaite, R et al. (2010). Vitamin D is associated with atheroprotective high-density lipoprotein profile in post-menopausal women. *Journal of Clinical Lipidology* 4(2): 113-9.

Kirsch, I (2010). *The emperor's new drugs: Exploding the antidepressant myth*. New York: Basic Books.

Kirsch, I et al. (2008). Initial severity and antidepressant benefits: A meta-analysis of data submitted to the Food and Drug Administration. *PLoS Medicine* 5(2) doi:10.1371/journal.pmed.0050045.

Kruman, II et al. (2002). Folic acid deficiency and homocysteine impair DNA repair in hippocampal neurons and sensitize them to amyloid toxicity in experimental models of Alzheimer's disease. *Journal of Neuroscience* 22(5): 1752-62.

Kohrt, W & Gonzansky, W (2006). Anti-aging strategies: Science or hype. *Menopause Management* 15(3): 12-8.

Lipovac, M et al. (2010). Improvement of postmenopausal depressive and anxiety symptoms after treatment with isoflavones derived from red clover extracts. *Maturitas* 65(3): 258-61.

Ma, J et al. (2006). US women desire greater professional guidance on hormone and alternative therapies for menopausal symptom management. *Menopause: The Journal of the North American Menopause Society* 13(3): 506-16.

Mahan, K et al. (2004). *Krause's food, nutrition & diet therapy*, 11th ed. Philadelphia: Elsevier.

Maki, PM et al. (2009). Effects of botanicals and combined hormone therapy on cognition in postmenopausal women. *Menopause: The Journal of North American Menopause Society* 16(6): 1167-77.

Mangialetti, N & Raso, J (1999). Should we thank God for Julian Whitaker? *American Council on Science and Health*. Available online: http://www.acsh.org/healthissues/newsID.901/healthissue_detail.asp

Maxwell, J & Mehlman, JD (2000). Nutraceuticals: Do they spell the end of FDA regulation of drugs? Available online: http://www.thedoctorwillseeyounow.com/articles/bios/bioethics.shtml

McAlindon, TE et al. (2000). Glucosamine and chondroitin for treatment of osteoarthritis: A systematic quality assessment and meta-analysis. *Journal of the American Medical Association* 283(11): 1469-75.

Medline Plus (2010). The Expert Group on Vitamins and Minerals [EVM] 2003 report, published by Food Standards Agency Publications. Medline Plus, a service of the US National Library of Medicine and the National Institute of Health.

Meisler, JG (2003). Towards optimal health: The experts discuss the use of botanicals by women. *Journal of Women's Health* 12(9): 847-52.

Meltzer, HM et al. (2004). Are vitamin and minerals supplements required for good health? *Journal of the Norwegian Medical Association* 124(12): 1646-9.

National Center for Complementary and Alternative Medicine (NCCAM) (2004). Workshop on the safety of black cohosh in clinical studies. NIH Office of Dietary Supplements. Available online: http://nccam.nih.gov/news/events/blackcohosh_mtngsumm.pdf

Natural Health Products Directorate (2007). *Black cohosh*. Available online: http://www.hc-sc.gc.ca/dhp-mps/alt_formats/hpfb-dgpsa/pdf/prodnatur/mono_cohosh-grappes_e.pdf

Nutrition Information Centre (NICUS). University of Stellenbosch. http://sun025.sun.ac.za/portal/page/portal/Health_Sciences/English/Centres%20and%20Institutions/Nicus/

Olshansky, SJ et al. (2002). Position statement on aging. *Scientific American Magazine and Journal of Gerontology* 57(8): B292-7. Available online: http://www.biomed.gerontology.org

Panay, N (2007). *Integrating complementary therapies (CAMS) with prescription medications: A conservative approach to vasomotor symptom management.* Royal College of Nursing.

Rachner TD et al. (2011). Osteoporosis: Now and the future. *The Lancet* 377(9773): 1276-87.

Reiter, E et al. (2009). Comparison of hormonal activity of isoflavone-containing supplements used to treat menopausal complaints. *Menopause: The Journal of North American Menopause Society* 16(5): 1049-60.

Sa, AM et al. (2003). Role of nutriceutical agents in cardiovascular diseases: An update – Part 1. *Cardiovascular Reviews & Reports* 24(7): 381-5, 391. Available online: http://www.medscape.com/viewarticle/460060

Santen RJ et al. (2010). Executive summary. Postmenopausal hormone therapy: An Endocrine Society scientific statement. *Journal of Clinical Endocrinology & Metabolism* 95(1 Suppl.): S1-66.

Scambia, G & Gallo, G (2006). The role of phytochemicals in menopause: A new actor on the scene of alternative treatment options. *Menopause: The Journal of the North American Menopause Society* 13(5): 724-6.

Scott, GN & Elmer, GW (2002). Update on natural product drug interactions. *American Journal Health System Pharmacy* 59(4): 339-47. Available online: http://www.ajhp.org/cgi/content/abstract/59/4/339

Shea, MK et al. (2009). Genetic and non-genetic correlates of vitamins K and D. *European Journal of Clinical Nutrition* 63(4): 458-64.

Singh, RB et al. (2003). Effect of coenzyme Q10 on risk of atherosclerosis in patients with recent myocardial infarction. *Molecular Cell Biochemistry* 246(1-2): 75-82.

Solomen, P et al. (2002). Ginkgo for memory enhancement: A randomized controlled trial. *Journal of the American Medical Association* 288(7): 835-40.

Stuenkel, CA (2007). Isoflavones and cardiovascular risk in postmenopausal women: No free lunch. *Menopause: The Journal of the North American Menopause Society* 14(4): 606-8.

Taylor, DA (2004). Botanical supplements: Weeding out the health risks. *Environmental Health Perspective* 12(13): A750A753. Available online: http://www.medscape.com/viewpublication/1084_index

Tice, JA et al. (2003). Phytoestrogen supplements for the treatment of hot flashes: the Isoflavone Clover Extract (ICE) Study – a randomized controlled trial. *Journal of the American Medical Association* 290(2): 207-14.

Turunen, M et al. (2004). Metabolism and function of coenzyme Q. *Biochimica et Biophysica Acta* 1660(1-2): 171-99.

Unfer, V et al. (2004). Endometrial effects of long-term treatment with phytoestrogens: A randomized, double-blind, placebo-controlled study. *Fertility and Sterility* 82(1): 145-8.

Vupadhyayula, PM et al. (2009). Effects of soy protein isolate on bone mineral density and physical performance indices in postmenopausal women: A 2-year randomized, double-blind, placebo-controlled trial. *Menopause: The Journal of the North American Menopause Society* 16(2): 320-8.

Walter, P (2001). Towards ensuring the safety of vitamins and minerals. *Toxicology Letters* 120(1-3): 83-7.

Wandel, S et al. (2010). Effects of glucosamine, chondroitin, or placebo in patients with osteoarthritis of hip or knee: Network meta-analysis. *BMJ* 341: c4675.

Weil, A (2000). *Eating well for optimum health.* London: Little, Brown and Company.

Wilburn, AJ et al. (2004). The natural treatment of hypertension. *Journal of Clinical Hypertension* 6(5): 242-8.

Wing, RR & Phelan, S (2005). Long-term weight loss maintenance. *American Journal of Clinical Nutrition* 82 (Suppl.): S222-5.

Witham, MD et al. (2010). The effect of different doses of vitamin D(3) on markers of vascular health in patients with type 2 diabetes: A randomised controlled trial. *Diabetologia* 53(10): 2112-9.

Wu, J et al. (2007). Possible role of equal status in the effects of isoflavone on bone and fat mass in postmenopausal Japanese women: A double-blind, randomized controlled trial. *Menopause: The Journal of the North American Menopause Society* 14(5): 866-74.

Wuttke, W et al. (2006). Effects of black cohosh (Cimcifuga racemosa) on bone turnover, vaginal mucosa, and various blood parameters in postmenopausal women: A double-blind placebo-controlled, and conjugated estrogens-controlled study. *Menopause: The Journal of the North American Menopause Society* 13(2): 185-96.

Xiao, OS et al. (2009). Soy food intake and breast cancer survival. *Journal of the American Medical Association* 302(22): 2437-43.

Available online

http://dietary-supplements.info.nih.gov/factsheets/dietarysupplements.asp
http://health.allrefer.com/alternative-medicine/dietary-supp-4.html

http://innerself.com/
http://iom.edu/~/media/Files/Activity%20Files/Nutrition/DRIs/DRI_Elements.pdf
http://iom.edu/~/media/Files/Activity%20Files/Nutrition/DRIs/DRI_Vitamins.pdf
http://nccam.nih.gov/health/
http://nccam.nih.gov/health/supplements.htm
http://ods.od.nih.gov/
http://www.biochem.northwestern.edu/holmgren/Glossary/Definitions/Def-V/vitamin.html
http://www.bodyand tness.com/Information/Health/Research/minerals.htm
http://www.cfsan.fda.gov/~dms/supplmnt.html
http://www.diagnose-me.com/glossary/G668.html
http://www.dietandbody.com/article1143.html
http://www.dietandbody.com/article1145.html
http://www.drugdigest.org/DD/Home/AllAboutDrugs/0,4081,,00.html
http://www.food.gov.uk/healthiereating/vitaminsminerals
http://www.food.gov.uk/multimedia/pdfs/vitmin2003.pdf
http://www.healthatoz.com/healthatoz/Atoz/dc/cen/cam/altdicnew.html
http://www.healthcentral.com/mhc/top/000339.cfm
http://www.nlm.nih.gov/medlineplus
http://www.nlm.nih.gov/medlineplus/ency/article/002399.htm http://www.oasisfoods.com/wild_life/health_
    guides/nutrition_ glossary_n.html
http://www.quackwatch.org/index.html
http://www.urbanext.uiuc.edu/thriftyliving/index.html

Chapter 6

Aiello, EJ et al. (2004). Effect of a year long, moderate-intensity exercise intervention on the occurrence and severity of menopausal symptoms in postmenopausal women. *Menopause: The Journal of the North American Menopause Society* 11(4): 369-71.

Aydin, Z (2010). Determinants of age at natural menopause in the Isparta Menopause and Health Study: Premenopausal body mass index gain rate and episodic weight loss. *Menopause: The Journal of the North American Menopause Society* 17(3): 494-505.

Balfour, RP (1999). Laparoscopic assisted vaginal hysterectomy, 190 cases: Complications and training. *Journal of Obstetrics and Gynaecology* 19(2): 164-6.

Blue Cross and Blue Shield Association, the Technology Evaluation Center (2008). *CYP2D6 Pharmacogenomics of tamoxifen treatment.* http://www.bcbs.com/blueresources/tec/vols/23/cyp2d6-pharmacogenomics-of.html

Boggia, J et al. (2011). Ambulatory BP monitoring in 9357 subjects from 11 populations highlights missed opportunities for CV prevention in women. *Hypertension* 57(3): 397-405.

Bordeleau, L et al. (2007). Therapeutic options for the management of hot flashes in breast cancer survivors: An evidence-based review. *Clinical Therapeutics* 29(2): 230-41.

Borud, EK et al. (2010). The Acupuncture on Hot Flashes Among Menopausal Women Study: Observational follow-up results at 6 and 12 months. *Menopause: The Journal of the North American Menopause Society* 17(2): 262-8.

Brunner, RL et al. (2010). Menopause symptom experience before and after stopping estrogen therapy in the Women's Health Initiative randomized placebo-controlled trial. *Menopause: The Journal of the North American Menopause Society* 17(5): 946-54.

Carmody, J et al. (2006). A pilot study of mindfulness-based stress reduction for hot flashes. *Menopause: The Journal of the North American Menopause Society* 13(5): 760-9.

Carmody, JF (2011). Mindfulness training for coping with hot flashes: Results of a randomized trial. *Menopause: The Journal of the North American Menopause Society* 18(6): 611-20.

Carpenter, JS et al. (2004). Hot flashes, core body temperature and metabolic parameters in breast cancer survivors. *Menopause: The Journal of the North American Menopause Society* 11(4): 375-81.

Chattha, R et al. (2008). Treating the climacteric symptoms in Indian women with integrated approach of yoga therapy: A randomized control study. *Menopause: The Journal of the North American Menopause Society* 15(5): 862-70.

Col, NF et al. (2009). Duration of vasomotor symptoms in middle-aged women: A longitudinal study. *Menopause: The Journal of the North American Menopause Society* 16(3): 453-7.

Crisafulli, A et al. (2004). Effects of genistein on hot flushes in early postmenopausal women: A randomised, double-blind EPT and placebo controlled study. *Menopause: The Journal of the North American Menopause Society* 11(4): 400-4.

Debernardo, RL (2005). *Fibroid tumours.* Department of *Obstetrics & Gynecology,* Massachusetts General Hospital, Boston, MA. Review provided by VeriMed Healthcare Network. Available online: https://ssl.adam. com/content.aspx?productId=10&pid=10&gid=000529&site=morehead2.adam.Com&login=MORE6662

Deecher, DC et al. (2006). Desvenlafaxine succinate: A new serotonin and norepinephrine reuptake inhibitor. *Journal of Pharmacology and Experimental Therapeutics* 318(2): 657-65.

Elkind-Hisch, K (2004). Cooling off hot flashes: Uncoupling of the circadian pattern of core body temperature and hot flash frequency in breast cancer survivors. *Menopause: The Journal of the North American Menopause Society* 11(4): 369-71.

Evans, ML et al. (2005). Management of postmenopausal hot flushes with venlafaxine hydrochloride: A randomized, controlled trial. *Journal of Obstetrics and Gynaecology* 105(1): 161-6.

Fitzpatrick, LA & Santen, RJ (2002). Hot flashes: The old and the new, what is really true? Mayo Clinic Proceedings 77(11): 1155-8. *Mayo Foundation for Medical Education and Research.*

Freedman, RR (2001). Physiology of hot flashes. *American Journal of Human Biology* 13(4): 453-64.

Freedman, RR et al. (1995). Core body temperature and circadian rhythm of hot flashes in menopausal women. *Journal of Clinical Endocrinology and Metabolism* 80(8): 2354-8.

Freeman, EW et al. (2011). Duration of menopausal hot flashes and associated risk factors. *Obstetrics & Gynecology* 117(5):1095-104.

Garreau, JR et al. (2006). Side effects of aromatase inhibitors versus tamoxifen: The patients' perspective. *American Journal of Surgery* 192(4): 496-8.

Gordon, P et al. (2006). Sertraline to treat hot flashes: A randomized controlled, double-blind, crossover trial in a general population. *Menopause: The Journal of the North American Menopause Society* 13(4): 568-75.

Gould, SA et al. (1999). Emergency obstetric hysterectomy an increasing incidence. *Journal of Obstetrics and Gynaecology* 19(6): 580-3.

Guttuso, T et al. (2003). Gabapentin's effects on hot flashes in postmenopausal women: A randomized controlled trial. *Obstetrics and Gynaecology* 101(2): 337-45.

Haimovich, S et al. (2008). Treatment of endometrial hyperplasia without atypia in peri- and postmenopausal women with a levonorgestrel intrauterine device. *Menopause: The Journal of the North American Menopause Society* 15(5): 1002-7.

Haney, AF & Wilde, RA (2007). Options for hormone therapy in women who have had a hysterectomy. *Menopause: The Journal of the North American Menopause Society* 14(3): 592-7.

Hervik, J & Mjaland, O (2009). Acupuncture for the treatment of hot flashes in breast cancer patients: A randomized, controlled trial. *Breast Cancer Research and Treatment* 116(2): 311-6.

Hickey, M et al. (2010). The multidisciplinary management of menopausal symptoms after breast cancer: A unique model of care. *Menopause: The Journal of the North American Menopause Society* 17(4): 727-33.

Horn, JR & Hansten, P (2009). Drug interactions: Beware of CYP2D6 inhibitors in patients taking tamoxifen. *Pharmacy Times.* Available online: http://www.pharmacytimes.com/publications/ issue/2009/2009-03/2009-03-10041

Ingelsson, E (2011). Hysterectomy and risk of cardiovascular disease: A population-based cohort study. *European Heart Journal* 32(6): 745-50.

Kerwin, J et al. (2007). The variable response of women with menopausal hot flashes when treated with sertraline. *Menopause: The Journal of the North American Menopause Society* 14(5): 841-5.

Lacroix, AZ et al. (2011). Health outcomes after stopping conjugated equine estrogens among postmenopausal women with prior hysterectomy: A randomized controlled trial. *Journal of the American Medical Association* 305(13): 1305-14.

Lermer, MA et al. (2011). Somatic and affective anxiety symptoms and menopausal hot flashes. *Menopause: The Journal of the North American Menopause Society* 18(2): 129-32.

Lindh-Astrand, L et al. (2009). Vasomotor symptoms usually reappear after cessation of postmenopausal hormone therapy: A Swedish population-based study. *Menopause: The Journal of the North American Menopause Society* 16(6): 1213-7.

Loprinzi, CL (2010). Phase III, randomized, double-blind, placebo-controlled evaluation of pregabalin for alleviating hot flashes N07C1. *Journal of Clinical Oncology* 28(4): 641-7.

Loprinzi, CL et al. (2009). Newer antidepressants and gabapentin for hot flashes: An individual patient pooled analysis. *Journal of Clinical Oncology* 27(17): 2831-7.

Maki, PM (2011). New data on mindfulness-based stress reduction for hot flashes: How do alternative therapies compare with selective serotonin reuptake inhibitors? *Menopause: The Journal of the North American Menopause Society* 18(6): 596-8.

Miller, ER et al. (2004). Meta-analysis: High dose vitamin E supplementation may increase all-cause mortality. *Annuals of Internal Medicine* 142(1): 37-46.

Nelson, HD et al. (2005). *Management of menopause related symptoms.* Agency of Healthcare Research and Quality, Evidence Report/Technology assessment No. 120. US Department of Health and Human Services, Rockville, MD.

Nelson, HD et al. (2006). Non-hormonal therapies for menopausal hot flashes: Systematic review and meta-analysis. *JAMA* 295(17): 2057-71.

North American Menopause Society. (2003). *Menonote* No. 32. http://www.menopause.org/

North American Menopause Society. (2010). *Menopause practice: A clinician's guide*, 4th ed. NAMS, Cleveland, OH.

North American Menopause Society (2004). Position statement on the treatment of menopause-associated vasomotor symptoms. *Menopause: The Journal of the North American Menopause Society* 11(1): 11-33.

Obermeyer, C et al. (2004). Therapeutic decisions for menopause: Results of the DAMES project in central Massachusetts. *Menopause: The Journal of the North American Menopause Society* 11(4): 456-65.

Parente, RC et al. (2008). The relationship between smoking and age at the menopause: A systematic review. *Maturitas* 61(4): 287-98.

Parker, WH & Manson, JE. (2009). Oophorectomy and cardiovascular mortality: Is there a link? Editorial. *Menopause: The Journal of the North American Menopause Society* 16(1): 1-2.

Parsanezhad, ME et al. (2010). Fertility: A randomized, controlled clinical trial comparing the effects of aromatase inhibitor (Letrozole) and gonadotropin-releasing hormone agonist (Triptorelin) on uterine leiomyoma volume and hormonal status. *Fertility & Sterility* 93(1): 192-8.

Pinkerton, JV & Pastore, LM (2007). Perspective on menopausal vasomotor symptoms, CAM and SWAN. *Menopause: The Journal of the North American Menopause Society* 14(4): 601-5.

Pinkerton, JV et al. (2011). Desvenlafaxine efficacy vs placebo for the treatment of menopausal vasomotor symptoms. Poster presented at the 59th Annual Clinical Meeting of the American College of Obstetricians and Gynecologists (ACOG), 30 April – 3 May 2011, Washington, DC.

Politi, MC et al. (2008). Revisiting the duration of vasomotor symptoms of menopause: A meta-analysis. *Journal of General Internal Medicine* 23(9): 1507-13.

Reddy, SY et al. (2006). Gabapentin, estrogen, and placebo for treating hot flushes: A randomized controlled trial. *Obstetrics and Gynecology* 108(1): 41-8.

Rivera, C et al. (2009). Increased cardiovascular mortality following early bilateral oophorectomy. *Menopause: The Journal of the North American Menopause Society,* 16(1): 15-23.

Seritan, AL et al. (2010). Self-reported anxiety, depressive, and vasomotor symptoms: A study of perimenopausal women presenting to a specialized midlife assessment center. *Menopause: The Journal of the North American Menopause Society* 17(2): 410-5.

Shanafelt, TD et al. (2002). Pathophysiology and treatment of hot flashes. *Mayo Clinic Proceedings* 77(11): 1207-18. Mayo Clinic Foundation for Medical Education and Research.

Shuster, LT et al. (2010). Premature menopause or early menopause: Long-term health consequences. *Maturitas* 65(2): 161-6.

Sicat, BL & Brokaw, DK (2004). Non-hormonal alternatives for the treatment of hot flashes. *Pharmacotherapy* 24(1): 79-93.

Soares, CN (2011). In the heat of the moment: Assessing anxiety and hot flashes in postmenopausal women. Editorial. *Menopause: The Journal of the North American Menopause Society* 18(2): 121-2.

Stearns, V et al. (2003). Controlled release in the treatment of menopausal hot flashes: A randomized controlled trial. *Journal of the American Medical Association* 289(21): 2827-34.

Stuenkel, CA. (2011). Checking the pulse of the menopausal hot flash: Feeling the heat and saving the beat. *Menopause: The Journal of the North American Menopause Society* 18(6): 593-5.

The HOPE and HOPE-TOO Trial Investigators (2005). Effects of long-term vitamin E supplementation on cardiovascular events and cancer: A randomized trial. *Journal of the American Medical Association* 293(11): 1338-47.

Thurston, R et al. (2007). SSRIs for menopausal hot flashes: A promise yet to be delivered. *Menopause: The Journal of the North American Menopause Society* 14(5): 820-2.

Van Dole, KB et al. (2010). Longitudinal association of vasomotor symptoms and psychosocial outcomes among postmenopausal women in the United States: A population-based study. *Menopause: The Journal of the North American Menopause Society* 17(5): 917-23.

Walker, EM et al. (2010). Acupuncture versus venlafaxine for the management of vasomotor symptoms in patients with hormone receptor-positive breast cancer: A randomized controlled trial. *Journal of Clinical Oncology* 28(4): 634-40.

Wegman, P et al. (2005). Genotype of metabolic enzymes and the benefit of tamoxifen in postmenopausal breast cancer patients. *Breast Cancer Research* 7(3): R284-90.

Whiteman, MK et al. (2003). Smoking, body mass and hot flashes in midlife women. *Obstetrics and Gynaecology* 101(2): 264-72.

Wilde, RA (2007). Introduction to special issue on surgical menopause. *Menopause: The Journal of the North American Menopause Society* 14(3): 556-61.

Available online

http://sharedjourney.com/dene/endometriosis.html

http://www.breastcancer.org/tips/menopausal/facing/hot_flashes.jsp

http://www.chclibrary.org/micromed/004820.htm

http://www.dyspareunia.org/html/uterine_prolapse.htm

http://www.nlm.nih.gov/medlineplus/ency/article/000914.htm

Chapter 7

Adolphe, A et al. (2009). A cross-sectional study of intima-media thickness, ethnicity, metabolic syndrome, and cardiovascular risk in 2268 study participants. *Mayo Clinic Proceedings* 84(3): 221-8.

Alam, MU et al. (2009). Calcification is associated with loss of functional calcium-sensing receptor in vascular smooth muscle cells. *Cardiovascular Research* 81(2): 260-8.

Alberti, KG et al. (2009). Harmonizing the metabolic syndrome. A joint interim statement of the International Diabetes Federation Task Force on Epidemiology and Prevention: National Heart, Lung and Blood Institute, American Heart Association, World Heart Federation, International Atherosclerosis Society and International Association for the Study of Obesity. *Circulation* 120(16): 1640-5.

Allison, MA (2010). Vasomotor symptoms and coronary artery calcium in postmenopausal women. Editorial. *Menopause: The Journal of the North American Menopause Society* 17(6): 1136-45.

American Health Association (2004). AHA guidelines: Evidence based guidelines for cardiovascular disease prevention in women. *Circulation* 109: 672-93.

American Heart Association (2003). *Heart disease and stroke statistics.* http://www.americanheart.org

Armitage, JM et al. (2010). Effects of homocysteine lowering with folic acid plus vitamin B12 vs placebo on mortality and major morbidity in myocardial infarction survivors: A randomized trial. Study of the Effectiveness of Additional Reductions in Cholesterol and Homocysteine (SEARCH) Collaborative Group. *Journal of the American Medical Association* 303(24): 2486-94.

Astma, F et al. (2006). Postmenopausal status and early menopause independent risk factors for cardiovascular disease: A metaanalysis. *Menopause: The Journal of the North American Menopause Society* 13(2): 256-79.

Barclay, L (2004). Many type 2 diabetics should take statins. *Medscape Medical News.* Available online: http://www.medscape.com/viewarticle/474426_print

Barnes, J et al. (2005). Effects of two continuous hormone therapy regimens on C-reactive protein and homocysteine. *Menopause: The Journal of the North American Menopause Society* 12(1): 92-8.

Barrett-Connor, E (2007). Hormones and heart disease in women: The timing hypothesis. *American Journal of Epidemiology* 166(5): 506-10.

Bechlioulis, A et al. (2010). Endothelial function, but not carotid intima-media thickness, is affected early in menopause and is associated with severity of hot flushes. *Journal of Clinical Endocrinology & Metabolism* 95(3): 1199-1206.

Becker, DJ et al. (2009). Red yeast rice for dyslipidemia in statin-intolerant patients: A randomized trial. *Annals of Internal Medicine* 150(12): 830-9.

Berg, G et al. (2004). Lipid and lipoprotein profile in menopausal transition: Effects of hormone, age and fat distribution. *Hormone & Metabolic Research* 36(4): 215-20.

Boggia, J et al. (2011). Ambulatory BP monitoring in 9357 subjects from 11 populations highlights missed opportunities for CV prevention in women. *Hypertension* 57(3): 397-405.

Bolland, MJ et al. (2010). Effect of calcium supplements on risk of myocardial infarction and cardiovascular events: Meta-analysis. *BMJ* 341: c3691.

Brien, SE et al. (2011). Effect of alcohol consumption on biological markers associated with risk of coronary heart disease: Systematic review and meta-analysis of interventional studies. *BMJ* 342: d636.

Brinton, EA (2010). Hot flashes and hormone use: harbingers of heart disease? *Menopause: The Journal of the North American Menopause Society* 17(2): 223-5.

Brookes, L (2004). The British Guidelines – plus race, alcohol, exercise and more. *Medscape Cardiology* 8(1): 1-8. Available online: http://www.medscape.com/viewarticle/473321

Brookes, L (2004). Update of US National Cholesterol Education Program (NCEP), Adult Treatment Panel (ATP) III Guidelines: An expert interview with Christie M Ballantyne, MD. *Medscape Cardiology* 8(1). Available online: http://www.medscape.com/viewarticle/491820

Caboral, M (2004). Women: The target of the New American Heart Association guidelines in cardiovascular prevention. *Topics in Advanced Nursing Journal* 4(3). Available online: http://www.medscape.com/viewarticle/487462

Cagnacci, A et al. (2011). Increased cortisol: A possible link between climacteric symptoms and cardiovascular risk factors. *Menopause: The Journal of the North American Menopause Society* 18(3): 273-8.

Canonico, M et al. (2007). Hormone therapy and venous thromboembolism among postmenopausal women: Impact of the route of estrogen administration and progestogens. *Circulation* 115(7): 840-5.

Carels, R et al. (2004). Reducing cardiovascular risk factors in postmenopausal women through a lifestyle intervention. *Journal of Women's Health* 13(4): 412-26.

Centers for Disease Control and Prevention (CDC) (2010). Vital signs: State-specific obesity prevalence among adults – United States. *MMWR Morbidity and Mortality Weekly Report* 59(30): 951-5.

Chataigneau, T et al. (2004). Chronic treatment with progesterone but not medroxyprogesterone acetate restores the endothelial control of vascular tone in the mesenteric artery of ovariectomized rats. *Menopause: The Journal of the North American Menopause Society* 11(3): 255-63.

Chen, ST et al. (2010). The effect of dietary patterns on estimated coronary heart disease risk: Results from the Dietary Approaches to Stop Hypertension (DASH) trial. *Circulation: Cardiovascular Quality and Outcomes* 3(5): 484-9.

Chlebowski, RT et al. (2010). Estrogen plus progestin and breast cancer incidence and mortality in postmenopausal women. *Journal of American Medical Association* 304(15): 1684-92.

Cheung, BMY & Lam, KSL (2010). Is intensive LDL-cholesterol lowering beneficial and safe? *The Lancet* 376(9753): 1622-4.

Cholesterol definition and glossary of related terms for cholesterol.com © Pfizer Inc.

Cholesterol Treatment Trialists (CTT) Collaboration (2010). Efficacy and safety of intensive LDL-cholesterol lowering therapy: A meta-analysis of data from 170 000 participants in 26 randomised trials. *The Lancet* 376(9753): 1670-81.

Clarke, R et al. (2010). Effects of lowering homocysteine levels with B vitamins on cardiovascular disease, cancer, and cause-specific mortality: Meta-analysis of 8 randomized trials involving 37 485 individuals. *Archives of Internal Medicine* 170(18): 1622-31.

Clarkson, TB & Kaplan, JR (2007). Stage of reproductive life, atherosclerosis progression and estrogen effects on coronary artery atherosclerosis. *Menopause: The Journal of the North American Menopause Society* 14(3): 785-93.

Clearfield, M (2004). Coronary heart disease risk reduction in postmenopausal women: The role of statin therapy and hormone replacement therapy. *Preventative Cardiology* 7(3): 131-6.

Cleveland Clinic (2011). *Questions and answers about C-reactive protein: JUPITER study changes doctors' approach to heart disease prevention – the key: your CRP*. Review by Dr Leslie Cho. http://my.clevelandclinic.org/heart/news/hot/crp.aspx

Diercks, DB et al. (2010). Gender differences in time to presentation for myocardial infarction before and after a National Women's Cardiovascular Awareness Campaign: A temporal analysis from the Can Rapid Risk Stratification of Unstable Angina Patients Suppress Adverse Outcomes with Early Implementation (CRUSADE) and the National Cardiovascular Data Registry Acute Coronary Treatment and Intervention Outcomes Network – Get with the Guidelines (NCDR ACTION Registry, GWTG). *American Heart Journal* 160(1): 80-7.

Gast, GC et al. (2010). Vasomotor symptoms, estradiol levels and cardiovascular risk profile in women. *Maturitas* 66(3): 285-90.

Gast, GC et al. (2011). Vasomotor symptoms are associated with increased risk of coronary heart disease. *Menopause: The Journal of the North American Menopause Society* 18(2): 146-51.

Gordon, RY et al. (2010). Marked variability of monacolin levels in commercial red yeast rice products: Buyer beware! *Archives of Internal Medicine* 170(19): 1722-7.

Greenland, P et al. (2010). ACCF/AHA guidelines for assessment of cardiovascular risk in asymptomatic adults: Executive summary. A report from the American College of Cardiology Foundation/American Heart Association Task Force on Practice Guidelines. *Circulation* 122(25): 2748-64.

Halbert, SC et al. (2010). Tolerability of red yeast rice (2,400 mg twice daily) versus pravastatin (20 mg twice daily) in patients with previous statin intolerance. *American Journal of Cardiology* 105(2): 198-204.

Hardy, R. (2011). Vasomotor menopausal symptoms and risk of coronary artery heart disease: A life course perspective. *Menopause: The Journal of the North American Menopause Society* 18(2): 127-8.

Healy, K & Mosca, L (2004). New strategies to prevent and treat coronary heart disease in women. *Menopause Management* 13(4): 12-21.

Helfand, M et al. (2009). Emerging risk factors for coronary heart disease: A summary of systematic reviews conducted for the US Preventive Services Task Force. *Annals of Internal Medicine* 151(7): 496-507.

Herrington, DM et al. (1999). *Completed and ongoing trials of women and heart disease: PEPI and HERS*. 48th Annual Scientific Session, American College of Cardiology. Available online: http://www.medscape.com/viewarticle/439518

Hoikkala, H et al. (2010). Association between vasomotor hot flashes and heart rate variability in recently postmenopausal women. *Menopause: The Journal of the North American Menopause Society* 17(2): 313-20.

Holick, MF (2010). The D-bate: Do calcium and vitamin D affect cardiovascular health? Editorial. *Menopause: The Journal of the North American Menopause Society* 17(4): 667-8.

Hsia, J et al. (2007). Calcium/vitamin D supplementation and cardiovascular events. *Circulation* 115(7): 846-54.

Hunter, MS. (2011). Cortisol, hot flashes, and cardiovascular risk. Editorial. *Menopause: The Journal of the North American Menopause Society* 18(3): 251-2.

Jeon, GH et al. (2010). Association between serum estradiol level and coronary artery calcification in postmenopausal women. *Menopause: The Journal of the North American Menopause Society* 17(5): 902-7.

Kabalak-Ziembicka, A (2010). The role of carotid intima-media thickness assessment in cardiovascular risk evaluation in patients with polyvascular atherosclerosis. *Atherosclerosis* 209(1): 125-30.

Karas, RH (2007). Mechanisms of action of estrogen on the cardiovascular system. In Lobo RA (Ed.), *Treatment of the postmenopausal woman: Basic and clinical aspects*, 3rd ed. Burlington, MA: Elsevier, 453-69.

Khor, LL et al. (2004). Sex- and age-related differences in the prognostic value of C-reactive protein in patients with angiographic coronary artery disease. *American Journal of Medicine* 117(9): 657-64.

Kopernik, G & Shoham, Z (2004). Tools for making the correct decisions regarding hormone therapy. Part II: Organ response and clinical applications. *Fertility and Sterility* 81(6): 1447-57.

Kullo, IJ & Ballantyne, CM (2005). Conditional risk factors for atherosclerosis. *Mayo Clinic Proceedings* 80(2): 219-30. Available online: http://www.mayoclinicproceedings.com/inside.asp?AID=681&UID=

Kurtz, EG et al. (2011). Oral postmenopausal hormone therapy, C-reactive protein, and cardiovascular outcomes. *Menopause: The Journal of the North American Menopause Society* 18(1): 23-9.

Lammers, C (2003). *Novel risk factors are now being used to identify new culprits in heart disease*. Available online: http://www.mayoclinic.org/news2003-rst/1885.html

Little, MP et al. (2010). Review and meta-analysis of epidemiological associations between low/moderate doses of ionizing radiation and circulatory disease risks, and their possible mechanisms. *Radiation and Environmental Biophysics* 49(2): 139-53.

Lobo, R (2007). Surgical menopause and cardiovascular risks. *Menopause: The Journal of the North American Menopause Society* 14(3): 562-6.

Lobo, RA & Clarkson, TB (2011). Different mechanisms for benefit and risk of coronary heart disease and stroke in early post menopausal women: A hypothetical explanation. *Menopause: The Journal of the North American Menopause Society* 18(2): 237-40.

Lorenz, MW et al. (2010). Is carotid intima media thickness useful for individual prediction of cardiovascular risk? Ten-year results from the Carotid Atherosclerosis Progression Study (CAPS). *European Heart Journal* 31(16): 2041-8.

Mann, E & Hunter, MS (2011). Concordance between self-reported and sternal skin conductance measures of hot flushes in symptomatic perimenopausal and postmenopausal women: A systematic review. (Published online ahead of print, 12 February 2011). *Menopause PMID* 21326119.

Manson, JE (2010). Calcium/vitamin D supplementation and coronary artery calcification in the Women's Health Initiative. *Menopause: The Journal of the North American Menopause Society* 17(4): 683-91.

Manson, JE (2011). Calcium and heart attack risk: Ending the confusion. *Medscape Ob/Gyn & Women's Health* Posted 01 November 2011. Available online: http://www.medscape.com/viewarticle/735444

Martins, D et al. (2007). Prevalence of cardiovascular risk factors and the serum levels of 25-hydroxyvitamin D in the United States: Data from the Third National Health and Nutrition Examination Survey. *Archives of Internal Medicine* 167(11): 1159-65.

Mayo Foundation for Medical Education and Research (2004). *Aspirin: From pain relief to preventive medicine*. January 09 2004 HQ00269. Available online: http://www.mayoclinic.com/invoke.cfm?id=HQ00269

Meinert, CL et al. (2000). Gender representation in trials. *Controlled Clinical Trials* 21(5): 462-75.

Miller, VM et al. (2009). Using basic science to design a clinical trial: Baseline characteristics of women enrolled in the Kronos Early Estrogen Prevention Study (KEEPS). *Journal of Cardiovascular Translational Research* 2(3): 228-9.

Miller, M et al. (2011). Triglycerides and cardiovascular disease. *Circulation*. doi: 10.1161/CIR.0b013c3182160726.

Mohandas, B & Jawahar, LM (2007). Lessons from hormone replacement therapy trials for primary prevention of cardiovascular disease. *Current Opinion in Cardiology* 22(5): 434-42.

Mookadam, F et al. (2010). Subclinical atherosclerosis: Evolving role of carotid intima-media thickness. *Preventative Cardiology* 13(4): 186-97.

Morch, LS et al. (2009). Hormone therapy and ovarian cancer. *Journal of the American Medical Association* 302(3): 298-305.

Mosca, L et al. (2011). Effectiveness-based guidelines for the prevention of cardiovascular disease in women – 2011 update: A guideline from the American Heart Association. *Circulation* 123(11): 1243-62.

Mumford, SL et al. (2010). A longitudinal study of serum lipoproteins in relation to endogenous reproductive hormones during the menstrual cycle: Findings from the BioCycle study. *Journal of Clinical Endocrinology & Metabolism* 95(9): E80-E85.

Naftolin, F et al. (2004). The Women's Health Initiative could not have detected cardioprotective effects of starting hormone therapy during the menopausal transition. *Fertility and Sterility* 81(6): 1498-501.

Nainggolan, L (2007).Oral contraceptives increase risk of plaques. *Medscape Medical News*. Available online: http://www.medscape.org/viewarticle/565874

Nainggolan, L (2007). *WHI substudy: Estrogen reduces coronary calcification in younger postmenopausal women*. Available online: http://www.theheart.org/article/797797.do

Nandur, R et al. (2004). Cardiovascular actions of selective estrogen receptor modulators and phytoestrogens. *Preventative Cardiology* 7(2): 73-9.

National Institute of Health (2003). *The National Institute of Health and the Expert Group on Vitamins and Minerals* (EVM) Report. Published by the Food Standards Agency.

Ozkaya, E et al. (2011). Comparison of the effects of surgical and natural menopause on carotid intima media thickness, osteoporosis, and homocysteine levels. *Menopause: The Journal of the North American Menopause Society* 18(1): 73-6.

Parashar, S et al. (2010). Early menopause predicts angina after myocardial infarction. *Menopause: The Journal of the North American Menopause Society* 17(5): 938-45.

Pettee, KK (2007). The relationship between physical activity and lipoprotein subclasses in postmenopausal women: The influence of hormone therapy. *Menopause: The Journal of the North American Menopause Society* 14(1): 115-22.

Pokwryka, GS (2010). Menopause e-consult, 6(1). http://www.menopause.org/ME0110.pdf

Polotsky, AJ & Santoro, N (2007). Menopause and cardiovascular disease: Endogenous reproductive hormone exposure affects risk factors. *Menopause Management* 16(2): 21-6.

Reid IR et al. (2010). Does calcium supplementation increase cardiovascular risk? *Clinical Endocrinology (Oxford)* 73(6): 689-95.

Rietzschel, E (2007). American Heart Association 2007 Scientific Sessions. Abstracts 3537 and 3614 presented 6 November 2007.

Ronksley, PE et al. (2011). Association of alcohol consumption with selected cardiovascular disease outcomes: A systematic review and meta-analysis. *BMJ* 342: d671.

Salagame, U et al. (2011). An epidemiological overview of the relationship between hormone replacement therapy and breast cancer. *Expert Review of Endocrinology & Metabolism* 6(3): 397-409.

Sanada, M et al. (2004). Substitution of transdermal estradiol during oral estrogen-progestin therapy in postmenopausal women: Effects on hypertriglyceridemia. *Menopause: The Journal of the North American Menopause Society* 11(3): 331-6.

Scarabin, P et al. (2003). Differential association of oral and transdermal oestrogen-replacement therapy with venous thromboembolism risk. *The Lancet* 362(9382): 428-32.

Simoncini, T et al. (2005). Activation of nitric oxide synthesis in human endothelial cells by red clover extracts. *Menopause: The Journal of the North American Menopause Society* 12(1): 69-77.

Study of the Effectiveness of Additional Reductions in Cholesterol and Homocysteine (SEARCH) Collaborative Group (2010). Intensive lowering of LDL cholesterol with 80 mg vs 20 mg simvastatin daily in 12 064 survivors of myocardial infarction: A double-blind randomised trial. *The Lancet* 376(9753): 1658-69.

Stuenkel, CA (2008). Does the yardstick of cardiovascular risk assessment really measure up? *Menopause: The Journal of the North American Menopause Society* 15(2): 212-4.

Stuenkel, CA (2011). Checking the pulse of the menopausal hot flash: Feeling the heat and saving the beat. 18(6): 593-5.

Stuenkel, C (2011). Hold, raise, or fold: C-reactive protein, hormone therapy, and cardiovascular risk. Editorial. *Menopause: The Journal of the North American Menopause Society* 18(1): 8-10.

Szmuilowicz ED et al. (2011). Vasomotor symptoms and cardiovascular events in postmenopausal women. *Menopause: The Journal of the North American Menopause Society* 18(6): 603-10.

Szmuilowicz, ED & Manson, JE (2011). Menopausal vasomotor symptoms and cardiovascular disease. Editorial. *Menopause: The Journal of the North American Menopause Society* 18(4): 345-7.

Tackett, AH et al. (2010). Hormone replacement therapy among postmenopausal women presenting with acute myocardial infarction: Insights from the GUSTO-III trial. *American Heart Journal* 160(4): 678-84.

Taylor, F et al. (2011). Statins for the primary prevention of cardiovascular disease. *Cochrane Database System Review*, 1 (CD004816). Cochrane Library.

The Merck Manual, Second Home Edition. Melanoma. In Chapter 216, Skin cancer. USA: Merck & Co Inc. Available online: http://www.merck.com/mmhe/sec08/ch113/ch113d.html

Thurston, RC (2010). Getting to the heart of things: Is endogenous estradiol associated with coronary artery calcification? Editorial. *Menopause: The Journal of the North American Menopause Society* 17(5): 887-8.

Thurston, RC et al. (2010). History of hot flashes and aortic calcification among postmenopausal women. *Menopause: The Journal of the North American Menopause Society* 17(2): 256-61.

Thurston, RC et al. (2010). Hot flashes and vagal control: A link to cardiovascular risk? *Menopause: The Journal of the North American Menopause Society* 17(3): 456-63.

Tice, JA (2010). The vital amines: Too much of a good thing? Comment on: Effects of lowering homocysteine levels with B vitamins on cardiovascular disease, cancer and cause specific mortality. *Archives of Internal Medicine* 170(18): 1631-3.

Tuomikoski, P et al. (2010). Hot flushes and biochemical markers for cardiovascular disease: A randomized trial of hormone therapy. *Climacteric* 13(3): 457-66.

Vega, CP (2010). Calcium supplements and myocardial infarction: The evidence grows . Best evidence review. *Medscape Ob/Gyn & Women's Health* Posted: 10/22/2010. Available online: http://www.medscape.com/viewarticle/730536

Welty, F (2004). Preventing clinically evident coronary heart disease in the postmenopausal woman. *Menopause: The Journal of the North American Menopause Society* 11(4): 484-94.

Wilde, RA (2007). Endogenous androgens and cardiovascular risk. *Menopause: The Journal of the North American Menopause Society* 14(4): 609-10.

Woodard, GA et al. (2010). Lipids, menopause, and early atherosclerosis in study of Women's Health across the Nation Heart Women. *Menopause: The Journal of the North American Menopause Society* 18(4): 376-84.

Woods, NN et al. (2009). Cortisol levels during the menopausal transition and early postmenopause: Observations from the Seattle Midlife Women's Health Study. *Menopause: The Journal of the North American Menopause Society* 16(4): 708-18.

Writing Group for the PEPI Trial (1995). Effects of estrogen or estrogen/progestin regimens on heart disease risk factors in postmenopausal women: The Postmenopausal Estrogen/Progestin Interventions (PEPI) Trial. *Journal of the American Medical Association* 273(3): 199-208. Erratum in: *Journal of the American Medical Association*, 1995, 274(21): 1676.

Yin, WH et al. (2004). Independent prognostic value of elevated high-sensitivity C-reactive protein in chronic heart failure. *American Heart Journal* 147(5): 931-8. Available online: http://www.medscape.com/viewarticle/477549

Zouridakis, E et al. (2004). Markers of inflammation and rapid coronary artery disease progression in patients with stable angina pectoris. *Circulation* 110(13): 1747-53.

Available online

http://en.wikipedia.org/wiki/Circulatory_system
http://quitsmoking.about.com/od/tobaccostatistics/a/heartdiseases.htm
http://www.ahrq.gov/clinic/tp/menopstp.htm
http://www.altvetmed.com/face/8304-cholesterol-and-ldl.html
http://www.answers.com/cardiovascular+disease&r=67
http://www.answers.com/cholesterol&r=67
http://www.answers.com/homocysteine&r=67

http://www.answers.com/phytochemicals&r=67
http://www.cancer.org
http://www.clevelandclinicmeded.com/diseasemanagement/cardiology/vthromboembolism/vthrombembolism.htm
http://www.fda.gov/fdac/features/2003/503_aspirin.html
http://www.forcholessterol.com/cwp/appmanager/for_cholessterolDesktop?_nfpb=true&_pageLabel=FC_glossary
http://www.goredforwomen.org/index.aspx
http://www.healthcentral.com
http://www.healthcentral.com/mhc/top/000171.cfm
http://www.hyperdictionary.com/medical/cholesterol
http://www.lifeclinic.com/focus/blood/whatisit.asp
http://www.mayoclinic.com/health/fat/NU00262
http://www.mayoclinic.com/invoke.cfm?id=HQ00269
http://www.medicinenet.com/script/main/hp.asp
http://www.neurologychannel.com/stroke/
http://www.uihealthcare.com/reports/cardiovascular/011203cholesterol.html
http://www.wordreference.com/definition/fibrinogen

Chapter 8

Allen, TL et al. (2010). The breast self-examination controversy: What providers and patients should know. *Journal for Nurse Practitioners* 6(6): 444-51.

American Association for Cancer Research (AACR) (2010). Ninth Annual AACR Frontiers in Cancer Prevention Research Conference, Philadelphia, 7 November 2010.

American Cancer Society (2005). *Overview: Breast cancer. What causes breast cancer?* http://www.cancer.org

American College of Obstetricians and Gynecologists (ACOG) (2009). ACOG Committee on Practice Bulletins – Gynecology: Cervical cytology screening. ACOG Practice Bulletin No. 109. *Obstet Gynecol* 114: 1409-20.

Archer, DF (2011). The gynecologic effects of lasofoxifene, an estrogen agonist/antagonist, in postmenopausal women. Editorial. *Menopause: The Journal of the North American Menopause Society* 18(1): 6-7.

Arnould, L et al. (2006). Trastuzumab-based treatment of HER2-positive breast cancer: An antibody dependent cellular cytotoxicity mechanism? *British Journal of Cancer* 94(2): 259-67.

Arnould, L et al. (2006). Trastuzumab for the adjuvant treatment of early-stage HER2-positive breast cancer. *National Institute for Health and Clinical Excellence* (NICE).

Azar, B (1999). Probing links between stress, cancer. APA *Monitor Online* 30(6). Available online: http://www.intensivenutrition.com/stress.pdf

Baer, HJ et al. (2010). Body fatness at young ages and risk of breast cancer throughout life. *American Journal of Epidemiology* 171(11): 1183-94.

Bakkum-Gamez, JN et al. (2011). Challenges in the gynecologic care of premenopausal women with breast cancer. *Mayo Clinic Proceedings* 86(3): 229-40.

Banerjee, S & Smith, IE (2010). Management of small HER2-positive breast cancers *Lancet Oncology* 11(12): 1193-9.

Barclay, L & Vega, C (2004). MRI more sensitive than mammography in women at high risk of breast cancer. *Medscape Medical News.* Available online: http://www.medscape.com/viewarticle/484354

Baselga, J et al. (2011). *First results of the NeoALTTO trial (BIG 01-06 / EGF 106903): A phase III, randomized, open label, neoadjuvant study of lapatinib, trastuzumab, and their combination plus paclitaxel in women with HER2-positive primary breast cancer.* 33rd Annual San Antonio Breast Cancer Symposium. Abstract S3-3 presented 10 December 2011.

Baum, M (2004). Current status of aromatase inhibitors in the management of breast cancer and critique of the NCIC MA-17 trial. *Cancer Control* 11(4): 217-21. Available online: http://www.moftt.usf.edu/pubs/ccj/v11n4/pdf/217.pdf

Baumgart, J et al. (2011). Urogenital disorders in women with adjuvant endocrine therapy after early breast cancer. *American Journal of Obstetrics and Gynecology* 204(1): 26e1-7

Bezuhly, M (2010). The finding comes from an analysis of the US National Cancer Institute Surveillance, Epidemiology, and End Results (SEER) registry database, which looked at cases of breast cancer between 1998 and 2003. Joint Annual Scientific Meeting of the American Society of Plastic Surgery (ASPS) and the Canadian Society of Aesthetic Plastic Surgery (CSAPS). Presented 3 October 2010.

BIG 1-98 Collaborative Group (2009). Letrozole therapy alone or in sequence with tamoxifen in women with breast cancer. *New England Journal of Medicine* 361(8): 766-77.

Blunt, S et al. (1999). Aromatase in aging women. *Seminars in Reproductive Medicine* 17(4): 349-58.

Bond, B et al. (2002). Women like me: Reflections on health and hormones from women treated for breast cancer. *Journal of Psychosocial Oncology* 20(3): 39-57.

Burstein, HJ et al. (2010). *American Society of Clinical Oncology* clinical practice guideline: Update on adjuvant endocrine therapy for women with hormone receptor-positive breast cancer. *Journal of Clinical Oncology* 28(23): 3784-96.

Buzdar, A (2010). *Breast cancer survival has improved steadily over past 6 decades.* Breast Cancer Symposium. Abstract 172 presented 2 October 2010.

Cairns, B (2004). *The five steps of a breast self exam.* Available online: http://www.healtharticles.org/breast_self_exam_070904.html

Cameron, D et al. (2008). A phase III randomized comparison of lapatinib plus capecitabine versus capecitabine alone in women with advanced breast cancer that has progressed on trastuzumab: Updated efficacy and biomarker analyses. *Breast Cancer Research and Treatment* 112(3): 533-43.

Chlebowski, RT et al. (2010). Estrogen plus progestin and breast cancer incidence and mortality in postmenopausal women. *Journal of the American Medical Association* 302(15): 1684-92.

Cho, E et al. (2003). Premenopausal fat intake and risk of breast cancer. *Journal of the National Cancer Institute* 95(14): 1079-85.

Clemons, M & Vera, S (2003). Aromatase inhibitors in the treatment of early breast cancer: Highlights of the 26th Annual San Antonio Breast Cancer Symposium. *Medscape Hematology-Oncology* 6(2). Available online: http://www.medscape.com/viewarticle/467141

Committee on Gynecological Practice (2011). Colonoscopy and colorectal screening strategies. *Obstetrics & Gynecology* 117(3): 766-71.

Cummings, SR et al. (2010). Lasofoxifene in postmenopausal women with osteoporosis. *New England Journal of Medicine* 362(8): 686-96.

De Lingers, B (2002). Effects of progestogens on the postmenopausal breast. *Climacteric* 5: 229-35.

De Lingers, B et al. (2002). Combined hormone replacement therapy and risk of breast cancer in a French cohort study of 3175 women. *Climacteric* 5(4): 332-40.

Douchi, T (2007). Difference in segmental lean and fat mass components between pre- and postmenopausal women. *Menopause: The Journal of the North American Menopause Society* 14(5): 875-8.

Domchek, SM et al. (2010). Association of risk-reducing surgery in BRCA1 or BRCA2 mutation carriers with cancer risk and mortality. *Journal of the American Medical Association* 304(9): 967-75.

Eitan, A et al. (2010). Assessing women at high risk of breast cancer: A review of risk assessment models – assessing breast cancer over time. *Journal of the National Cancer Institute* 102(10): 680-91.

Ellis, GK et al. (2008). Randomized trial of denosumab in patients receiving adjuvant aromatase inhibitors for nonmetastatic breast cancer. *Journal of Clinical Oncology* 26(30): 4875-81.

ESHRE Capri Workshop Group (2005). Non-contraceptive health benefits of combined oral contraception. *Human Reproduction Update* 11(5): 513-25.

Evans, EM et al. (2007). Effects of soy protein isolate and moderate exercise on bone turnover and bone mineral density in postmenopausal women. *Menopause: The Journal of the North American Menopause Society* 14(3): 481-8.

Fabian, CJ et al. (2004). Breast cancer chemoprevention phase I: Evaluation of biomarker modulation by arzoxifene, a third generation selective estrogen receptor modulator. *Clinical Cancer Research* 10: 5403-17.

Fournier, A et al. (2008). Unequal risks for breast cancer associated with different hormone replacement therapies: Results from the E3N cohort study. *Breast Cancer Research Treatment* 107(1): 103-11.

Frankel, C & Palmieri, FM (2010). Lapatinib side-effect management. *Clinical Oncology Nursing* 14(2): 223-33.

Friedenreich, CM et al. (2010). Alberta Physical Activity and Breast Cancer Prevention Trial: Sex hormone changes in a year-long exercise intervention among postmenopausal women. *Journal of Clinical Oncology* 28(9): 1458-66.

Gainford, MC et al. (2005). A practical guide to the management of menopausal symptoms in breast cancer patients. *Support Care Cancer* 13(8): 573-8.

Gallicchico, L (2010). Ninth Annual American Association for Cancer Research (AACR) International Conference on Frontiers in Cancer Prevention Research, 7-10 November 2010.

Getting, G et al. (2006). Hormone therapy and breast cancer: What factors modify the association? *Menopause: The Journal of the North American Menopause Society* 13(2): 178-84.

Harms, SE et al. (2006). ACR Practice Guideline for the performance of magnetic resonance imaging (MRI) of the breast. *ACR Practice Guideline*, Res. 35.

Harper, DM (2009). Currently approved prophylactic HPV vaccines. *Expert Review of Vaccines* 8(12): 1663-79.

Harper, DM (2009). Prevention of human papillomavirus infections and associated diseases by vaccination: A new hope for global public health. *Public Health Genomics*, 10 August.

Hendrick, RE & Helvie, MA (2011). United States Preventive Services Task Force screening mammography recommendations: Science ignored. *AJR American Journal Roentgenology* 196(2): W112-6.

Howell, A et al. (2004). Comparison of fulvestrant versus tamoxifen for the treatment of advanced breast cancer in postmenopausal women previously untreated with endocrine therapy: A multinational, double-blind, randomized trial. *Journal of Clinical Oncology* 22(9): 1605-13.

Hughes, KS (2011). The complexity of breast cancer risk needs to be embraced, not oversimplified. *Menopause: The Journal of the North American Menopause Society* 18(6): 599-600.

Ingle, JN (2006). Evaluation of fulvestrant in women with advanced breast cancer and progression on prior aromatase inhibitor therapy: A phase II trial of the North Central Cancer Treatment Group. *Journal of Clinical Oncology* 24(7): 1052-6.

Jacoby, VL et al. (2011). Oophorectomy vs ovarian conservation with hysterectomy: Cardiovascular disease, hip fracture, and cancer in the Women's Health Initiative Observational Study. *Archives of Internal Medicine* 171(8): 760-8.

Jarvis, W (2004). *How quackery harms cancer patients*. Quackwatch home page at http:www.quackwatch.com

Joffe, H et al. (2010). Augmentation of venlafaxine and SSRIs with zolpidem improves sleep and quality-of-life in breast cancer patients with hot flashes: A randomized double-blind placebo controlled trial. *Menopause: The Journal of the North American Menopause Society* 17(5): 908-16.

Johnston, SRD (2006). *New approaches to preventing resistance to aromatase inhibitors*. Available online: http://www.medscape.org/viewarticle/520923

Kalager, M et al. (2010). Effect of screening mammography on breast-cancer mortality in Norway. *New England Journal of Medicine*, 363(13): 1203-10.

Kaunitz, AM (2010). *Reappraising the value of screening mammography*. Available online: http://www.medscape.com/viewarticle/729567

Keen, JD (2010). Promoting screening mammography: Insight or uptake? *Journal of the American Board of Family Medicine* 23(6): 775-82.

Kelly, CM et al. (2010). Selective serotonin reuptake inhibitors and breast cancer mortality in women receiving tamoxifen: A population based cohort study. *BMJ* 340: c693.

Kerlikowske, K et al. (2010). Breast cancer risk by breast density, menopause, and use of postmenopausal HRT. *Journal of Clinical Oncology* 28(24): 3830-7.

Komm, BS et al. (2005). Bazedoxifene acetate: A selective estrogen receptor modulator with improved selectivity. *Endocrinology* 146(9): 3999-4008.

Kopans, D & Vickers, AJ (2011). Mammography screening and the evidence: From one hominem to the other. Point-Counterpoint between Andrew Vickers, PhD, and Daniel Kopans, MD. *Medscape Internal Medicine* Available online: http://www.medscape.com/viewarticle/734977

Kopans, DB (2010). The 2009 US Preventive Services Task Force Guidelines ignore important scientific evidence and should be revised or withdrawn. *Radiology* 256(1): 15-20.

Kurian, AW et al. (2010). Survival analysis of cancer risk reduction strategies for BRCA1/2 mutation carriers. *Journal of Clinical Oncology* 28(2): 222-31.

Kubow, S et al. (2000). Lipid peroxidation is associated with the inhibitory action of all trans-retinoic acid on mammary cell transformation. *Anticancer Research* 20(2A): 843-8.

Kwan, ML et al. (2010). Alcohol and breast cancer recurrence and survival among women with early-stage breast cancer: The life after cancer epidemiology study. *Journal of Clinical Oncology* 28(29): 4410-6.

Lacroix, AZ et al. (2010). Breast cancer incidence in the randomized PEARL trial of lasofoxifene in postmenopausal osteoporotic women. *Journal of the National Cancer Institute* 102(22): 1706-15.

Lewis-Wambi, JS & Jordan, VC (2005-2006). Treatment of postmenopausal breast cancer with selective estrogen receptor modulators (SERMs). *Breast Disease* 24: 93-105.

Leyland-Jones, B et al. (2010). Outcome according to CYP 2D6 genotype among postmenopausal women with endocrine-responsive early invasive breast cancer randomized in the BIG 1-98 Trial. Abstract S1-8 presented at the 33rd Annual San Antonio Breast Cancer Symposium, San Antonio, TX, 8-12 December.

Li, CI et al. (2010). Alcohol consumption and risk of postmenopausal breast cancer by subtype: The Women's Health Initiative Observational Study. *Journal of the National Cancer Institute* 102(18): 1422-31.

Lurie, G et al. (2007). Association of estrogen and progestin potency of oral contraceptives with ovarian carcinoma risk. *Obstetrics and Gynaecology* 109(3): 597-607.

Mayo Clinic Staff (2011). *Monoclonal antibody drugs for cancer treatment: How they work.* January 2011 http://www.mayoclinic.com/health/monoclonal-antibody/CA00082

McLemore, MR (2006). Gardasil: Introducing the new human papilloma virus vaccine. *Clinical Journal of Oncology Nursing* 10(5): 559-60.

Menon, U et al. (2005). Prospective study using the risk of ovarian cancer algorithm to screen for ovarian cancer. *Journal of Clinical Oncology* 23(31): 7919-26.

Miglioretti, DL et al. (2010). Accuracy of screening mammography varies by week of menstrual cycle. *Radiology* 258(2): 372-9.

Moreira, C & Kaklamani, V (2010). Lapatinib and breast cancer: Current indications and outlook for the future. *Expert Review of Anticancer Therapy* 10(8): 1171-82.

Moreno, V et al. (2002). Effect of oral contraceptives on risk of cervical cancer in women with human papillomavirus infection: The IARC multicentric case-control study. *The Lancet* 359(9312): 1085-92.

Munoz, N et al. (2002). Role of parity and human papillomavirus in cervical cancer: The IARC multicentric case-control study. *The Lancet* 359(9312): 1093-101.

Musa, MA et al. (2007). Medicinal chemistry and emerging strategies applied to the development of selective estrogen receptor modulators (SERMs). *Current Medicinal Chemistry* 14(11): 1249-61.

Naieralski, J (1998). *Alcohol and the risk of breast cancer.* Program on Breast Cancer and Environmental Risk Factors, Cornell University (BCERF). Available online: http://envirocancer.cornell.edu/factsheet/diet/fs13. alcohol.cfm

Nandur, R et al. (2004). Cardiovascular actions of selective estrogen receptor modulators and phytoestrogens. *Preventative Cardiology* 9(2): 73-9.

Nelson, HD et al. (2009). Screening for breast cancer: An update for the US Preventive Services Task Force. *Annals of Internal Medicine* 151(10): 727-37, W237-742.

Nielsen, M et al. (2010). Breast density changes associated with postmenopausal hormone therapy: Post hoc radiologist- and computer-based analyses. *Menopause: The Journal of the North American Menopause Society* 17(4): 772-8.

Nolan, T et al. (2004). HRT and SERMS: New guidelines for patient management-Part 1. *Medscape Ob/Gyn & Women's Health.* Available online: http://www.medscape.com/viewarticle/448832_25

Olsen, O & Gøtzsche, PC (2001). Screening for breast cancer with mammography. *Cochrane Database of Systematic Reviews,* 4 (CD001877). doi: 10.1002/14651858.CD001877.

Oncology Channel. (2005). *Endometrial cancer.* http://www.healthcommunities.com/endometrial-cancer/overview.shtml

Peckham, C (2010). *More mammography studies – will they resolve the debate? A response from the ACR.* Interview with Carol H Lee, MD, Chair of the American College of Radiology Breast Imaging. Available online: http://www.medscape.com/viewarticle/730281

Perez, E et al. (2005). Women with early stage, HER2-positive breast cancer. *American Society of Clinical Oncology* Annual Meeting: 419-24.

Petitti, DB et al. (2010). Breast cancer screening: From science to recommendation. *Radiology* 256(1): 8-14.

Pinkerton, JV & Goldstein, SR (2010). Endometrial safety: A key hurdle for selective estrogen receptor modulators in development. Review article. *Menopause: The Journal of the North American Menopause Society* 17(3): 642-53.

Pinsky, RW & Helvie, MA (2010). Mammographic breast density: Effect on imaging and breast cancer risk. *NCCN –Journal of the National Comprehensive Cancer Network* 8(10): 1157-65.

Phipps, AI et al. (2011). Body size, physical activity, and risk of triple-negative and estrogen receptor-positive breast cancer. *Cancer Epidemiology, Biomarkers & Prevention* 20(3): 454-63.

Phipps, AI et al. (2011). Reproductive history and oral contraceptive use in relation to risk of triple-negative breast cancer. *Journal of the National Cancer Institute* 103(6): 470-7.

Pritchard, K (2004). *Impact of the Women's Health Initiative (WHI) on the practising oncologist: Putting the WHI results into perspective.* American Society of Clinical Oncology (ASCO) Annual Meeting. Available online: http://www.asco.org/ac/1,1003,12-002673-00_18-0026-00_19-00543-00_29-00E,00.asp

Radiological Society of North America (RSNA) (2010). *Yearly mammograms starting at age 40: Cut mastectomy risk in half.* 96th Scientific Assembly and Annual Meeting. Abstract SSQ01- 08 presented 2 December 2010.

Rae, JM et al. (2010). Lack of correlation between gene variants in tamoxifen metabolizing enzymes with primary endpoints in the ATAC trial. Abstract S1-7 presented at: 33rd Annual San Antonio Breast Cancer Symposium; San Antonio, TX, 8-12 December 2010.

Rebbeck, TR et al. (2009). Meta-analysis of risk reduction estimates associated with risk-reducing salpingo-oophorectomy in BRCA1 or BRCA2 mutation carriers. *Journal of the National Cancer Institute* 101(2): 80-7.

Richardson, LC et al. (2010). Vital signs: Breast cancer screening among women aged 50-74 years – United States, 2008. *Morbidity & Mortality Weekly Report* 59(26): 813-6.

Rodriguez, AC et al. (2010). Longitudinal study of human papillomavirus persistence and cervical intraepithelial neoplasia grade 2/3: Critical role of duration of infection. *Journal of the National Cancer Institute* 102(5): 315-24.

Rojas, M et al. (2005). Follow-up strategies for women treated for early breast cancer. *Cochrane Database Systems Review*, 1: CD001768.

Rossing, MA et al. (2010). Predictive value of symptoms for early detection of ovarian cancer. *Journal of the National Cancer Institute* 102(4): 222-9.

Salvador, S et al. (2009). The fallopian tube: Primary site of most pelvic high-grade serous carcinomas. *International Journal of Gynecological Cancer* 19(1): 58-64.

Saraiya, M et al. (2010). Cervical cancer screening with both human papillomavirus and Papanicolaou testing vs Papanicolaou testing alone: What screening intervals are physicians recommending? *Archives of Internal Medicine* 170(11): 977-86.

Saxena, T et al. (2010). Menopausal hormone therapy and subsequent risk of specific invasive breast cancer subtypes in the California Teachers' Study. *Cancer Epidemiology, Biomarkers and Prevention* 9(9): 2366-78.

Schueler, KM et al. (2008). Factors associated with mammography utilization: A systematic quantitative review of the literature. *Journal of Women's Health* 17(9): 1477-9.

Scott Lind, D (2004). Breast complaints ACS surgery. WebMD 5: 1-16. Available online: http://www.acssurgery.com:6200/wnis/acs_0604a.htm-66k

Shaver, JLF (2010). Ameliorating hot flashes/awakenings in the context of breast cancer treatments. Editorial. *Menopause: The Journal of the North American Menopause Society* 17(5): 889-91.

Smith, RA et al. (2004). The randomized trials of breast cancer screening: What have we learned? *Radiologic Clinics of North America* 42(5): 793-806.

Smith, RP et al. (2011). Breast cancer risk assessment: Positive predictive value of family history as a predictor of risk. *Menopause: The Journal of the North American Menopause Society* 18(6): 621-4.

Sporn, MB (2004). Commentary re CJ Fabian et al., Breast cancer chemoprevention phase I evaluation of biomarker modulation by arzoxifene, a third generation selective estrogen receptor modulator. *Clinical Cancer Research* 10(16): 5403-17.

Stefanek, ME et al. (2010). Mammography and women under 50: Déjà vu all over again? *Cancer Epidemiology Biomarkers & Prevention* 19(3): 635-9.

Strasser-Weippl, K & Goss, PE (2005). Advances in adjuvant hormonal therapy for postmenopausal Women. *Journal of Clinical Oncology* 23(8): 1751-9.

Tang, T (2003). Questions and answers about the CA-125 test. *John Hopkins Pathology*. Available online: http://www.ovariancancer.jhmi.edu/ca125qa.cfm

Telli, ML (2007). Trastuzumab-related cardiotoxicity: Calling into question the concept of reversibility. *Journal of Clinical Oncology* 25(23): 3525-33.

The Merck Manual Second Home Edition, Chapter 216: Paget's Disease skin cancer. USA: Merck & Co. Inc. Available online: http://www.merck.com/mmhe/sec08/ch113/ch113d.html

Trottier, H et al. (2010). Human papillomavirus infection and the role of sexual activity and natural immunity. *Cancer Research* 70(21): 8569-77.

Tsilidis, K on behalf of the EPIC collaborators. (2010). Menopausal hormone therapy and risk of ovarian cancer in the European Prospective Investigation into Cancer and Nutrition. Program and abstracts of the Ninth Annual American Association for Cancer Research Frontiers in Cancer Prevention Research Conference, Philadelphia, Pennsylvania, 7-10 November, 2010.

Tu, CM (2009). Trastuzumab (Herceptin)-associated cardiomyopathy presented as new onset of complete left bundle-branch block mimicking acute coronary syndrome: A case report and literature review. *American Journal of Emergency Medicine* 27(7): 903 e1-3.

US Preventive Services Task Force (2009). Screening for breast cancer: US Preventive Services Task Force recommendation statement. Agency for Healthcare Research and Quality, Rockville, Maryland. *Annals of Internal Medicine* 151(10): 716-26.

Van Veen, WA & Knottnerus, JA (2002). The evidence to support mammography screening. *Netherlands Journal of Medicine (Amsterdam)* 60(5): 200-6.

Vogel, VG (2006). Managing breast cancer risk in postmenopausal women. *Menopause Management* 16(s1): 19-21.

Vogel, VG et al. (2010). Update of the National Surgical Adjuvant Breast and Bowel Project Study of Tamoxifen and Raloxifene (STAR) P-2 Trial: Preventing breast cancer. *Cancer Prevention Research* 3(6): 696-706.

Widdice, LE & Kahn, JA (2006). Using the new HPV vaccines in clinical practices. *Cleveland Clinical Journal of Medicine* 73(10): 929-35.

Winer, EP (2005). *American Society of Clinical Oncology* technology assessment on the use of aromatase inhibitors as adjuvant therapy for postmenopausal women with hormone receptor-positive breast cancer: Status Report 2004. *American Society of Clinical Oncology* 23(3): 619-29.

Wu, Y et al. (2011). Impact of lapatinib plus trastuzumab versus single-agent lapatinib on quality of life of patients with trastuzumab-refractory HER2+ metastatic breast cancer. *Annals of Oncology*, 15 March 2011. [Epub ahead of print.]

Yu, B et al. (2007). Structural modulation of reactivity/activity in design of improved benzothiophene selective estrogen receptor modulators: Induction of chemopreventive mechanisms. *Molecular Cancer Therapeutics* 6(9): 2418-28.

Zebecchi, L et al. (2003). Comprehensive menopausal assessment: An approach to managing vasomotor and urogenital symptoms in breast cancer survivors. *Oncology Nursing Forum* 30(3): 393-405.

Zielinski, SL (2005). Hormone replacement therapy for breast cancer survivors: An unanswered question? *Journal of the National Cancer Institute*, 97(13): 955.

Available online

http://dictionary.laborlawtalk.com/

http://envirocancer.cornell.edu/factsheet/diet/fs13.alcohol.cfm

http://www.answers.com/ovarian%20cancer

http://www.answers.com/ovarian+cyst&r=67

http://www.cancer.org

http://www.cancerbackup.org.uk/Cancertype/Breast/Causes-diagnosis/HER2testing

http://www.cancer.gov/cancertopics/types/colon-and-rectal

http://www.cancer.org/Cancer/BreastCancer/OverviewGuide/index

http://www.cancer.org/Cancer/ColonandRectumCancer/index

http://www.cancer.org/docroot/CRI/content/CRI

http://www.cancer.gov/bcrisktool/about-tool.aspx#gailhttp://www.cochrane.org

http://www.cdc.gov/cancer/colorectal/basic_info/screening/guidelines.htm

http://www.drsuzman.com/procedureset.htm

http://www.girlzone.com?FEMedia?RareBreastCancer.html

http://www.infoforyourhealth.com/Cancer/ovarian%20cancer.htm

http://www.mayoclinic.com/health/breast-cancer/AN00495

http://www.medicinenet.com/endometriosis/page4.htm

http://www.medicinenet.com/ovaraian-cancer/article.htm

http://www.medicinenet.com/ovarian_cysts/index.htm

http://www.oncologychannel.com/ovariancancer/

http://www.positivehealth.com/permit/Articles/Nutrition/byrnes64.htm

Chapter 9

Adochi, JD & Cosman, F (2007). Osteoporosis: A disease across the skeleton. *Menopause Management* 16(1): 22-4.

Aftab, M et al. (2003). Effects of growth hormone replacement on parathyroid hormone sensitivity and bone mineral metabolism. *Journal of Clinical Endocrinology & Metabolism* 88(6): 2860-8.

Akesson, K et al. (1997). Rationale for active vitamin D analog therapy in senile osteoporosis. *Calcified Tissue International* 60(1): 100-5.

Al-Ghazal, SK et al. (2000). The psychological impact of immediate rather than delayed breast reconstruction. *European Journal of Surgical Oncology* 26(1): 17-9.

Aragon-Ching, JB (2011). Unravelling the role of denosumab in prostate cancer. *The Lancet* 377(9768):785-6.

Balasubramanyam, A (2005). *Osteoporosis: New insights and novel treatments.* Available online: http://www.medscape.com/viewarticle/510285

Barclay, L (2004). Exercise program improves osteoporosis. *Medscape Ob/Gyn & Women's Health.* Available online: http://www.medscape.com/viewarticle/478726

Barclay, L (2004). Long-term use of alendronate continues to protect against osteoporosis. *Medscape Medical News.* Available online: http://www.medscape.com/viewarticle/471934

Birge, S (2007). Non-vertebral osteoporotic fractures: A brain disease or bone disease. *Menopause: The Journal of the North American Menopause Society* 14(1): 1-2.

Bischoff-Ferrari, H (2007). How to select the doses of vitamin D in the management of osteoporosis. *Osteoporosis International* 18(4): 401-7.

Bischoff-Ferrari, HA et al. (2006). Effect of calcium supplementation on fracture risk: A double-blind randomized controlled trial. *Journal of Bone & Mineral Research* 21: s1-530.

Bischoff-Ferrari, HA et al. (2006). Estimation of optimal serum concentrations of 25-hydroxyvitamin D for multiple health outcomes. *American Journal of Clinical Nutrition* 84(1): 18-28.

Biskobing, DM et al. (2002). Novel therapeutic options for osteoporosis. *Current Opinion in Rheumatology* 14(4): 447-52.

Bjarnason, NH & Christiansen, C (2000). The influence of thinness and smoking on bone loss and response to hormone replacement therapy in early postmenopausal women. *Journal of Clinical Endocrinology and Metabolism* 85(2): 590-6.

Black, D (2004). *Which regions of spine and hip should be used to assess osteoporosis and/or risk of fracture?* Available online: http://www.medscape.com/viewarticle/470473

Bliuc, D et al. (2005). Barriers to effective management of osteoporosis in moderate and minimal trauma fractures: a prospective study. *Osteoporosis International* 16(8): 977-82.

Boonen, S et al. (2007). Need for additional calcium to reduce the risk of hip fracture with vitamin D supplementation: Evidence from a comparative meta-analysis of randomized controlled trials. *Journal of Clinical Endocrinology & Metabolism* 92(4): 1415-23.

Boonen, S et al. (2011). Treatment with denosumab reduces the incidence of new vertebral and hip fractures in postmenopausal women at high risk. *Journal of Clinical Endocrinology & Metabolism* 96(6): 1727-36.

Brooke-Wavell, K (1997). Brisk walking reduces calcaneal bone loss in post-menopausal women. *Clinical Science* 92(1): 75-80.

Brown, JP et al. (2009). Bone turnover markers in the management of postmenopausal osteoporosis. *Clinical Biochemistry* 42(10-11): 929-42.

Brown, S (1996). *Better bones, better body: Beyond estrogen and calcium – a comprehensive self-help program for preventing, halting and overcoming osteoporosis.* New Canaan, CT: Keats Publishing Inc.

Centers for Disease Control and Prevention (CDC) (2004). Awareness of family health history as a risk factor for disease – United States. *Morbidity & Mortality Weekly Report* 53(44): 1044-7.

Chambliss, KL et al. (2010). Non-nuclear estrogen receptor alpha signaling promotes cardiovascular protection but not uterine or breast cancer growth in mice. *Journal of Clinical Investigation*, 120(7): 2319-30.

Clegg, D et al. (2006). Glucosamine, chondroitin sulfate and the two in combination for painful knee osteoarthritis. *New England Journal of Medicine* 354(8): 795-808.

Coetzee, M & Kruger, MC (2004). Osteoprotegerin-receptor activator of nuclear factor [kappa] B lignan ratio: A new approach to osteoporosis treatment? *Southern Medical Journal* 97(5): 506-11.

Colon-Emeric, CS et al. (2004). The HORIZON Recurrent Fracture Trial: Design of a clinical trial in the prevention of subsequent fractures after low trauma hip fracture repair. *Current Medical Research Opinions* 20(6): 903-10.

Compston, JE (2001). Sex steroids and bone. *Physiological Reviews* 81(1): 419-47.

Cornuz, J et al. (1999). Smoking, smoking cessation, and risk of hip fracture in women. *American Journal of Medicine* 106(3): 311-4.

Cortet, B et al. (2004). Does quantitative ultrasound of bone reflect more bone mineral density than bone microarchitecture? *Calcified Tissue International* 74(1): 60-7.

Cosman, F (2003). Selective estrogen-receptor modulators. *Clinics in Geriatric Medicine* 19(2): 371-9.

Cosman, F (2007). Secondary causes of postmenopausal osteoporosis. *Menopause Management* 16(1): 22-4.

Cox, D et al. (2004). Effect of raloxifene on the incidence of elevated low-density lipoprotein (LDL) and achievement of LDL target goals in postmenopausal women. *Current Medical Research & Opinion* 20(7): 1049-55.

Crandall, C (2002). Combination treatment of osteoporosis: A clinical review. *Journal of Women's Health and Gender Based Medicine* 11(3): 211-24.

Cranney, A et al. (2006). Parathyroid hormone for the treatment of osteoporosis: A systematic review. *Canadian Medical Association Journal* 175(1): 52-9.

Crans, GG et al. (2004). Association of severe vertebral fractures with reduced quality of life: Reduction in the incidence of severe vertebral fractures by teriparatide. *Arthritis & Rheumatism* 50(12): 4028-34.

Cummings, SR et al. (2008). The effects of lasofoxifene on fractures and breast cancer: 3-year results from the PEARL trial. *Journal of Bone Mineral Research* 23(1 Suppl.): S81-4.

Cummings, SR et al., for the FREEDOM Trial (2009). Denosumab for prevention of fractures in postmenopausal women with osteoporosis. *New England Journal of Medicine* 361(8): 756-65.

Cummings, SR et al., for the LIFT Trial Investigators (2008). The effects of tibolone in older postmenopausal women. *New England Journal of Medicine* 1359(7): 697-708.

Davey, MR (2010). The role of hormone therapy in the treatment of osteoporosis: A review Article. *Journal of Endocrinology,* Metabolism and Diabetes of South Africa 15(1): 49-51.

Dawson Hughes, B & Mayer, J (2010). *New NOF guidelines.* USDA Human Nutrition Center on Aging. 3rd Plenary Symposium and 21st Annual Meeting of the North American Menopause Society, Chicago, IL, 6-9 October 2010.

Dennison, E (2003). Growth hormone predicts bone density in elderly women. *Bone* 32(4): 434-40.

Doggrell, SA (2003). Present and future pharmacotherapy for osteoporosis. *Drugs Today* 39(8): 633-57.

Dosa, L (2003). *Teriparatide reduces fracture-related back pain over long term.* Available online: http://www.medscape.com/viewarticle/463526

Edwards, BJ et al. (2010). Functional decline after incident wrist fractures study of osteoporotic fractures: Prospective cohort study. *BMJ* 341: c3324.

Emkey, R (2004). Alendronate and risedronate for the treatment of postmenopausal osteoporosis: Clinical profiles of the once-weekly and once-daily dosing formations. *Medscape General Medicine* 6(3). Available online: http://www.med-scape.com/viewarticle/480498_print

Farley, D (1997). *Bone builders: Support your bones with healthy habits.* US Food and Drug Administration, FDA Consumer, September – October.

Fielding, RA (1995). The role of progressive resistance training and nutrition in the preservation of lean body mass in the elderly. *Journal of American College Nutrition* 14(6): 587-94.

Fizazi, K et al. (2011). Denosumab versus zoledronic acid for treatment of bone metastases in men with castration-resistant prostate cancer: A randomised, double-blind study. *The Lancet* 377(9768): 813-22.

Follin, SL & Hansen, LB (2003). Current approaches to the prevention and treatment of postmenopausal osteoporosis. *American Journal Health System Pharmacy* 60(9): 883-901.

Gallagher, JC (2007). Effect of early menopause on bone mineral density and fractures. *Menopause: The Journal of the North American Menopause Society.* 14(3): 567-71.

Gallagher, JC & Sai, AJ (2010). Bone: Is screening for secondary causes of osteoporosis worthwhile. *Nature Reviews Endocrinology* 6(7): 360-2.

Gallagher, JC & Levine, P (2011). Preventing osteoporosis in symptomatic postmenopausal women. *Menopause: The Journal of the North American Menopause Society* 18(1): 109-18.

Gallagher, JC & Sai, AJ (2010). Molecular biology of bone remodeling: Implications for new therapeutic targets for osteoporosis. *Maturitas* 65(4): 301-7.

Germano, C & Cabot, M (1999). *The osteoporosis solution: New therapies for prevention and treatment.* New York: Kensington Books.

Geusens, P & Boonen, S (2002). Osteoporosis and the growth hormone-insulin-like growth factor axis. *Hormone Research* 58(3 Suppl.): 49-55.

Greenspan, SL et al. (2007). Effect of recombinant human parathyroid hormone (1-84) on vertebral fracture and bone mineral density in postmenopausal women with osteoporosis: A randomized trial. *Annals of Internal Medicine* 146(5): 326-39.

Gold, DT, Lee, LS & Tresolini, CP (Eds) (2001). *Working with patients to prevent, treat and manage osteoporosis: A curriculum guide for the health professions,* 3rd ed. Center for the Study of Aging and Human Development, Duke University, Durham.

Hadji, P et al. (2009). The effect of exemestane or tamoxifen on markers of bone turnover: Results of a German sub-study of the Tamoxifen Exemestane Adjuvant Multicentre (TEAM) trial. *Breast* 18(3): 159-64.

Harris, ST et al. (1999). Effects of risedronate treatment on vertebral and nonvertebral fractures in women with postmenopausal osteoporosis: A randomized controlled trial. Vertebral Efficacy with Risedronate Therapy (VERT) Study Group. *Journal of the American Medical Association* 282(14): 1344-52.

Hartard, M et al. (1996). Systematic strength training as a model of therapeutic intervention: A controlled trial in postmenopausal women with osteopenia. *American Journal of Physical Medicine & Rehabilitation* 75(1): 21-8.

Health Encyclopedia. Hip fracture. Available online: http://www.healthscout.com/ency/68/110/main.html.

Heaney, RP (2003). Long-latency deficiency disease: Insights from calcium and Vitamin D. *American Journal of Clinical Nutrition* 78(5): 912-9.

Henry, DH et al. (2011). Randomized, double-blind study of denosumab versus zoledronic acid in the treatment of bone metastases in patients with advanced cancer (excluding breast and prostate cancer) or multiple myeloma. *Journal of Clinical Oncology* 29(9): 1125-32.

Hill, AP (2007). Hormone therapy and oral health. *Menopause: The Journal of the North American Menopause Society* 16(3): 16-40.

Hodsman, A et al. (2003). Efficacy and safety of human parathyroid hormone (1-84) in increasing bone mineral density in postmenopausal osteoporosis. *Journal of Clinical Endocrinology & Metabolism* 88(11): 5212-20.

Hoidrup, S et al. (2000). Tobacco smoking and risk of hip fracture in men and women. International Journal of Epidemiology 29(2): 253-9.

Holick, M et al. (2011). Evaluation, treatment, and prevention of vitamin D deficiency: An Endocrine Society clinical practice guideline. *Journal of Clinical Endocrinology & Metabolism* 6 June: 38.

Holden, M (2005). PILATES: The best kept secret in back rehabilitation. Available online: http://www.medic8. com/health-guide/articles/pilates.html

Ives, JC & Sosnoff, J (2000). Beyond the mind-body exercise hype. *The Physician and Sports Medicine* 28(3): 67-81.

Jean Hailes Foundation for Women's Health (2004). *Definition of osteoporosis*. http://www.bonehealthforlife.org

Jean Hailes Foundation for Women's Health (2011). *Interpretation of DEXA measures*. http://www. bonehealthforlife.org

Kagan, R (2009). *After stopping HT bisphosphonates as prevention for prophylactic therapy?* NAMS Menopause e-Consult newsletter, 5(3).

Kanis, J et al. (2005). Assessment of fracture risk. *Osteoporosis International* 16(3): 581-9.

Karim, R et al. (2010). *Increase in incidence of hip fracture in postmenopausal women after cessation of hormone therapy: Data from a large health management organization.* Plenary Scientific Abstract Session, Abstract S-1. 21st Annual Meeting of the North American Menopause Society, Chicago, IL, 6-9 October 2010.

Kasukawa, Y et al. (2004). The anabolic effects of GH/IGF system on bone. *Current Pharmaceutical Design* 10(21): 2577-92.

Kauppenhein, M et al. (2002). Design, material and methods in the NORA study (Nordic Research on Ageing). *Aging Clinical and Experimental Research* 14(3 Suppl.): 5-9.

Katz, W & Sherman, C (1998). Exercise for osteoporosis. *The Physician and Sports Medicine* 26(2): 43.

Katz, WA & Sherman, C (1998). Osteoporosis: The role of exercise in optimal management. *The Physician and Sports Medicine* 26(2): 33-42.

Kelley, GA et al. (2001). Resistance training and bone mineral density in women: A meta-analysis of controlled trials. *American Journal of Physical and Medical Rehabilitation* 80(1): 65-77.

Krall, EA & Dawson-Hughes, B (1994). Walking is related to bone density and rates of bone loss. *American Journal of Medicine* 96(1): 20-6.

Kremer, C et al. (2000). Patient satisfaction with outpatient hysteroscopy versus day case hysteroscopy: Randomised controlled trial. *BMJ* 320(7230): 279-82.

Lang, T et al. (2004). Cortical and trabecular bone mineral loss from the spine and hip in long-duration space flight. *Journal of Bone & Mineral Research* 19(6): 1006-12.

Langsetmo, L et al. (2011). Dietary patterns and incident low-trauma fractures in postmenopausal women and men aged ≥50 y: A population-based cohort study. *American Journal of Clinical Nutrition* 93(1): 192-9.

Lemaire, V et al. (2004). Modeling the interactions between osteoblast and osteoclast activities in bone remodeling. *Journal of Theoretical Biology* 229(3): 293-309.

Lewiecki, EM et al. (2008). Santa Fe Bone Symposium: Update on osteoporosis. *Journal of Clinical Densitometry* 12(2): 135-57.

Lian, J, Gorski, J & Ott, S (2004). *Bone curriculum: Bone structure and function.* American Society for Bone Mineral Research.

Lindsay, R et al. (1997). Randomised controlled study of effect of parathyroid hormone on vertebral-bone mass and fracture incidence among postmenopausal women on oestrogen with osteoporosis. *The Lancet* 350(9077): 550-5.

Lindsay, R et al. (2002). Effect of lower doses of conjugated equine estrogens with and without medroxyprogesterone acetate in early postmenopausal women. *Journal of the American Medical Association* 287(20): 2668-76.

Lindsay, R et al. (2004). Sustained vertebral fracture risk reduction after withdrawal of teriparatide in postmenopausal women with osteoporosis. *Archives of Internal Medicine* 164(18): 2024-30.

Liu, J et al. (2009). Effect of long-term intervention of soy isoflavones on bone mineral density in women: A meta-analysis of randomized controlled trials. *Bone* 44(5): 948-53.

Liu-Ambrose, T et al. (2004). Resistance and agility training reduce fall risk in women aged 75 to 85 with low bone mass: A 6-month randomised controlled trial. *Journal of the American Geriatrics Society* 52(5): 657-65.

Luckey, MM. (2010). *FRAX update: Issues in practice*. 21st Annual Meeting of the North American Menopause Society, Chicago, IL, 6-9 October.

Manson, JE (2010). *Vitamin D: Spotlight on the sunshine vitamin*. 11th Plenary Symposium, 21st Annual Meeting of the North American Menopause Society, Chicago, IL, 6-9 October.

Maricic, M et al. (2002). Early effects of raloxifene on clinical vertebral fractures at 12 months in postmenopausal women with osteoporosis. *Archives of Internal Medicine* 162(10): 1140-3.

McClung, M et al. (2006). Prevention of bone loss in postmenopausal women treated with lasofoxifene compared with raloxifene. *Menopause: The Journal of the North American Menopause Society* 13(3): 377-86.

McLean, RR et al. (2004). High homocysteine levels linked to fracture risk in two reports. *New England Journal of Medicine* 350: 2042-9. First to Know, North American Menopause Society, released June 2004.

McTiernan, A et al. (2004). Effect of exercise on serum estrogens in postmenopausal women: A 12-month randomized clinical trial. *Cancer Research* 64(8): 2923-8.

Mendelsohn, ME & Karas, RH (2010). Rapid progress for non-nuclear estrogen receptor signaling. *Journal of Clinical Investigation* 120(7): 2277-9.

Meunier, PJ et al. (2004). The effects of strontium ranelate on the risk of vertebral fracture in women with postmenopausal osteoporosis. *New England Journal of Medicine* 350(5): 459-68.

Miller, L et al. (2004). Bone mineral density in postmenopausal women: Does exercise training make a difference? *The Physician and Sports Medicine* 32(2): 18-24.

National Institutes of Health (NIH) (1994). NIH Consensus Development Panel on optimal calcium intake. *Journal of the American Medical Association* 272(24): 1942-8.

National Osteoporosis Foundation (2008). *Clinician's guide to prevention and treatment of osteoporosis.*: National Osteoporosis Foundation, Washington DC.

North American Menopause Society (2006). Management of osteoporosis in postmenopausal women: Position statement of the North American Menopause Society. *Menopause: The Journal of the North American Menopause Society* 13(3): 340-67.

North American Menopause Society (2010). 21st Annual Meeting of the North American Menopause Society, Chicago, IL, 6-9 October.

North American Menopause Society (2010). Management of osteoporosis in postmenopausal women: Position statement of the North American Menopause Society. NAMS Continuing Medical Education Activity. *Menopause: The Journal of the North American Menopause Society* 17(1): 23-55.

Orenstein, B (2004). Lost in space: Bone mass. *Radiology Today* 5(6): 10.

Peck, P (2004). Ultra-low dose estradiol patch stops bone turnover, increases bone density. *Medscape Medical News*. Available online: http://www.medscape.com/viewarticle/475033

Pouilles, JM et al. (1995). Effect of menopause on femoral and vertebral bone loss. *Journal of Bone and Mineral Metabolism* 10(10): 1534-6.

Rachner ,TD et al. (2011). Osteoporosis: Now and the future. *The Lancet* 377(9773): 1276-87.

Rapuri, PB et al. (2000). Smoking and bone metabolism in elderly women. *Bone* 27(3): 429-36.

Reginster, JY et al. (2004). Strontium ranelate: A new paradigm in the treatment of osteoporosis. *Expert Opinion on Investigational Drugs* 13(7): 857-64.

Reginster, JY et al. (2005). Strontium ranelate reduces the risk of non-vertebral fractures in postmenopausal women with osteoporosis: TROPOS study. *Journal of Clinical Endocrinology & Metabolism* 90(5): 2816-22.

Richman, S et al. (2006). Low dose estrogen therapy for prevention of osteoporosis: Working our way back to monotherapy. *Menopause: The Journal of the North American Menopause Society* 13(1): 148-55.

Riera-Espinoza, G et al. (2004). Changes in bone turnover during tibolone treatment. *Maturitas* 47(2): 83-90.

Ringa, V (2004). Alternatives to hormone replacement therapy for menopause: An epidemiological evaluation. *Journal de Gynecologie, Obstetrique et Biologie de la Reproduction (Paris)* 33(3): 195-209.

Ross, AC et al. (2010). *DRI dietary reference intakes: Calcium, vitamin D*. Committee to Review Dietary Reference Intakes for Vitamin D and Calcium. Food and Nutrition Board. National Academies Press, Washington, DC.

Rowland, JH et al. (2000). Role of breast reconstructive surgery in physical and emotional outcomes among breast cancer survivors. *Journal of National Cancer Institute* 6 September, 92(17): 1422-9. Erratum in: *Journal of National Cancer Institute* 2001, 93(1): 68.

Rymer, J et al. (2002). Ten years of treatment with tibolone 2.5mg daily: Effects on bone loss in postmenopausal women. *Climacteric* 5(4): 390-8.

Sai, AJ et al. (2011). Relationship between vitamin D, parathyroid hormone, and bone health. *Journal of Clinical Endocrinology & Metabolism*. 96(3): E436-46.

Sambrook, PN et al. (2004). Alendronate produces greater effects than raloxifene on bone density and bone turnover in postmenopausal women with low bone density. *Journal of Internal Medicine* 255(4): 503-11.

Sartori, L et al. (2003). Injectable bisphosphonates in the treatment of postmenopausal osteoporosis. *Aging-Clinical & Experimental Research* 15(4): 271-83.

Sawicki, A et al. (2004). Strontium ranelate reduces the risk of vertebral fractures in postmenopausal women. *Calcified Tissue International* 74 (s84): 153.

Sawitzke, AD et al. (2010). Two-year GAIT study results: June 2010. *Annals of Rheumatic Diseases* 69(8): 1459-64.

Scott-Lind, D et al. (2004). Breast procedures. ACS Surgery: *Principles and Practice* (5): 1-16. Available online: http://www.acssurgery.com/sample/ACS0305.pdf

Seeman, E (2007). Is change in bone mineral density a sensitive and specific surrogate of anti fracture efficacy? *Bone* 41(3): 308-17.

Seeman, E et al. (2006). Strontium ranelate reduces the risk of vertebral and non-vertebral fractures in women eighty years or older. *Journal of Bone & Mineral Research* 21(7): 1113-20.

Shangold, M & Sherman, C (1998). Exercise and menopause: A time for positive changes. *The Physician and Sports Medicine* 26(12): 45-50.

Slipman, C et al. (2004). Osteoporosis (secondary). *eMedicine*. Available online: http://www.emedicine.com/pmr/topic95.htm

Ste-Marie, LS (2011). Novel study confirms strontium ranelate's bone-forming benefits. European Congress on Osteoporosis and Osteoarthritis. Abstract OC16 presented 24 March 2011.

Swegle, JM & Kelly, MV (2004). Tibolone: A unique version of hormone replacement therapy. *Annals of Pharmacotherapy* 38(5): 874-81.

Tekeoglu, I et al. (2005). Comparison of cyclic and continuous calcitonin regimens in the treatment of postmenopausal osteoporosis. *Rheumatology International*, 26(2): 157-61.

US Preventative Task Force (2011). Screening for osteoporosis: US Preventative Task Force recommendation statement. *Annals of Internal Medicine* 154(5): 356-64.

Ward, KD & Klesges, RC (2001). A meta-analysis of the effects of cigarette smoking on bone mineral density. *Calcified Tissue International* 68(5): 259-70.

Watts, NB et al. (2009). FRAX facts. *Journal of Bone and Mineral Research* 24(6): 975-9.

West, H (2011). Denosumab for prevention of skeletal-related events in patients with bone metastases from solid tumors: Incremental benefit, debatable value. *Journal of Clinical Oncology* 29(9): 1095-8.

Wilkins, EG et al. (2000). Prospective analysis of psychosocial outcomes in breast reconstruction: One-year postoperative results from the Michigan Breast Reconstruction Outcome Study. *Plastic Reconstructive Surgery* 106(5): 1014-25; discussion 1026-7.

World Health Organization (WHO) (2009). *FRAX: WHO risk assessment tool*. Collaborating Centre for Metabolic Bone Diseases. Available at: http://www.shef.ac.uk/FRAX; accessed 30 June 2009.

Ylikorkala, O & Metsa-Heikkila, M (2002). Hormone replacement therapy in women with a history of breast cancer. *Gynecological Endocrinology* 16(6): 469-78.

Yu, Z et al. (2004). Two to three years of hormone replacement therapy in healthy women have long term preventative effects on bone mass and osteoporotic fractures: The PERF study. *Bone* 34(4): 728-35.

Available online

http://arbl.cvmbs.colostate.edu/hbooks/pathphys/endocrine/thyroid/calcitonin.html
http://arbl.cvmbs.colostate.edu/hbooks/pathphys/endocrine/thyroid/pth.html
http://members.optushome.com.au/physio/glossa_m.html
http://www.4collegewomen.org/fact-sheets/osteoporosis.html
http://www.britannica.com/eb/article?tocId=9033466
http://www.earlymenopause.com/calcium.htm
http://www.e-ds.com/healthinfo_view/i_00000007B9./e-MedspatientEducationCalciumImbalance
http://www.emedicine.com/pmr/topic95.htm
http://www.fore.org/patients/bmd_testing.html
http://www.hersource.com/osteo/c1/smoking.cfm
http://www.hyperdictionary.com/medical/cytokines
http://www.infoaging.org/d-osteo-4-cause.html
http://www.meb.uni-bonn.de/cancer.gov/CDR0000062903.html
http://www.medicinenet.com/calcitonin/article.htm
http://www.medscape.com/viewarticle/510285

http://www.nlm.nih.gov/medlineplus/osteoporosis.html
http://www.nof.org/
http://www.opendoorclinic.org/hivglossary.htm
http://www.ozestuaries.org/indicators/Def_decomposition.html
http://www.phoenix5.org/glossary/bisphosphonates.html

Chapter 10

Abbott Labs (2010). Abbott to voluntarily recall Meridia® (sibutramine) in the US. Press release, 8 October 2010. Available online: http://www.abbott.com/global/url/pressRelease/en_US/60.5:5/Press_Release_0908.htm; accessed 28 September 2010.

Arterburn, LM et al. (2006). Distribution, inter conversion, and dose response of n-3 fatty acids in humans. *American Journal of Clinical Nutrition* 83 (Suppl.): S1467-76.

Artinian, NT et al. (2010). Interventions to promote physical activity and dietary lifestyle changes for cardiovascular risk factor reduction in adults: A scientific statement from the American Heart Association. *Circulation* 122(4): 406-11.

Aude, YW et al. (2004). The national cholesterol education program diet vs a diet lower in carbohydrates and higher in protein and monounsaturated fat: A randomized trial. *Archives of Internal Medicine* 164(19): 2141-6.

Avenell, A et al. (2004). What are the long-term benefits of weight reducing diets in adults? A systematic review of randomized controlled trials. *Journal of Human Nutrition and Dietetics* 17(4): 317-35.

Bantle, JP (2004). Weight management and type 2 diabetes. *Medscape Diabetes & Endocrinology* 6(1). Available online: http://www.medscape.com/viewarticle/473049

Barclay, L (2004). Obesity increases risk of false-positive mammograms. *Medscape General Medicine.* Available online: http://www.medscape.com/viewarticle/479111?src=mp

Barclay, L (2004). Relationship of obesity and fitness level to cardiovascular risk and diabetes. *Medscape Medical News.* Available online: http://www.medscape.com/viewarticle/488814_print

Barlovic, DP et al. (2010). Cardiovascular disease: What's all the AGE/RAGE about? *Cardiovascular & Hematological Disorders – Drug Targets* 10(1): 7-15.

Blackburn, GL (2004). Making scientific sense of different dietary approaches, Part 2: Evaluating the diets. *Medscape Diabetes & Endocrinology* 6(1). Available online: http://www.medscape.org/viewarticle/470747

Bravata, DM (2003). Efficacy and safety of low-carbohydrate diets. *Journal of the American Medical Association* 289(14): 1837-46.

Bravata, DM et al. (2007). Using pedometers to increase physical activity and improve health: A systematic review. *Journal of the American Medical Association* 298(19): 2296-2304.

Bray, G (2000). Physiology and consequences of obesity. *Medscape Ob/Gyn & Women's Health.* Available online: http://www.medscape.com/viewprogram/707

Brehm, BJ (2003). A randomized trial comparing a very low carbohydrate diet and a calorie-restricted low fat diet on body weight and cardiovascular risk factors in healthy women. *Journal of Clinical Endocrinology & Metabolism* 88(4): 1617-23.

Canadian Diabetes Association (2011). *Type 2 diabetes: Things you should know.* Available online: http://www.diabetes.ca/diabetes-and-you/living/insulin/should-know/

Carnethon, MR et al. (2004). Risk factors for the metabolic syndrome: The Coronary Artery Risk Development in Young Adults (CARDIA) study, 1985-2001. *Diabetes Care* 27(11): 2707-15.

Carney, PI (2010). Obesity and reproductive hormone levels in the transition to menopause. Editorial. *Menopause: The Journal of the North American Menopause Society* 17(4): 678-9.

Carroll, S & Dudeld, M (2004). What is the relationship between exercise and metabolic abnormalities? A review of the metabolic syndrome. *Sports Medicine* 34(6): 371-418.

Centres for Disease Control and Prevention (2011). Body Mass Index (BMI): About BMI for adults. Department of Health and Human Services. Available online: http://www.cdc.gov/healthyweight/assessing/bmi/adult_bmi/index.html

Cercato, C et al. (2009). A randomized double-blind placebo-controlled study of the long-term efficacy and safety of diethylpropion in the treatment of obese subjects. *International Journal of Obesity (London)* 33(8): 857-65.

Cohen, S et al. (2009). Obesity and screening for breast, cervical, and colorectal cancer in women: A review. *Cancer* 112(9): 1892-904.

Crowther, NJ (2004). The clinical relevance of fasting serum insulin levels in obese subjects. *South African Medical Journal* 94(7): 519-20.

Deon, T & Braun, B (2002). The roles of estrogen and progesterone in regulating carbohydrate and fat utilization at rest and during exercise. *Journal of Women's Health* & Gender Based Medicine 11(3): 225-37.

Douchi, T et al. (2007). Difference in segmental lean and fat mass components between pre- and postmenopausal women. *Menopause: The Journal of the North American Menopause Society* 14(5): 875-8.

Egan, BM et al. (2010). Does dark chocolate have a role in prevention and management of hypertension? Commentary on the evidence. *Hypertension* 55(6): 1289-95.

Engler, MB et al. (2004). Flavonoid-rich dark chocolate improves endothelial function and increases plasma epicatechin concentrations in healthy adults. *Journal of the American College of Nutrition* 23(3): 197-204.

Fayerman, P (2011). A weighty issue: How much sugar is too much? *Vancouver Sun*, 14 March 2011.

Foster, GD et al. (2003). A randomized trial of a low-carbohydrate diet for obesity. *New England Journal of Medicine* 348(21): 2082-90.

Fox, M (2004). Low-carb fad seen as unhealthy and a rip-off. *Reuters Health Information*, 22 June 2004.

Freeman, EW et al. (2010). Obesity and reproductive hormone levels in the transition to menopause. *Menopause: The Journal of the North American Menopause Society* 17(4): 718-26.

Fung, TT et al. (2004). Prospective study of major dietary patterns and stroke risk in women. *Stroke* 35(9): 2014-9.

Fung Low, TT et al. (2010). Carbohydrate diets and all-cause and cause-specific mortality: Two cohort studies. *Annals of Internal Medicine* 153(5): 289-98.

Gallagher, EJ et al. (2008). The metabolic syndrome: From insulin resistance to obesity and diabetes. *Endocrinology Metabolism Clinics of North America* 37(3): 559-79.

Gambacciani, M et al. (1999). *Climacteric* modifications in body weight and fat tissue distribution. *Climacteric* 2(1): 37-44.

Gambacciani, M et al. (2001). Prospective evaluation of body weight and body fat distribution in early postmenopausal women with and without hormonal replacement therapy. *Maturitas* 39(2): 125-32.

Greenway, FL et al. (2010). Effect of naltrexone plus bupropion on weight loss in overweight and obese adults (COR-I): A multicentre, randomised, double-blind, placebo-controlled, phase 3 trial. *The Lancet* 376(9741): 595-605.

Grundy, S et al. (2004). Definition of metabolic syndrome. Report of the National Heart, Lung and Blood Institute/American Heart Association Conference on scientific issues related to definition. *Circulation* 109(3): 433-8.

Hagey, AR & Warren, MP (2006). Exercise and menopause: Positive effects. *Menopause Management* 15(3): 19-25.

Harvard Health Publications (2005). *Answering your questions on trans fats*. Harvard Medical School. Available online: http://www.health.harvard.edu/healthbeat/HEALTHbeat_030205.htm

He, K (2004). Fish consumption and incidence of stroke: A metaanalysis of cohort studies. Stroke 35(7): 1538-42.

HealthCentral.com (2001). *What are the exercise basics?* Available online: http://www.healthcentral.com/fitorfat/408/42759.html

Hendricks, EJ et al. (2009). How physician obesity specialists use drugs to treat obesity. *Obesity* 17(9): 1730-5.

Homehealth.uk.com (2007). What is a healthy balanced diet? Available online: http://www.homehealth-uk.com/medical/healthybalanceddiet.htm

Huang, AJ et al. for the Program to Reduce Incontinence by Diet and Exercise (PRIDE) (2010). An intensive behavioral weight loss intervention and hot flushes in women. *Archives of Internal Medicine* 170(13): 1161-7.

James, WP et al. (2010). Effect of sibutramine on cardiovascular outcomes in overweight and obese subjects. *New England Journal of Medicine* 363(10): 905-17.

Kerr, M (2004). Incidence of metabolic syndrome low when weight is stable. *Medscape Medical News*, *Medscape General Medicine*. Available online: http://www.medscape.com/viewarticle/493446

Knowles, W et al. (2002). Reduction in the incidence of type 2 diabetes with lifestyle intervention or metformin. *New England Journal of Medicine* 346(6): 393-403.

Kulie, T et al. (2011). Obesity and women's health: An evidence-based review. *Journal of the American Board of Family Medicine* 24(1): 75-85.

Kuller, LH et al. (2006). Lifestyle intervention and coronary heart disease risk factor changes over 18 months in postmenopausal women: The Women on the Move Through Activity and Nutrition (WOMAN study) clinical trial. *Journal of Women's Health* 15(8): 962-74.

Larsen, TM et al. for the Diet, Obesity, and Genes (Diogenes) Project. (2010). Diets with high or low protein content and glycemic index for weight loss maintenance. *New England Journal of Medicine* 363(23): 2102-13.

László, B (2003). Central and peripheral fat mass have contrasting effect on the progression of aortic calcification in postmenopausal women. *European Heart Journal* 24(16): 1531-7.

Lemoine, S et al. (2007). Effect of weight reduction on quality of life and eating behaviors in obese women. *Menopause: The Journal of the North American Menopause Society* 14(3): 432-40.

Lewis, JE (2006). A randomized controlled trial of the effect of dietary soy and flaxseed muffins on quality of life and hot flashes during menopause. *Menopause: The Journal of the North American Menopause Society* 13(4): 631-42.

Lichtenstein, A et al. (2006). Diet and lifestyle recommendations revision 2006: A scientific statement from the American Heart Association Nutrition Committee. *Circulation* 114(1): 82-96.

Lovejoy, JC (1998). The influence of sex hormones on obesity across the female life span. *Journal of Women's Health* 7(10): 1247-56.

Marco, M et al. (2006). Menopause, insulin resistance and risk factors for cardiovascular disease. *Menopause: The Journal of the North American Menopause Society* 13(5): 809-19.

Mayo Clinic (2004). *Low-carbohydrate diets: Are they safe and effective?* Available online: http://www.atkinsexposed.org/atkins/99/mayo_clinic.htm

McAuley, KA (2005). Comparison of high-fat and high-protein diets with a high-carbohydrate diet in insulin-resistant obese women. *Diabetologia* 48(1): 8-16.

Meckling, KA et al. (2004). Comparison of a low-fat diet to a low-carbohydrate diet on weight loss, body composition, and risk factors for diabetes and cardiovascular disease in free- living, overweight men and women. *Journal of Clinical Endocrinology & Metabolism* 89(6): 2717-23.

MedicineNet.com (1996-2005). Low carb-state of mind. http://www.medicinenet.com/mental_health/article.htm

Milewicz, A et al. (2001). Menopausal obesity: Myth or fact? *Climacteric* 4(4): 273-83.

Moller, SE (1992). Serotonin, carbohydrates, and atypical depression. *Pharmacology & Toxicology* 71(1): 61-71.

Morgan, T et al. (2004). Acute effects of nicotine on serum glucose insulin growth hormone and cortisol in healthy smokers. *Metabolism* 53(5): 578-82.

Mottillo, S et al. (2010). The metabolic syndrome and cardiovascular risk: A systematic review and meta-analysis. *Journal of the American College of Cardiology* 56(14): 1113-32.

Mursu, J (2004). Dark chocolate consumption increases HDL cholesterol concentration and chocolate fatty acids may inhibit lipid peroxidation in healthy humans. *Free Radical Biology and Medicine* 37(9): 1351-9.

National Cancer Institute. *Obesity and cancer: Questions and answers.* http://www.cancer.gov/cancertopics/factsheet/Risk/obesity

National Institutes of Health (NIH) (2004). *Insulin resistance and pre-diabetes.* NIH Publication No. 04-4893, May 2004.

Norman, R et al. (1999). Oestrogen and progestogen hormone replacement therapy for perimenopausal and post-menopausal women: Weight and body fat distribution. *Cochrane Database of Systematic Reviews* 3(CD001018). doi: 10.1002/14651858.CD001018.

Nutrition Education for the Public Dietetic Practice Group (2000). Wholegrains for healthful eating. Edited by NCND staff. *Journal of the American Dietetic Association,* 1 September 2001.

Partnership for Essential Nutrition (2004). http://www.essentialnutrition.org/

Peck, P (2004). Both uphill, downhill exercise help lipid and glucose metabolism. *Medscape General Medicine.* Available online: http://www.medscape.com/viewarticle/493323

Pittas, AG (2003). Nutrition interventions for prevention of type 2 diabetes and the metabolic syndrome. *Nutrition in Clinical Care* 6(2): 79-88.

Rao, G (2001). Insulin resistance syndrome. *American Family Physician* 63(6): 1159-63, 1165-6.

Raynor, HA et al. (2004). Relationship between changes in food group variety, dietary intake, and weight during obesity treatment. *International Journal of Obesity & Related Metabolic Disorders* 28(6): 813-20.

Ried, K et al. (2010). Chocolate and blood pressure: Chocolate dose may be too much. *BMJ* 341: c4176.

Ried, K et al. (2010). Does chocolate reduce blood pressure? A meta-analysis. *BMC Medicine* 8: 39.

Robinson, JR & Niswender, KD (2009). What are the risks and the benefits of current and emerging weight-loss medications? *Current Diabetes Reports* 9(5): 368-75.

Rolls, BJ et al. (2004). What can intervention studies tell us about the relationship between fruit and vegetable consumption and weight management? *Nutrition Abstracts & Reviews* 62(1): 1-17.

Rose, DP & Vona-Davis, L (2010). Interaction between menopausal status and obesity in affecting breast cancer risk. *Maturitas* 66(1): 33-8.

Salodof, MJ (2004). Weight loss maintenance program keeps pounds off. *Medscape General Medicine.* Available online: http://www.medscape.com/viewarticle/494143?src=mp

Salodof MacNeil, J (2004). High and low carb diets produce similar results. *Medscape General Medicine*. Available online: http://www.medscape.com/viewarticle/494078

Salodof MacNeil, J (2004). Water-rich diet more effective than low-fat regimen for weight loss. *Medscape General Medicine*. Available online: http://www.medscape.com/viewarticle/494144?src=mp

Sattelmair, JR (2010). Physical activity and risk of stroke in women. *Stroke: Journal of the American Heart Association* 41(6): 1243-50.

Shi, H & Clegg, DJ (2009). Sex differences in the regulation of body weight. *Physiology & Behavior* 97(2): 199-204.

Shipp, T (2005). Does ultrasound have a role in the evaluation of postmenopausal bleeding and among postmenopausal women with endometrial cancer? *Menopause: The Journal of the North American Menopause Society* 12(1): 8-11.

Simkin-Silverman, LR et al. (2003). Lifestyle intervention can prevent weight gain during menopause: Results from a 5-year randomized clinical trial. *Annals of Behavioral Medicine* 26(3): 212-20.

Song, Y et al. (2004). A prospective study of red meat consumption and type 2 diabetes. *Diabetes Care* 27(9): 2108-15.

Sørenson, MB (2002). Changes in body composition at menopause: Age, lifestyle or hormone deficiency? *Journal of the British Menopause Society* 8(4): 137-40.

South, J (2002). L-Tryptophan: Nature's answer to Prozac. *Off-shore Pharmacy*. Available online: http://www.smart-drugs.com/JamesSouth-tryptophan.htm

Staropoli, CA et al. (1998). Predictors of menopausal hot flashes. *Journal of Women's Health* 7(9): 1149-55.

Stern, L et al. (2004). The effects of low-carbohydrate versus conventional weight loss diets in severely obese adults: One-year follow-up of a randomized trial. *Annals of Internal Medicine* 10: 778-85.

Sternfeld, B et al. (2004). Physical activity and changes in weight and waist circumference in midlife women: Findings from the Study of Women's Health Across the Nation. *American Journal of Epidemiology* 160(9): 912-22.

St-Onge, MP & Heymsfeld, SB (2004). Reducing CVD risk through appropriate weight management. *Medscape General Medicine*. Available online: http://www.medscape.com/viewprogram/3118

Storti, KL et al. (2010). Physical activity and coronary artery calcification in two cohorts of women representing early and late post-menopause. *Menopause: The Journal of the North American Menopause Society* 17(6): 1146-51.

Stuenkel, CA (2010). Taking steps (literally) toward a healthier heart. Editorial. *Menopause: The Journal of the North American Menopause Society* 17(6): 111-3.

Sue, LY et al. (2010). Body Mass (BMI), change in BMI, and postmenopausal breast cancer risk in the Prostate, Lung, Colorectal, and Ovarian Cancer Screening Trial (PLCO) Cohort. Presented at the 101st Annual Meeting of the American Association for Cancer Research, 20 April 2010.

Tanko, LB & Christiansen, C (2004). An update on the antiestrogenic effect of smoking: A literature review with implications for researchers and practitioners. *Menopause: The Journal of the North American Menopause Society* 11(1): 104-9.

Teff, KL et al. (2009). Endocrine and metabolic effects of consuming fructose- and glucose-sweetened beverages with meals in obese men and women: Influence of insulin resistance on plasma triglyceride responses. *Journal of Clinical Endocrinology and Metabolism* 94(5): 1562-9.

Thompson, D et al. (2004). Relationship between accumulated walking and body composition. *Medicine & Science in Sports & Exercise* 36(5): 911-4.

Till, A. *The GI factor*. ©Anne Till & Associates, Registered Dieticians, Johannesburg.

US Department of Health and Human Services (HHS) and the US Department of Agriculture (USDA) (2010). *Dietary guidelines for Americans*. http://www.health.gov/dietaryguidelines/

Utian, W et al. (2004). Body mass index does not influence response to treatment, nor does body weight change with lower doses of conjugated estrogens and medroxyprogesterone acetate in early post menopausal women. *Menopause: The Journal of the North American Menopause Society* 11(3): 306-14.

Vasanti, SM et al. (2010). Sugar-sweetened beverages and risk of metabolic syndrome and type 2 diabetes: A meta-analysis. *Diabetes Care* 33(11): 2477-83.

Volek, JS et al. (2004). Comparison of energy-restricted very low-carbohydrate and low-fat diets on weight loss and body composition in overweight men and women. *Nutrition & Metabolism* (London) 1: 13.

Wasnich, R (2004). Changes in bone density and turnover after alendronate or estrogen withdrawal. *Menopause: The Journal of the North American Menopause Society* 11(6): 622-30.

Welsh, JA (2010). Caloric sweetener consumption and dyslipidemia among US adults. *Journal of the American Medical Association* 303(15): 1490-7.

Wildman, RP et al. (2004). Healthy life style diet and exercise slow atherosclerosis in menopausal women. *Journal of the American College of Cardiology* 44(3): 579-85.

Wing, R (2004). North American Association for the Study of Obesity (NAASO) Annual Scientific Meeting. Abstract 96-OR presented 17 November 2004.

Wing, R et al. (1991). Weight gain at the time of menopause. *Archives of Internal Medicine* 151(1): 97-102.

Wurtman, RJ & Wurtman, JJ (1996). Brain serotonin, carbohydrate-craving, obesity and depression. *Advances in Experimental Medicine & Biology* 398: 35-41.

Yancy, WS et al. (2004). Low-carbohydrate, ketogenic diet versus a low-fat diet to treat obesity and hyperlipidemia: A randomized, controlled trial. *Annals of Internal Medicine* 140(10): 769-77.

Yancy, WS et al. (2010). Animal, vegetable, or … clinical trial? Editorial. *Annals of Internal Medicine* 153(5): 337-9.

Available online

http://syndromex.stanford.edu/InsulinResistance.htm
http://www.answers.com/topic/carbohydrate
http://www.answers.com/topic/metabolism
http://www.caloriecontrol.org/metricconversion.html
http://www.cdc.gov/nccdphp/dnpa/bmi/bmi-adult-formula.htm
http://www.goredforwomen.org/pdf/hhaaa/quitting_and_weight_gain.pdf
http://www.healthyeatingclub.com/info/articles/body-shape/lowcarbevidence.htm
http://www.mindbodyhealth.com/lowfatdietmyth.htm
http://www.schering.de/scripts/en/20_busareas/gyn_andro/index.php
http://www.women.fitness.net/

Chapter 11

Alster, T et al. (2004). *The aging face: More than skin deep.* Discovery Institute of Medical Education.

Alvarez, G & Ayas, N (2004). The impact of daily sleep duration on health: A review of the literature. *Progress in Cardiovascular Nursing* 19(2): 56-9.

American Heritage® Dictionary of the English Language, 4th ed. (2004). G-spot. Houghton Mifflin Company. Available online: http://www.answers.com/topic/g-spot

Anderson, M et al. (2004). Are vaginal symptoms ever normal? A review of the literature. *Medscape General Medicine* 6(4). Available online: http://www.medscape.com/viewarticle/490226

Aydin, ZD (2010). Determinants of age at natural menopause in the Isparta Menopause and Health Study: Premenopausal body mass index gain rate and episodic weight loss. *Menopause: The Journal of the North American Menopause Society* 17(3): 494-505.

Bancroft, J et al. (2003). Distress about sex: A national survey of women in heterosexual relationships. *Archives of Sexual Behavior* 32(3): 193-211.

Basson, R (2007). Recent conceptualization of women's sexual response. *Menopause Management* 16(3): 16-27.

Benca, RM (2005). Diagnosis and treatment of chronic insomnia: A review. *Psychiatric Services* 56(3): 332-43.

Berkow, R & Beers, M (1999). Melanoma. *The Merck Manual of Diagnosis and Therapy*, 17th ed. USA: Merck & Co.

Beyene, Y et al. (2007). I take the good with the bad, and I moisturize. *Menopause: The Journal of the North American Menopause Society* 14(4): 734-41.

Briden, ME (2004). Alpha-hydroxyacid chemical peeling agents: Case studies and rationale for safe and effective use. *Cutis* 73(2 Suppl.): 18-24.

Cahill, K et al. (2010). Nicotine receptor partial agonists for smoking cessation. *The Cochrane Database of Systematic Reviews* 8(12): CD006103.

Carruthers, J et al. (2004). Consensus recommendations on the use of botulinum toxin type A in facial aesthetics. *Plastic & Reconstructive Surgery* 114(6 Suppl.): S1-22.

Conen, D et al. (2011). Smoking, smoking cessation, and risk for symptomatic peripheral artery disease in women: A cohort study. *Annals of Internal Medicine* 154(11): 719-26.

Chiu, A & Kimball, AB (2003). Topical vitamins, minerals and botanical ingredients as modulators of environmental and chronological skin damage. *British Journal of Sports Medicine* 149(4): 681-91.

Christen, WG et al. (2011). Dietary omega-3 fatty acid and fish intake and incident age-related macular degeneration in women. *Archives of Ophthalmology*. Published online 14 March 2011. doi: 10.1001/archophthalmol.2011.34.

Directoryskincare.com (2002-3). *A skin care directory: Skin care & beauty glossary* ©2002–2003. http://www.
directoryskincare.com/

Fuchs, KO et al. (2003). The effects of an estrogen and glycolic acid cream on the facial skin of postmenopausal
women: A randomized histologic study. *Cutis* 71(6): 481-8.

Garay, M & Rigel, DS (2011). *Pollution may aggravate skin damage*. 69th Annual Meeting of the American
Academy of Dermatology, New Orleans, 4-8 February 2011.

Gladstone, HB (2000). Efficacy of hydroquinone cream (USP 4%) used alone or in combination with salicylic
acid peels in improving photodamage on the neck and upper chest. *Dermatologic Surgery* 26(4): 333.

Goodson, JM et al. (2005). Tooth whitening: Tooth color changes following treatment by peroxide and light.
Journal of Clinical Dentistry 16(3): 78-82.

Hays JT et al. (2008). Efficacy and safety of varenicline for smoking cessation. *American Journal of Medicine*
121(4 Suppl. 1): S32-42.

Hurt, RD (2009). *Is it true that smoking causes wrinkles?* Nicotine Dependence Center, Mayo Clinic. http://www.
mayoclinic.com/health/smoking/AN00644

Lahmann, C et al. (2001). Matrix metalloproteinase-1 and skin ageing in smokers. *The Lancet* 357(9260):
935-6.

Lasovich, D (2010). Indoor tanning and risk of melanoma: A case-control study in a highly exposed population.
Cancer Epidemiology, Biomarkers and Prevention 19(6): 1557-68.

Lewis, DM & Cachelin, FM (2001). Body image, body dissatisfaction, and eating attitudes in midlife and elderly
women. *Eating Disorders: Journal of Treatment & Prevention* 9(1): 29-39.

Luk, K et al. (2004). Effect of light energy on peroxide tooth bleaching. *Journal of the American Dental
Association* 135(2): 194-201.

Monheit, GD (2004). Chemical peels. *Skin Therapy Letter* 9(2): 6-11. Available online: http://www.
skintherapyletter.com

National Cancer Institute (n.d.). *Skin cancer*. US National Institutes of Health. Available online: http://www.
cancer.gov/cancertopics/types/skin

National Cancer Institute (2010). Sun protection. *Cancer Trends Progress Report*, 2009/10 Update. Accessed 1
November 2010.

Natural Medicines (2005). *Kinetin*. Monograph. Natural Medicines Comprehensive Database, 10 March 2005.
Available online: http://www.naturaldatabase.com

Pray, WS (2001). Self-treatment for minor eye conditions. *US Pharmacist* 26(12). Available online: http://www.
medscape.com/viewarticle/421501

Rosenbaum, JT (2008). The eye and rheumatoid arthritis. In Firestein, GS et al., *Kelley's textbook of
rheumatology*, 8th ed. Philadelphia, PA: Saunders Elsevier, Chapter 46.

Sall, K et al. (2000). Two multicenter, randomized studies of the efficacy and safety of cyclosporine ophthalmic
emulsion in moderate to severe dry eye disease. *Ophthalmology* 107(4): 631-9.

Sørensen, LT et al. (2009). Effect of smoking, abstention, and nicotine patch on epidermal healing and
collagenase in skin transudate. *Wound Repair and Regeneration* 17(3): 347-53.

Sørensen, LT et al. (2009). Acute effects of nicotine and smoking on blood flow, tissue oxygen, and aerobe
metabolism of the skin and subcutis. *Journal of Surgical Research* 152(2): 224-30.

Stern, RS (2010). Prevalence of a history of skin cancer in 2007: Results of an incidence-based model. *Archives
of Dermatology* 146(3): 279-82.

Suzuki, T et al. (2004). Mechanisms involved in apoptosis of human macrophages induced by lipopolysaccharide
from *Actinobacillus actinomycetemcomitans* in the presence of cycloheximide. *Infection & Immunity* 72(4):
1856-65.

Thyssen, JP et al. (2010). The effect of tobacco smoking and alcohol consumption on the prevalence of self-
reported hand eczema: A cross-sectional population based study. *British Journal of Dermatology* 162(3):
619-26.

Tredwin, CJ et al. (2006). Hydrogen peroxide tooth-whitening (bleaching) products: Review of adverse effects
and safety issues. *British Dental Journal* 200(7): 371-6.

Vartanian, AJ & Dayan, SH (2005). Complications of botulinum toxin: A use in facial rejuvenation. *Facial Plastic
Surgery Clinics of North America Journal* 13(1): 1-10.

Vegeto, E et al. (2004). Regulation of the lipopolysaccharide signal transduction pathway by 17â-estradiol in
macrophage cells. *Journal of Steroid Biochemistry & Molecular Biology* 91(1-2): 59-66.

Xi, ZX (2010). Preclinical pharmacology, efficacy and safety of varenicline in smoking cessation and clinical
utility in high risk patients. *Journal of Drug Healthcare and Patient Safety* 1(2): 39-48.

Available online

http://en.mimi.hu/beauty/glycolic_acid.html
http://www.againstsmoking.co.za
http://www.cdc.gov/tobacco/
http://www.citihealth.com/forsha/neova_.htm
http://www.lungusa.org/stop-smoking/
http://www.sjorgrens.org/home/about-sjorgrens-syndrome
http://www.webmd.com/melanoma-skin-cancer/slideshow-sun-damaged-skin
http://www.webmd.com/smoking-cessation/

Chapter 12

Abdo, CHN et al. (2010). Hypoactive sexual desire disorder (HSDD) in a population-based study of Brazilian women: Associated factors classified according to their importance. *Menopause: The Journal of the North American Menopause Society* 17(6): 1114-21.

Alder, J et al. (2008). Sexual dysfunction after premenopausal stage I and II breast cancer: Do androgens play a role? *Journal of Sexual Medicine* 5(8): 1898-1906.

American Heritage® Dictionary of the English Language (2002). Dyspareunia in women. Houghton Mifflin Company.

Avis, NE et al. (2005). Correlates of sexual function among multi-ethnic middle-aged women: Results from the Study of Women's Health Across the Nation (SWAN). *Menopause: The Journal of the North American Society* 12(4): 385-98.

Badr, MS (2010). Central sleep apnea syndrome: Risk factors, clinical presentation, and diagnosis. http://www.uptodate.com/home/index.html; accessed 13 April 2010.

Basson, R (2008). Testosterone supplementation to improve women's sexual satisfaction: Complexities and unknowns. *Annals of Internal Medicine* 148(8): 620-1.

Basson, R (2010). Is it time to move on from hypoactive sexual desire disorder? Editorial. *Menopause: The Journal of the North American Menopause Society* 17(6): 1097-8.

Basson, R et al. (2010). Role of androgens in women's sexual dysfunction. *Menopause: The Journal of the North American Menopause Society* 17(5): 962-71.

Berman, L et al. (2003). Seeking help for sexual function complaints: What gynecologists need to know about the female patient's experience. *Fertility & Sterility* 79(3): 572-6.

Brandenburg, U & Bitzer, J (2009). The challenge of talking about sex: The importance of patient-physician interaction. *Maturitas* 63(2): 124-7.

Braunstein, GD et al. (2005). Safety and efficacy of a testosterone patch for the treatment of hypoactive sexual disorder in surgically menopausal women: A randomized placebo controlled trial. *Archives of Internal Medicine* 165(14): 1582-9.

Buster, J et al. (2005). Testosterone patch for low sexual desire in surgically menopausal women: A randomized trial. *Obstetrics and Gynecology* 105(5 Pt 1): 944-52.

Cameron, D & Braunstein, G (2005). Androgen replacement therapy in women. *Fertility and Sterility* 8(2): 273-89.

Clayton, AH et al. (2009). Validation of the Decreased Sexual Desire Screener (DSDS): A brief diagnostic instrument for generalized acquired female hypoactive sexual desire disorder (HSDD). *Journal of Sexual Medicine* 6(3): 730-8.

Davis, SR et al. (2005). Circulating androgen levels and self-reported sexual function in women. *Journal of the American Medical Association* 294(8): 91-6.

Davison, SL & Davis, SR (2003). Androgens in women. *Journal of Steroid Biochemistry & Molecular Biology* 85(2-5): 363-6.

Davison, SL et al. (2005). Androgen levels in adult females: Changes with age, menopause and oophorectomy. *Clinical Endocrinology and Metabolism* 90(7): 3847-53.

Dickerson, LM et al. (2003). Premenstrual syndrome. *American Family Physician* 67(8): 1743-52.

Dragisic, KG & Milad, MP (2004). Sexual functioning and patient expectations of sexual functioning after hysterectomy. *American Journal of Obstetrics & Gynecology* 190(5): 1416-8.

El-Toukhy, TA et al. (2004). The effect of different types of hysterectomy on urinary and sexual functions: A prospective study. *Journal of Obstetrics & Gynaecology* 24(4): 420-5.

Farrell, SA & Kieser, K (2000). Sexuality after hysterectomy. *Obstetrics & Gynecology* 95 (6 Part 2): 1045-51.

Freedman, R & Roehrs, T (2007). Sleep disturbances in menopause. *Menopause: The Journal of the North American Menopause Society* 14(5): 826-9.

Fugate, WN (2004). Prostate cancer: A family affair. *Menopause Management* 13(3): 12-3.

Gracis, C et al. (2004). Predictors of decreased libido in women during the late reproductive years. *Menopause: The Journal of the North American Menopause Society* 11(2): 144-50.

Goldstein, I (2010). Recognizing and treating urogenital atrophy in postmenopausal women. *Journal of Women's Health* (Larchmt) 19(3): 425-32.

Holms, KJ & Goa, KL (2000). Zolpidem: An update of its pharmacology, therapeutic efficacy and tolerability in the treatment of insomnia. *Drugs* 59(4): 865-89.

Hung, M (2003). Low dose DHEA increases androgen, estrogen levels in menopause. *Medscape General Medicine*. Available online: http://www.medscape.com/viewarticle/465827

Joffe, H et al. (2010). Augmentation of venlafaxine and selective serotonin reuptake inhibitors with zolpidem improves sleep and quality of life in breast cancer patients with hot flashes: A randomized, double-blind, placebo-controlled trial. *Menopause: The Journal of the North American Menopause Society* 17(5): 908-16.

Joffe, H et al. (2010). Eszopiclone improves insomnia and depressive and anxious symptoms in perimenopausal and postmenopausal women with hot flashes: A randomized, double-blinded, placebo-controlled crossover trial. *American Journal of Obstetrics & Gynecology* 202(2): 171, e1-e171, e11.

Juska, J (2003). *A round-heeled woman: My late-life adventures in sex and romance*. London: Chatto & Windus.

Katz, A (2002). Sexuality after hysterectomy. *JOGN Nursing: Journal of Obstetric, Gynecologic & Neonatal Nursing* 31(3): 256-62.

Kim, DH et al. (2003). Alteration of sexual function after classic intrafascial supracervical hysterectomy and total hysterectomy. *Journal of the American Association of Gynecologic Laparoscopists* 10(1): 60-4.

Kingsberg, S (2006). Prevalence of hypoactive sexual desire disorder in postmenopausal women: Results from the WISHeS Trial. *Menopause: The Journal of the North American Menopause Society* 13(1): 10-1.

Kingsberg, SA (2004).Helping couples cope with prostate cancer: The role of the gynaecologist. *Menopause Management* 3: 14-7.

Komisaruk, BR & Whipple, B (1998). Love as sensory stimulation: Physiological consequences of its deprivation and expression. *Psychoneuroendocrinology* 23(8): 927-44.

Krystal, AD (2004). Gonadal hormone-related insomnia in women. *Medscape Primary Care* 6(1). Available online: http://www.medscape.com/viewarticle/478995

Krystal, AD et al. (2003). Sustained efficacy of eszopiclone over 6 months of nightly treatment: Results of a randomized, doubleblind, placebo-controlled study in adults with chronic insomnia. *Sleep* 26(7): 793-9.

Labrie, F et al. (2009). Androgen glucuronides, instead of testosterone, as the new markers of androgenic activity in women. *Journal of Steroid Biochemistry and Molecular Biology* 99(4-5): 182-8.

Leiblum, S et al. (1983). Vaginal atrophy in the postmenopausal woman: The importance of sexual activity and hormones. *Journal of the American Medical Association* 249(2): 195-8.

Leiblum, S et al. (2006). Hypoactive sexual desire disorder in postmenopausal women: US results from the Women's International Study of Health and Sexuality (WISHeS). *Menopause: The Journal of the North American Menopause Society* 13(1): 46-56.

Lukacs, JL et al. (2004). Midlife women's response to a hospital sleep challenge: Age and menopause effects on sleep architecture. *Journal of Women's Health* 13(3): 333-40.

MacBride, MB et al. (2010). Vulvovaginal atrophy. *Mayo Clinic Proceedings*. 85(1): 87-94.

Mazza, E et al. (1999). Dehydroepiandrosterone sulfate levels in women: Relationships with age, body mass index and insulin levels. *Journal of Endocrinological Investigation* 22(9): 681-7.

Medscape (2005). Medscape Conference Coverage, based on selected sessions at the International Society for Sexual Impotence Research, 11th World Congress (ISSIR) on Female Sexual Dysfunction. *Medscape General Medicine*. Available online: http://www.medscape.com/viewprogram/3515

Moore, AA (2010). Addressing vaginal atrophy with your patients: Modifying an existing therapeutic approach – Part 1. *Medscape Education Ob/Gyn & Women's Health* CE released 24 June 2010.

Morales, AJ et al. (1998). The effect of six months' treatment with a 100 mg daily dose of dehydroepiandrosterone (DHEA) on circulating sex steroids, body composition and muscle strength in age-advanced men and women. *Clinical Endocrinology* (Oxford) 49(4): 421-32.

Morin, CM et al. (2009). Cognitive behavioral therapy, singly and combined with medication, for persistent insomnia: A randomized controlled trial. *Journal of the American Medical Association* 301(19): 2005-15.

Morley, JE & Kaiser, FE (2003). Female sexuality. *Medical Clinics of North America* 87(5): 1077-90.

Palacios, S (2011). Hypoactive sexual desire disorder and current pharmacotherapeutic options in women. *Women's Health (London)* 7(1): 95-107.

Pillai-Friedman, S (2010). Barriers to communications about female sexual health: Tips for successful dialogue with patients CME/CE. *Medscape CME Ob/Gyn & Women's Health*, 21 May 2010.

Politi, MC et al. (2009). Patient-provider communication about sexual health among unmarried middle-aged and older women. *Journal of General Internal Medicine* 24(12): 511-6.

Regestein, QR (2006). Hot flashes and sleep. *Menopause: The Journal of the North American Menopause Society* 13(4): 549-52.

Regenstein, QR et al. (2004). Self reported sleep in postmenopausal women. *Menopause: The Journal of the North American Menopause Society* 11(2): 198-207.

Resnick, SM & Maki, PM (2001). Effects of hormone replacement therapy on cognitive and brain aging. *Annals of the New York Academy of Sciences* 949: 203-14.

Rhodes, JC et al. (1999). Hysterectomy and sexual functioning. *Journal of the American Medical Association* 282(20): 1934-41.

Roussis, NP et al. (2004). Sexual response in the patient after hysterectomy: Total abdominal versus supracervical versus vaginal procedure. *American Journal of Obstetrics & Gynecology* 90(5): 1427-8.

Sarrel, P (2006). Testosterone therapy for postmenopausal decline in sexual desire: Implications for a new study. *Menopause: The Journal of the North American Menopause Society* 13(3): 328-30.

Schover, LR (2008). Androgen therapy for loss of desire in women: Is the benefit worth the breast cancer risk? *Fertility and Sterility* 90(1): 129-40.

Shaver, JL (2009). The interface of depression, sleep and menopausal symptoms. *Menopause: The Journal of the North American Menopause Society* 16(4): 626-9.

Shaver, JLF (2010). Sleep difficulties: Due to menopause status, age, other factors, or all of the above? Editorial. *Menopause: The Journal of the North American Menopause Society* 17(6): 1104-7.

Snabes, MC & Simes, SM (2009). Approved hormonal treatments for HSDD: An unmet medical need. *Journal of Sexual Medicine* 6(7): 1846-9.

Sturdee, DW & Panay, N (2010). Recommendations for the management of postmenopausal vaginal atrophy. *Climacteric* 13(6): 509-22.

Suckling, J et al. (2004). Local oestrogen for vaginal atrophy in postmenopausal women. Cochrane Review in *The Cochrane Library* 3. Chichester: John Wiley & Sons.

Thomas, HM et al. (2011). Dyspareunia is associated with decreased sexual frequency of intercourse in the menopausal transition. *Menopause: The Journal of the North American Society* 18(2): 152-7.

Toates, F (2009). An integrative theoretical framework for understanding sexual motivation, arousal, and behaviour. *Journal of Sexual Research* 46(2-3): 168-93.

Tom, SE (2010). Self-reported sleep difficulty during the menopausal transition: Results from a prospective cohort study. *Menopause: The Journal of the North American Menopause Society* 17(6): 1128-35.

Tuohy, W (2003). Sexual healing in life's autumn. *The Age*. Available online: http://www.theage.com.au

Utian, W (2005). Problems with desire and arousal in surgically menopausal women: Advances in assessment, diagnosis and treatment. *Menopause Management* 14(1): 10-22.

Women's Sexual Health Foundation (2004). *Hysterectomy and your sexual response*. Available online: http://www.twshf.com/pdf/Hysterectomy_Brochure_5.pdf

Wylie, K & Mimoun, S (2009). Sexual response models in women. *Maturitas*.63(2): 112-5.

Wysocki, S (2010). An expert interview with Susan Wysocki: Addressing vaginal atrophy with your patients – restarting estrogen therapy after the WHI studies. *Medscape Education Ob/Gyn & Women's Health*, CE released 27 July 2010.

Wysocki, SJ et al. (2010). Addressing vaginal atrophy with your patients: Restarting estrogen therapy. *Medscape Education Ob/Gyn & Women's Health* CME released 27 July 2010.

Yazbeck, C (2004). Sexual function following hysterectomy. *Gynecology Obstetrique & Fertilité* 32(1): 49-54.

Zee, P (2004). Expert column: Insomnia and menopause. *Medscape Ob/Gyn & Women's Health*. Available online: http://www.medscape.com/viewarticle/484767

Zobbe, V et al. (2004). Sexuality after total vs. subtotal hysterectomy. *Acta Obstetricia et Gynecologica Scandinavica* 83(2): 191-6.

Available online

http://www.menopause.org/sex.aspx
Sleep apnoea: http://www.nhlbi.nih.gov/health/dci/Diseases/SleepApnea/SleepApnea_WhoIsAtRisk.html
Sleep apnoea: http://www.ninds.nih.gov/disorders/sleep_apnea/sleep_apnea.htm

Chapter 13

Ancelin, ML et al. (2010). Hormones won't cut menopause depression risk. *Journal of Clinical Psychiatry*, 10 August.

Beatty, MN & Blumenthal, PD (2009). The levonorgestrel-releasing intrauterine system: Safety, efficacy, and patient acceptability. *Journal of Therapeutics and Clinical Risk Management* 5(3): 561-74.

Berent-Spillson, A (2010). Early menopausal hormone use influences brain regions used for visual working memory. *Menopause: The Journal of the North American Menopause Society* 17(4): 692-9.

Berga, SL (2009). Beyond the obvious: Why behavioral interventions matter. *Menopause: The Journal of the North American Menopause Society* 16(2): 229-30.

Bigal, ME et al. (2009). Migraine and cardiovascular disease: Possible mechanisms of interaction. *Neurology* 72(21): 1864-71.

Brandes, JL (2006). The influence of estrogen on migraine. *Journal of the American Medical Association* 295(15): 1824-30.

Chawla, J (2011). Migraine headache. *Medscape Reference*. Available online: http://emedicine.medscape.com/article/1142556-overview

Diener, HC et al. (2010) Onabotulinum toxin A for treatment of chronic migraine: Results from the double-blind, randomized, placebo-controlled phase of the PREEMPT 2 trial. *Cephalagia* 30(7): 804-14.

Elavsky, S (2009). Physical activity, menopause and quality of life: The role of affect and self-worth across time. *Menopause: The Journal of the North American Menopause Society* 16(2): 265-71.

Erickson, KI et al. (2010). A cross-sectional study of hormone treatment and hippocampal volume in postmenopausal women: Evidence for a limited window of opportunity. *Neuropsychology* 24(1): 68-76.

Fleisher, AS et al. (2008). Volumetric MRI vs clinical predictors of Alzheimer's disease in mild cognitive impairment. *Neurology* 70(3): 191-9.

Gudmundsson, LS et al. (2010). Migraine with aura and risk of cardiovascular and all cause mortality in men and women: Prospective cohort study. *BMJ* 24 August, 341: c3966.

Henderson, VW (2009). Aging, estrogens, and episodic memory in women. *Cognitive and Behavioral Neurology* 22(4): 205-14.

Henderson, VW (2009). Estrogens, episodic memory, and Alzheimer's disease: A critical update. *Seminars in Reproductive Medicine* 27(3): 283-93.

Henderson, VW & Popat, RA (2011). Effects of endogenous and exogenous estrogen exposures in midlife and late-life women on episodic memory and executive functions. *Neuroscience*, 6 June [Epub ahead of print].

Hillman, CH et al. (2008). Be smart, exercise your heart: Exercise effects on brain and cognition. *Nature Reviews Neuroscience* 9(1): 58-65.

Hillman, CH et al. (2009). The effect of acute treadmill walking on cognitive control and academic achievement in preadolescent children. *Neuroscience* 159(3): 1044-54.

Huppert, FA & Van Niekerk, JK (2007). Dehydroepiandrosterone (DHEA) supplementation for cognitive function. *Cochrane Review Abstract*, 18 July (2): CD000304.

Kabat-Zin, J (2005). *Wherever you go, there you are: Mindfulness meditation in everyday life*. Hyperion Books, New York.

Kabat-Zin, J (2009). *Letting everything become your teacher: 100 lessons in mindfulness*. Dell Publishing Company, New York.

Kalantaridou, SN et al. (2004). Reproductive functions of corticotropin-releasing hormone: Research and potential clinical utility of antalarmins (CRH receptor type 1 antagonists). *American Journal of Reproductive Immunology* 51(4): 269-74.

Kang, J et al. (2004). Postmenopausal hormone therapy and risk of cognitive decline in community-dwelling women. *Neurology* 63(1): 101-7.

Kennan, RP et al. (2005). Human cerebral blood flow and metabolism in acute insulin-induced hypoglycemia. *Journal of Cerebral Blood Flow & Metabolism* 25(4): 527-34.

Kerwin, D et al. (2011). Interaction between body mass index and central adiposity and risk of cognitive impairment and dementia: Results from the Women's Health Initiative Memory Study. *Journal of the American Geriatrics Society* 59(1): 107-12.

Kerwin, J et al. (2007). The variable response of women with menopausal hot flushes when treated with sertraline. *Menopause: The Journal of the North American Menopause Society* 14(5): 841-5.

Knechtle, B (2004). Influence of physical activity on mental well-being and psychiatric disorders. Schweizerische Rundschau Fuer Medizin. *Praxis* 93(35): 1403-11.

Kockler, D & McCarthy, M (2004). Antidepressants as a treatment for hot flashes in women. *American Journal of Health System Pharmacy* 61(3): 287-92.

Kocoska-Maras, L et al. (2011). A randomized trial of the effect of testosterone and estrogen on verbal fluency, verbal memory, and spatial ability in healthy postmenopausal women. *Fertility and Sterility* 95(1): 152-7.

Kok, H et al. (2006). Cognitive function across the life course and the menopausal transition. *Menopause: The Journal of the North American Menopause Society* 13(1): 19-27.

Kornstein, S et al. (2010). The influence of menopause status and postmenopausal use of hormone therapy on presentation of major depression in women. Special section: Menopause, cognition and mental health. *Menopause: The Journal of the North American Menopause Society* 17(4): 828-39.

Landy, S (2004). Migraine throughout the life cycle: Treatment through the ages. *Neurology* 62(5): S2-8.

LeBlanc, E (2004). Hormone therapy with oestrogen or oestrogen plus progesterone decreases cognitive function in older postmenopausal women. *Evidence-based Healthcare and Public Health* 8(6): 398-401.

LeBlanc, E et al. (2007). Hot flashes and estrogen therapy do not influence cognition in early menopausal women. *Menopause: The Journal of the North American Menopause Society* 14(2): 191-202.

Lautenschlager, NT et al. (2008). Effect of physical activity on cognitive function in older adults at risk for Alzheimer disease: A randomized trial. *Journal of the American Medical Association* 300(9): 1027-37.

Lermer, MA (2011). Somatic and affective anxiety symptoms and menopausal hot flashes. *Menopause: The Journal of the North American Menopause Society* 18(2): 129-32.

Lokuge, S et al. (2010). The rapid effects of estrogen: A mini-review. *Behavioural Pharmacology* 21(5-6): 465-72.

Loucks, T & Berga, SL (2009). Does postmenopausal estrogen confer menopausal protection. *Seminars in Reproductive Medicine* 27(3): 260-74.

Loprinzi, CL (2006). New anti-depressants inhibit hot flashes. *Menopause: The Journal of the North American Menopause Society* 13(4): 546-8.

Lowry, F (2010). Migraine with aura linked to increased mortality. *Medscape Medical News.* Available online: http://www.medscape.com/viewarticle/727498

MacGregor, EA (2008). Menstrual migraine. *Current Opinion Neurology* 21(3): 309-15.

MacLennan, A et al. (2006). Hormone therapy, timing of intervention, and cognition in women older than 60 years: The REMEMBER pilot study. *Menopause: The Journal of the North American Menopause Society* 13(1): 28-36.

Manson, JAE (2010). Preventing cognitive decline: How can we help our patients? *Medscape Ob/Gyn Women's Health.* Available online: http://www.medscape.com/viewarticle/730541

Marks, SJ et al. (2002). Estrogen replacement therapy for cognitive benefits: Viable treatment or forgettable senior moment? *Heart Disease & Stroke* 4(1): 26-32.

Martin, VT & Behbehani, M (2006). Ovarian hormones and migraine headaches: Understanding mechanisms and pathogenesis – Part 2. *Headache* 46(3): 365-86.

Meyer, PM et al. (2003). A population-based longitudinal study of cognitive functioning in the menopausal transition. *Neurology* 61(6): 801-6.

Mitchell, JL et al. (2003). Postmenopausal hormone therapy and its associations with cognitive impairment. *Archives of Internal Medicine* 163(20): 2485-90.

Moeller, MC (2010). Effects of testosterone and estrogen replacement on memory function. *Menopause: The Journal of the North American Menopause Society* 17(5): 983-9.

Morrison, MF et al. (2004). Lack of efficacy of estradiol for depression in postmenopausal women: A randomized controlled trial. *Biology & Psychiatry* 55(4): 406-12.

Muller, EE (2001). Steroids, cognitive processes and aging. *Recenti Progressi in Medicina* 92(5): 362-72.

Nappi, RE (2006). Different effects of tibolone and low dose EPT in the management of postmenopausal women with primary headaches. *Menopause: The Journal of the North American Menopause Society* 13(5): 818-25.

Newhouse, PA et al. (2010). Estrogen treatment impairs cognitive performance after psychosocial stress and monoamine depletion in postmenopausal women. *Menopause: The Journal of the North American Menopause Society* 17(4): 860-73.

Nilsson, LG et al. (2004). A prospective cohort study on memory, health and aging. *Aging Neuropsychology & Cognition* 11(3): 134-48.

Nordberg, A (2003). Toward an early diagnosis and treatment of Alzheimer's disease. *International Psychogeriatrics* 15(3): 223-37.

Obermeyer, CM & Sievert, L (2007). Cross-cultural comparisons: Midlife aging and menopause. *Menopause: The Journal of the North American Menopause Society* 14(4): 663-7.

Owens, JF et al. (2002). Cognitive function effects of suppressing ovarian hormones in young women. *Menopause: The Journal of the North American Menopause Society* 9(4): 221-3.

Pine, A (2006). The healing properties of exercise. *Menopause: The Journal of the North American Menopause Society* 13(4): 544-5.

Regestein, QR (2010). Antidepressant treatment. Editorial. *Menopause: The Journal of the North American Menopause Society* 17(4): 627-75.

Rusanen, MA (2010). Heavy smoking in midlife and long-term risk of Alzheimer disease and vascular dementia. *Archives of Internal Medicine* 171(4): 333-9.

Shaver, JLF (2010). Sleep difficulties: Due to menopause status, age, other factors, or all of the above? *Menopause: The Journal of the North American Menopause Society* 17(4): 627-75.

Schorr, M (2004). Coenzyme Q10 may ward off migraine attacks. *Medscape Ob/Gyn & Women's Health*. Available online: http://www.medscape.com/viewarticle/474831?src=mp

Schumacher, M et al. (2003). Steroid hormones and neurosteroids in normal and pathological aging of the nervous system. *Progress in Neurobiology (Oxford)* 71(1): 3-29.

Schwarz, S (2007). Menopause and determinants of quality of life in women at midlife and beyond: The Study of Health in Pomerania (SHIP). *Menopause: The Journal of the North American Menopause Society* 14(1): 123-34.

Shifren, JL & Avis, NE (2007). Surgical menopause: Effects on psychological well-being and sexuality. *Menopause: The Journal of the North American Menopause Society* 14(3): 586-91.

Shumaker, SA et al. (2004). Conjugated equine estrogens and incidence of probable dementia and mild cognitive impairment in postmenopausal women: Women's Health Initiative Memory Study. *Journal of the American Medical Association* 291(24): 2947-8.

Shumaker, SA et al. (2004). Hormone therapy does not prevent cognitive decline or dementia in older women: WHIMS data. *NAMS First to Know*. Part B. Available online: http://www.menopausemgmt.com/issues/13-05/MM13-5_First2Know.pdf

Soares, CN & Maki, PM (2010). Menopausal transition, mood, and cognition: An integrated view to close the gaps. *Menopause: The Journal of the North American Menopause Society* 17(4): 812-4.

Soares, CN et al. (2010). Desvenlafaxine and escitalopram for the treatment of postmenopausal women with major depressive disorder. *Menopause: The Journal of the North American Menopause Society* 17(4): 700-11.

Stearns, V & Hayes, DF (2002). Cooling off hot flashes. *Journal of Clinical Oncology* 20(6): 1436-8.

Thurston, R et al. (2006). Physical activity and risk of vasomotor symptoms in women with and without a history of depression: Results from the Harvard Study of Moods and Cycles. *Menopause: The Journal of the North American Menopause Society* 13(4): 553-60.

Tom, SE et al. (2010). Self-reported sleep difficulty during the menopausal transition: Results from a prospective cohort study. *Menopause: The Journal of the North American Menopause Society* 17(6): 1128-35.

Toran-Allerand, CD (2004). Estrogen and the brain: Beyond ER-alpha and ER-beta. *Experimental Gerontology* 1052: 136-44.

Vermeer, S et al. (2003). Silent brain infarcts and the risk of dementia and cognitive decline. *New England Journal of Medicine* 348(13): 1215-22.

Weill-Engerer, S et al. (2002). Neurosteroid quantification in human brain regions: Comparison between Alzheimer's and nondemented patients. *Journal of Clinical Endocrinology & Metabolism* 87(11): 5138-43.

Weill-Engerer, S et al. (2003). In vitro metabolism of dehydroepiandrosterone (DHEA) to 7alpha-hydroxy-DHEA and Delta5-androstene-3®, 17®-diol in specific regions of the aging brain from Alzheimer's and non-demented patients. *Brain Research* 969(1-2): 117-25.

Weuve, J et al. (2004). Physical activity, including walking, and cognitive function in older women. *Journal of the American Medical Association* 292(4): 1454-61.

Whitmer RA et al. (2011). Timing of hormone therapy and dementia: The critical window theory revisited. *Annals of Neurology* 69(1): 163-9.

Wolf, OT (2003). Cognitive functions and sex steroids. *Annales dEndocrinologie (Paris)* 64(2): 158-61.

Woods, NF et al. (2000). Memory functioning among midlife women: Observations from the Seattle Midlife Women's Health Study. *Menopause. Journal of the North American Menopause Society* 7(4): 257-65.

Ystad, MA et al. (2009). Hippocampal volumes are important predictors for memory function in elderly women. *BMC Medical Imaging* 9: 17.

Available online

Migraine triggers: http://uhs.berkeley.edu/home/healthtopics/pdf/triggers.pdf
The American Institute of Stress: http://www.stress.org/topic-effects.htm

Index

Desvenlafaxine: 129, 130

DEXA (Dual energy X-ray absorptiometry): 211-3, 219, 220, 224, 225, 306, 309

DHEA: 19, 25-6, 59, 73-4, 274

DHEA-S: 25, 26

Diabetes: 26, 111, 128, 148, 149, 153, 158, 171, 197, 229, 230, 231, 232, 235, 261, 295

DIEP flap: 192

Diet: 239-41

Dilation and curettage (D&C): 196

Diphenhydramine: 130

Diuretics: 154, 272

Dixarit: 126

Dong Quai: 109

Dopamine: 247

Double-blind: 37, 38, 64, 106

Double-blind randomised controlled study/trial: 34, 104, 106, 108, 142, 145, 238, 309

Drospirenone: 62. See also Progestogen

Ductal carcinoma in situ (DCIS): 166, 309. See also Invasive ductal carcinoma (IDC)

Ducts: 160, 162, 163, 166, 203, 310

Duloxetine: 130

DXA: 211. See also DEXA

Dydrogesterone: 62. See also Progestogen

Dyspareunia: 269

Effexor: 129, 130. See also Venlafaxine

Egg unit: 8, 10, 11, 13

Elastin: 235, 254, 258, 309

ELITE (Early versus Late Intervention Trial with Estrogen): 72, 145

Embolisation: 131, 138, 140, 309

Embolism: 186, 188, 309. See also Stroke

Embolus: 148

'Empty nest': 28, 294

Endocrine Society: 83, 219

Endocrine system: 10, 19, 133, 309

Endogenous estrogen: 60, 75, 310

Endometrial ablation: 65, 131, 136, 137, 140, 310

Endometrial cancer: 23, 32, 33, 84, 131, 134, 161, 173, 186, 187, 195-7

Endometrial hyperplasia: 32, 310

Endometriosis: 132, 133, 136, 138-9, 310

Endometriotic cysts: 201

Endometrium: 10, 12, 32, 65, 137, 138, 195, 310

Endorphins: 120, 255

Endothelial cells: 242, 270, 310

Endothelium: 63, 157, 310

Enzymes: 20, 92, 93, 98, 99, 100

Equilin: 32, 60, 309. See also Conjugated equine estrogen

Equilenin: 32, 309. See also Conjugated equine estrogen

Escitalopram: 129, 130

Estradiol (E2) and 17-estradiol: 11, 13, 14, 15, 19, 20, 21, 22, 23, 26, 27, 33, 44, 46, 48, 49, 50, 53, 57, 59, 60, 61, 63, 68, 69, 76, 77, 141, 146, 174, 185, 187, 188, 209, 268

Estradiol-hemihydrate: 60, 132

Estradiol-releasing vaginal ring: 18. See also Vaginal ring

Estriol: 20, 33, 50, 53, 59, 60, 61, 68, 69, 81, 82, 187

Estrogen: 6, 8, 10-4, 18, 19, 20, 21-2, 23, 24, 25, 30-4, 43-6, 48, 49, 50-2, 54, 56, 57, 59-61, 62, 63, 65, 66, 68, 70, 71, 72, 73, 75, 76, 77, 80, 82, 83, 85, 86, 104, 106, 107, 109, 114, 118, 119, 121, 123, 124, 125, 127, 131, 132, 134, 135, 136, 141-6, 148, 154, 156, 170, 175, 177, 179, 180, 181, 185- 8, 195-6, 197, 204, 205-7, 209, 210, 214, 215, 220, 222, 223, 228, 244, 257, 259, 263, 269, 270-1, 272, 273-4, 275, 282, 283, 285, 286, 289, 290-1, 292, 293, 294, 295, 296, 308, 310, 312, 313

Estrogen agonist/antagonist (Eaa): 65, 185, 186, 188, 310. See also SERMs; Bazedoxifene; Lasofoxifene

Estrogen and Thromboembolism Risk (ESTHER) study: 76, 148

Estrogen, low-dose: 64, 77, 81, 85, 282

Estrogen-only therapy: 39, 40, 41, 46, 51, 52, 65, 143, 144, 148, 175, 195, 196

Estrogen plus progestin or progestogen therapy: 45, 46, 77, 82, 142, 143, 179

Estrogen receptor modulators: 65, 83, 107, 119, 185, 313. See also SERMs

Estrogen receptor-negative: 59, 175, 181, 310

Estrogen receptor-positive: 59, 82, 84, 175, 180, 181, 182, 185, 223, 310

Estrogen receptors: 21, 22, 59, 79, 84, 90, 177, 185, 186, 187, 188, 211, 259

Estrogen, transdermal: 63, 74-6, 77, 85, 125, 145, 148

Estrone: 11, 19, 20, 21, 32, 33, 59, 60, 61, 68, 69, 309

Estrone sulfate: 60, 61, 75, 76

Evidence-based medicine: 2, 38, 42, 43, 44, 125, 310

Evista: 185, 222. See also Raloxifene

Exemestane: 186

Exercise: 27, 38, 43, 72, 79, 113, 123, 124, 139, 141, 145, 148, 151, 152, 181, 199, 215-7, 224, 226, 227, 229, 230, 231, 232, 243-5, 246, 248, 251, 252, 253, 255, 257, 264, 269, 278, 287, 290, 292, 293, 296, 300, 302

Exogenous estrogen: 310

Magnesium: 98, 154, 278, 287. *See also* Minerals

Magnetic Resonance Imaging (MRI): 143, 167, 312

Malignant: 59, 163, 169, 193, 195, 201, 308, 311, 312, 314

Mammogram: 33, 53, 57, 71,79, 86, 160, 161, 164, 165-70, 172, 176, 179, 180, 197, 199, 204, 206, 306, 311

Mammography, digital: 168

Manganese: 92, 100, 104. *See also* Minerals

Maxalt: 287

Medicine and Healthcare Products Regulatory Agency (MHRA): 89

Medicines Control Council (MCC) and regulatory boards: 60, 68, 69, 71, 73, 78, 83, 89, 127, 152, 174, 295, 312

Melanoma: 257, 311

Melatonin: 278

Memory: 25, 26, 91, 114, 221, 229, 282, 289, 290, 291, 306, 309, 311

Memory loss: 1, 13, 74, 113, 231, 283, 288, 289, 290, 291-4

Menopause and perimenopause, symptoms: 1, 2, 5, 6, 7, 8, 10, 11, 12-3, 14-5, 17, 25, 26, 28, 29, 36, 39, 57, 58, 59, 63, 64, 68, 69, 72, 74, 76, 78, 79, 80, 83, 84, 86, 87, 102, 104, 105,106, 107, 108, 109, 113, 115, 118-21, 124, 125, 126, 131-2, 139, 141, 143, 144, 157, 158, 174-5, 186-8, 205, 219, 221, 227, 271, 275, 282, 283, 294, 295, 296, 298, 304-5, 314

Menopause, early: 1, 57, 58, 107, 156, 174, 214, 219, 222

Menopause, premature: 39, 57, 58, 131, 135, 136, 175, 210, 292

Menopause, surgical: 73, 132, 134, 139, 145, 150, 175, 210, 214, 274, 285, 292

Menopause testing: 10, 13, 14, 15, 57, 205

Menstrual cycle: 5, 8, 9, 10, 11, 13, 15, 17, 23, 137, 167, 202, 312

Meta-analysis: 110, 128, 155, 156

Metabolic syndrome: 27, 226, 227, 231-2, 233, 243, 312. *See also* Insulin resistance

Metastasis: 166, 312

Metformin: 27. *See also* Glucophage

Methyltestosterone: 72, 274. *See also* Implant

Microadenoma: 27

Migraine: 7, 10, 56, 58, 76, 111, 127, 159, 284-6, 287-8, 302, 304, 305

Mindfulness: 124, 300

Mindfulness-based stress reduction programme: 125, 300

Minerals and trace minerals: 88, 89, 90, 91, 92, 93, 94, 98-100, 113, 197, 209, 210, 218, 240, 251, 312

Moderate carbohydrate diet: 241

Molybdenum: 100, 104. *See also* Minerals

Mono-unsaturated fat: 236, 312

Mood swings: 1, 7, 22, 132, 141, 174, 283, 294, 305

MPA (medroxyprogesterone acetate): 32, 62, 77

Myocardial infarction: 142, 312

Myomectomy: 131, 138, 140, 312

NAMS Certified Menopause Practitioner (NCMP): 3, 55, 315

National Centre for Complementary and Alternative Medicine (NCCAM): 113, 116

Needle biopsy: 169, 170, 309, 310

Neoplasm: 188, 312

Neurontin: 127

Neurotransmitters: 22, 120. *See also* Dopamine; Norepinephrine; Serotonin

Niacin (B3): 96, 149. *See also* Vitamins

Night sweats: 1, 7, 48, 58, 86, 101, 107, 108, 119, 124, 125, 126, 128, 129, 140, 141, 143, 156, 157, 180, 186, 187, 223, 227, 282, 283, 294, 304, 314

Nipple stimulation: 26

Nonbenzodiazepine: 278

Norepinephrine: 120, 121, 128, 129, 312

North American Menopause Society (NAMS): 3, 55, 65, 76, 122, 315

Nutraceutical: 91, 312

Off-label: 126, 127, 128, 129, 187, 287, 295, 312

Omega-3 fatty acid: 111-4, 115, 143, 149, 236, 263, 312. *See also* Fatty acids

Omega-6 fatty acid: 111-12, 236, 312

Omentectomy: 203

OnabotulinumtoxinA: 287

Onco-reconstructive breast surgery: 190

Oophorectomy: 133, 135, 136, 140, 185, 195, 285, 308

Orgasm: 268, 269, 276-7, 281. *See also* G-spot

Osteoblasts: 22, 207, 209, 220, 223, 224, 312

Osteoclasts: 207, 208, 209, 210, 214, 220, 221, 222, 223, 224, 308, 312

Osteocytes: 209, 312

Osteopenia: 211. *See also* Low bone density

Osteoporosis: 2, 18, 39, 56, 58, 64, 82, 83, 84, 89, 171, 205-24, 206, 207, 210, 211, 212, 213, 214, 215, 217, 219, 220, 221, 222, 223, 224, 225, 240, 243, 244, 263

Ovarian cancer: 126, 133, 134, 135, 161, 172, 173, 174, 175, 200-3

Ovarian cysts: 131, 133, 134, 146, 201, 202

Ovaries: 8, 11, 12, 13, 15, 16, 19, 20, 21, 23, 24, 25, 58, 59, 68, 73, 78, 119, 126, 132, 133,